Beating Mast Cell Activation Syndrome Naturally

Scott A. Johnson

Beating Mast Cell Activation Syndrome Naturally / Scott A. Johnson

Cover design: Scott A. Johnson

ISBN-13: 979-8988720690

Published by Scott A. Johnson Professional Writing Services, LLC: Orem, UT

Discover more books by Scott A. Johnson at authorscott.com/shop/

DISCLAIMERS OF WARRANTY AND LIMITATION OF LIABILITY

The author provides all information on an "as is" and "as available" basis and for informational purposes only. The author makes no representations or warranties of any kind, expressed or implied, as to the information, materials, or products mentioned. Every effort has been made to ensure accuracy and completeness of the information contained; however, it is not intended to replace any medical advice or to halt proper medical treatment, nor diagnose, treat, cure, or prevent any health condition or disease. Always consult a qualified medical professional before using any dietary supplement or natural product, engaging in physical activity, or modifying your diet; and seek the advice of your physician with any questions you may have regarding any medical condition.

Always consult your OB/GYN if you are pregnant or think you may become pregnant before using any dietary supplement or natural product, and to ensure you are healthy enough for exercise or any dietary modifications. The information contained in this book is for educational and informational purposes only, and it is not meant to replace medical advice, diagnosis, or treatment in any manner. Never delay or disregard professional medical advice. Use the information solely at your own risk; the author accepts no responsibility for the use thereof. This book is sold with the understanding that neither the author nor publisher shall be liable for any loss, injury, or harm allegedly arising from any information or suggestion in this book.

The Food and Drug Administration (FDA) has not evaluated the statements contained in this book. The information and materials are not meant to diagnose, prescribe, or treat any disease, condition, illness, or injury. You are encouraged to seek the most current information and medical care from your healthcare professional.

Contents

CHAPTER 1

Mast Cells 101

Your Body's Ancient Guardians—and What Happens When They Stop Trusting the World

The Day Everything Changed

Her name was Claire. She was thirty-four years old, a middle-school art teacher with a gift for making kids believe they could create something beautiful. She had always been what her mother called "a sensitive soul"—prone to headaches, stomach trouble, and what the family chalked up to nerves. But in the spring of her thirty-second year, something shifted.

It started with hives. Not the dramatic, throat-closing kind you see on medical dramas—just persistent, maddening welts that appeared on her forearms whenever she got too warm, too stressed, or ate certain foods. Her doctor prescribed antihistamines. The hives improved. But something else crept in: a racing heart on ordinary Tuesday afternoons, a bone-deep fatigue that sleep couldn't fix, brain fog so thick she once forgot a student's name mid-sentence. Her gut hurt most of the time. Scented candles—the ones she used to love—now sent her into sneezing fits that lasted an hour.

Over the next two years, Claire saw eleven specialists. She was tested for lupus, celiac disease, thyroid dysfunction, and anxiety. Some tests were slightly abnormal; most were unremarkably normal. She was told, in various kindly or not-so-kindly ways, that her symptoms didn't quite fit anything. One physician mentioned that she might be "a little sensitive." Another suggested stress management.

She wasn't imagining things. And she wasn't simply anxious.

Claire had mast cell activation syndrome (MCAS)—a condition in which tiny immune cells scattered throughout her body had gone from vigilant protectors to hair-trigger alarms, reacting to stimuli that posed no real threat. Once she understood what was happening inside her, everything changed. Not overnight. Not perfectly. But profoundly.

Although fictional, this story mirrors the frustrating journey of many people who suffer from MCAS. This chapter is where we begin to understand why.

✦ ✦ ✦

What Is a Mast Cell, Anyway?

Before we can talk about what goes wrong with mast cells, we need to appreciate what they are supposed to do. And honestly, when they're functioning normally, mast cells are nothing short of remarkable.

Mast cells are white blood cells—specialized members of your immune system that take up permanent residence in your body's tissues rather than simply circulating in the blood. You'll find them clustered precisely where your body meets the outside world: in the skin, the lining of the gut, the respiratory tract, the bladder, and the spaces surrounding blood vessels and nerves. This positioning is strategic. Mast cells are your body's first responders, stationed at the borders, watching for trouble.

Think of them as a combination between a smoke detector and a first-aid kit. When a genuine threat appears—a bacterium, a parasite, a splinter, a venomous sting—mast cells detect it, sound the alarm, and release a cascade of chemical signals that recruit the rest of the immune system, dilate local blood vessels to allow immune cells to pour in, trigger inflammation to wall off the danger, and begin the healing process. In this context, the mast cell's dramatic response is not just appropriate; it is life-saving.

> **Key Insight:** *Mast cells aren't the enemy. In a healthy immune system, they are indispensable guardians that have protected the human body for millennia of interaction with the outside world.*

Each mast cell contains hundreds of tiny granules—microscopic sacs packed with powerful chemical mediators. The most well-known of these is histamine, but the full roster is far more complex. Mast cells can release more than two hundred different mediators, including the following:

- Histamine—A mediator that triggers inflammation, itching, increased vascular permeability, and the contraction of smooth muscle.
- Tryptase—An enzyme that activates other inflammatory pathways and serves as a measurable marker of mast cell activity.
- Prostaglandins—Hormone-like compounds that regulate pain, blood vessel tone, and fever.

- Leukotrienes—Potent inflammatory mediators that are involved in airway constriction and mucus production.
- Cytokines—Signaling proteins that coordinate broader immune responses, including interleukins and tumor necrosis factor (TNF)
- Heparin—A natural blood thinner that is released during certain reactions
- Serotonin—A neurotransmitter that, when released by mast cells in the gut, influences motility and pain signaling

This chemical arsenal gives mast cells extraordinary reach. Depending on which mediators are released and in what combination, a single mast cell activation event can affect the skin, the gut, the cardiovascular system, the brain, and the nervous system—all at once.[1] This explains, in large part, why mast cell disorders look so different from person to person and why they so often baffle doctors trained to think in single-organ terms.

✦ ✦ ✦

The Art of Activation: Normal vs. Abnormal

"Activation" simply means that a mast cell has received a signal to release its mediators. In healthy immune function, this process is tightly regulated. The mast cell activates in response to a legitimate trigger—an allergen, a pathogen, a physical injury—releasing the correct mediators in the appropriate amounts before returning to a resting state.

Imagine a fire station in a well-run city. When an alarm sounds, the firefighters respond with speed and precision. They assess the scene, apply the right resources, extinguish the fire, and return to the station to await the next call. The system works because the alarm is calibrated correctly—it goes off when there's a real fire, not when someone lights a birthday candle.

In MCAS, the alarm system has become miscalibrated. Mast cells activate in response to stimuli that shouldn't trigger a full emergency response: certain foods,[2] temperature changes,[3] fragrances,[4] stress,[5] hormonal fluctuations,[6,7] nervous system dysregulation and neuropeptides,[8,9] gut disorders,[10,11] physical pressure,[12] environmental toxins,[13] heavy metals,[14] or sometimes no identifiable trigger at all. And rather than a measured, targeted response, they may release mediators excessively, in unusual combinations, or repeatedly without adequate recovery time.

Indeed, MCAS isn't usually driven by a single cause. It's typically a multi-trigger, cumulative condition where mast cells become overly sensitive and reactive. Think of it as an overloaded alarm system rather than a single "on/off" condition.

A leading major root trigger category is infections. Chronic infections can quietly keep the body's immune system stuck in "on" mode, which is a major driver of mast cell activation. Certain bacterial infections—like Lyme disease,[15] Bartonella,[16] and Mycoplasma[17]—can linger in the body and continuously stimulate the immune system. This ongoing fight leads to the release of inflammatory signals (called cytokines) that make mast cells more sensitive and easier to trigger. Some of these microbes also form protective layers called biofilms, which allow them to hide and persist, fueling long-term inflammation.

Viral infections such as Epstein-Barr virus (EBV),[18] human herpesvirus 6 (HHV-6),[19] cytomegalovirus (CMV),[20] and even COVID-19 can have a similar effect.[21] They may disrupt normal immune balance and reactivate during times of stress, increasing histamine and inflammation in the body. On top of that, fungal and yeast overgrowth—like *Candida* or mold living in the sinuses or gut—can produce toxins, damage the gut lining, and directly activate mast cells. Together, these hidden infections can keep the immune system in a constant state of irritation, making symptoms more intense and harder to calm.

To make things more complex, not all mast cells in the body behave the same way. Research—particularly the work of Dr. Lawrence Afrin and his colleagues—suggests that in MCAS, a subset of mast cells has acquired abnormal characteristics, likely through somatic mutations (genetic changes that occur in individual cells over a lifetime rather than being inherited). These mutated mast cells behave unpredictably, like smoke detectors with faulty wiring; they may stay silent through genuine emergencies and then blare at the scent of someone's perfume.

> **Analogy:** *Normal mast cell activation is a precision response—targeted, proportionate, time-limited. MCAS is the same system in chaos, responding to the wrong signals, at the wrong intensity, at the wrong time.*

✦ ✦ ✦

Deeper Dive: The Biology of Mast Cell Activation

For the Science-Minded Reader

Mast cells originate in the bone marrow as progenitor cells and then migrate to peripheral tissues, where they complete their maturation. Unlike most blood cells, which are relatively short-lived, mature mast cells can survive for months to years in their home tissues. This longevity has important implications: a population of dysfunctional mast cells isn't simply flushed out and replaced quickly.

Mast cell activation occurs through several distinct pathways, which is one reason MCAS is so heterogeneous (a condition that has multiple variations in symptoms and severity among different individuals).

IgE-Mediated Activation – The classical allergic pathway. IgE antibodies, produced during prior sensitization to an allergen, bind to high-affinity receptors (FcεRI) on the mast cell surface. When the allergen reappears and cross-links these IgE molecules, the mast cell degranulates rapidly. This is the mechanism behind classic anaphylaxis and many food allergies.

Non-IgE Receptor-Mediated Activation – Mast cells possess a remarkable array of surface receptors—some estimates suggest more than three hundred—that allow them to respond to complement proteins, neuropeptides, hormones, physical stimuli, and microbial components. In MCAS, it is often these non-IgE pathways that are dysregulated. The MRGPRX2 receptor, for instance, can trigger mast cell activation in response to certain drugs, neuropeptides, and even physical forces like pressure or vibration.

Stem Cell Factor (SCF) and Kit Signaling – SCF binds to the c-Kit receptor on mast cells and is essential for their survival, proliferation, and activation threshold. Mutations in c-Kit (most notably D816V) are the hallmark of systemic mastocytosis, but emerging research suggests that subtler variations in Kit signaling may contribute to MCAS pathology.

Neurogenic Activation – Mast cells are in intimate anatomical contact with nerve fibers and can be activated by neuropeptides such as substance P, calcitonin gene-related peptide (CGRP), and nerve growth factor. This neuro-immune cross-talk is bidirectional; activated mast cells, in turn, sensitize and stimulate surrounding neurons. This loop helps explain the visceral hypersensitivity, widespread pain, and neuropsychiatric symptoms many MCAS patients experience.

When a mast cell activates, it can release its mediators through three mechanisms: degranulation (rapid release of preformed mediators stored in granules), de novo synthesis (production of new lipid mediators like prostaglandins and leukotrienes), and cytokine secretion (a slower, more sustained release of signaling proteins). Different triggers tend to favor different release patterns, which is why MCAS presentations can vary so dramatically—not just from person to person, but from flare to flare in the same person.

Histamine, once released, acts on four receptor types (H1, H2, H3, H4) distributed throughout the body. H1 receptors mediate classic allergy symptoms—itching, hives, nasal congestion, and bronchoconstriction. H2 receptors are concentrated in the stomach lining and influence acid secretion. H3 receptors in the central nervous system modulate neurotransmitter release and circadian rhythms. H4 receptors are found on immune cells and influence inflammatory responses. This receptor distribution explains why histamine excess can simultaneously cause a runny nose, heartburn, disrupted sleep, brain fog, and immune dysregulation.

> **Note for Practitioners:** *MCAS is now broadly understood to involve dysregulated mast cell activation leading to excess mediator release, but the specific mediators released—and the downstream pathways affected—vary between individuals. This explains why no single symptom profile or biomarker is universal, and why individualized treatment approaches are necessary.*

✦ ✦ ✦

What This Means for You

Understanding mast cell biology isn't just an academic exercise. It changes the way you relate to your own symptoms—and that shift in understanding is genuinely therapeutic.

When you feel a rush of heat, a sudden drop in blood pressure, or an inexplicable wave of anxiety after eating a tomato or walking into a fragrant shop, your body is not betraying you. Your mast cells are doing exactly what they were designed to do—just with a trigger threshold that has become far too sensitive. Knowing this doesn't make the symptoms less real or less difficult, but it transforms the narrative from "something is mysteriously wrong with me" to "I understand the mechanism, and there are meaningful things I can do about it."

Here are three foundational understandings to carry with you as we move through this book:

1. Your symptoms are connected. The seemingly unrelated collection of problems—gut issues, skin reactions, heart palpitations, brain fog, fatigue—are not a mysterious constellation of separate disorders. They are different expressions of the same underlying process: mast cells releasing mediators that affect multiple organ systems simultaneously.

2. Triggers are cumulative. Mast cells don't activate in isolation from your life circumstances. Stress, poor sleep, hormonal fluctuations, dietary choices, environmental toxins, and infections all influence your mast cell reactivity. We'll explore this "bucket theory" in depth in Chapter 5, but for now, recognize that small, consistent interventions—reducing your total trigger load—can have outsized effects.

3. Healing is possible—and it happens in layers. Because mast cell dysfunction involves multiple systems and root causes, recovery rarely follows a straight line. The goal of this book is not to offer a single protocol that works for everyone. It is to help you understand your unique biology, identify your personal triggers and root causes, and build a layered approach to healing that is sustainable and genuinely supportive.

Claire, the art teacher we met at the beginning of this chapter, eventually found her way to a functional medicine practitioner who understood MCAS. It took time, patience, and a willingness to experiment. But when she began addressing her mast cell reactivity as the unifying thread running through all of her symptoms—rather than treating each symptom in isolation—she began to improve. Her hives quieted. Her heart found a steadier rhythm. The fog began to lift.

Her story is not exceptional. It is, in fact, increasingly common—and increasingly possible.

✦ ✦ ✦

Chapter 1 at a Glance

What to Remember:

- Mast cells are ancient, tissue-resident immune cells positioned at the body's borders—skin, gut, respiratory tract, and blood vessels—where they function as first responders to genuine threats.
- When activated, mast cells release more than two hundred chemical mediators, the most familiar being histamine. These mediators can simultaneously affect multiple organ systems, which explains MCAS's diverse and confusing symptom picture.
- In MCAS, mast cells activate in response to triggers that don't represent true danger—foods, fragrances, temperature, stress—and often release mediators excessively or in abnormal combinations.
- Activation occurs through multiple pathways: IgE-mediated (classic allergy), non-IgE receptor-mediated (including the MRGPRX2 receptor), Kit signaling, and neurogenic pathways. This diversity is why MCAS presents differently in different people.
- Histamine acts on four receptor types throughout the body, explaining why excess histamine affects the skin, gut, brain, cardiovascular system, and immune function simultaneously.
- Understanding the mast cell mechanism changes your relationship to your symptoms—from frightening mystery to comprehensible biology, from helplessness to informed action.
- MCAS symptoms are connected, triggers are cumulative, and healing happens in layers. These three principles will guide everything that follows.

Coming Up in Chapter 2:

Now that we understand mast cells themselves, we turn to the full clinical picture of mast cell activation syndrome—what it looks and feels like, why it so often masquerades as other conditions, and what the diagnostic journey typically involves. If you've ever felt dismissed or misunderstood by the medical system, Chapter 2 is for you.

CHAPTER 2

What Is MCAS?

Naming the Storm—Symptoms, Misdiagnosis, and the Long Road to Recognition

The Thousand-Faced Condition

Marcus was forty-one when his body began sending signals he couldn't decode. It started after a particularly brutal flu that never quite resolved. He recovered from the acute infection—or so it seemed—but what followed was a slow unraveling. His digestion, previously reliable, became unpredictable. He developed dark circles under his eyes that no amount of sleep erased. His skin, especially on his chest and neck, would flush crimson for no apparent reason. Crowds made him anxious in a way he hadn't experienced since adolescence. Exercise, once his stress valve, now left him flat for days.

His primary care physician ran a standard panel of blood work. Mostly normal, aside from a mildly elevated inflammatory marker. He was referred to a gastroenterologist who diagnosed irritable bowel syndrome. A cardiologist ruled out structural heart disease. A dermatologist offered a cream for the flushing. A psychiatrist suggested that the anxiety and fatigue might be generational trauma surfacing after the illness. Everyone was doing their best, yet no one saw the whole picture—a casualty of a fragmented system that treats symptoms in isolation rather than the patient as a whole.

What Marcus had—what connects the digestion, the flushing, the fatigue, the anxiety, the post-viral collapse—is mast cell activation syndrome. His case is not unusual. In fact, it is maddeningly typical.

MCAS is what physicians call a multi-system disorder, meaning it doesn't respect the specialty boundaries that medicine has drawn around the body. It crosses into gastroenterology, cardiology, dermatology, neurology, psychiatry, immunology, and rheumatology simultaneously. And because most doctors are trained to find single explanations for clusters of symptoms, MCAS—which is the single explanation—tends to be the last one considered.

This chapter is about recognizing the full face of MCAS: what it looks like across body systems, why it wears so many disguises, what the diagnostic process involves, and why getting a diagnosis is not the end of the road—it's the beginning of a more useful map.

✦ ✦ ✦

A Storm Across Body Systems: The Symptom Landscape

If you were to ask a hundred people with MCAS to list their symptoms, you would get a hundred somewhat different lists. That variability is a feature of the condition, not a flaw in the people reporting it. Recall from Chapter 1 that mast cells reside throughout the body and that different mediators affect different organ systems. The specific combination of symptoms any given person experiences reflects which mediators their mast cells are releasing most abundantly, which tissues are most affected, and how their individual nervous system and other organ systems respond.

With that said, there are common themes. Here is what MCAS can look like across the major body systems:

Skin

The skin is perhaps the most visible arena for MCAS activity, because mast cells are densely concentrated in the dermis. Common skin manifestations include:

- **Urticaria (hives)** – Hives are raised, itchy welts that may come and go rapidly, appear in different locations, and are often disproportionate to apparent triggers.
- **Angioedema** – A deeper swelling beneath the skin, often affecting the lips, eyelids, hands, or throat—potentially dangerous when it involves the airway.
- **Dermatographism** – Stroking or scratching the skin produces a raised wheal along the path of contact, sometimes called "skin writing."
- **Flushing** – A sudden redness and warmth, most often in the face, neck, and chest, which may be triggered by heat, exertion, certain foods, alcohol, or emotional stress.
- **Pruritus (itching)** – A generalized or localized itching without a visible rash.
- **Rashes and skin sensitivity** – Seen as various presentations, including eczema-like patches, hypersensitivity to clothing textures, and easy bruising.

Gastrointestinal System

Given that the gut lining is one of the most mast-cell-rich environments in the body, it's not surprising that gastrointestinal symptoms are among the most prevalent in MCAS:

- **Nausea and vomiting** – It is often unpredictable and not clearly tied to specific foods.
- **Abdominal pain and cramping** – This is frequently misdiagnosed as IBS or functional (no identifiable physical cause) abdominal pain.
- **Diarrhea, constipation, or alternating patterns** – Can be driven by mast-cell-mediated effects on gut motility and secretion.
- **Bloating and gas** – This can be partly related to dysbiosis and partly to mast-cell-driven changes in intestinal permeability.
- **Gastroesophageal reflux (GERD)** – Histamine stimulates gastric acid secretion via H2 receptors, worsening reflux.
- **Food sensitivities** – Reactions to an expanding list of foods, often confusingly inconsistent—the same food may be tolerated one day and not the next, depending on the patient's overall mast cell load.

Cardiovascular System

Mast cells in vascular tissue and the heart play significant roles in regulating blood vessel tone and cardiac function. Their dysregulation can produce:

- **Palpitations and tachycardia** – Rapid or irregular heartbeat often occurs at rest or with minimal exertion.
- **Hypotension (low blood pressure)** – Mast-cell-released mediators cause vasodilation (widening of the blood vessels); in severe cases this progresses to anaphylaxis.
- **Orthostatic intolerance** – Dizziness or near-fainting when standing, often overlapping with POTS (postural orthostatic tachycardia syndrome) is a connection we explore further in Chapter 3.
- **Chest pain and pressure** – Without cardiac cause, may relate to esophageal spasm or direct mast cell effects on cardiac tissue.
- **Temperature dysregulation** – Difficulty maintaining normal body temperature; feeling excessively hot or cold without external cause.

Neurological and Cognitive Symptoms

Mast cells are present in the meninges (protective membranes that cover the brain and spinal cord) and at the blood-brain barrier, and their mediators can cross into the central nervous system, producing a range of neurological and psychiatric effects:

- **Brain fog** – Brain fog is the cardinal cognitive complaint: difficulty concentrating, word-finding problems, memory lapses, and a sense of mental "static" that worsens with triggers.
- **Headaches and migraines** – These are often histamine-driven—may be positional, weather-related, or triggered by certain foods and scents.
- **Anxiety and panic** – Mast-cell-mediated release of corticotropin-releasing hormone (CRH) and direct nervous system sensitization can produce anxiety that feels physiological rather than psychological.
- **Depression and mood instability** – Neuroinflammation driven by mast cell mediators disrupts neurotransmitter balance, contributing to depressive symptoms
- **Sleep disturbances** – Histamine is a wakefulness-promoting neurotransmitter; excess histamine disrupts sleep architecture, particularly the transition to and maintenance of deep sleep.
- **Sensory hypersensitivity** – Heightened sensitivity to light, sound, smell, and touch results from the nervous system turned up too high.
- **Neuropathic symptoms** – Tingling, burning, or numbness is often related to small-fiber neuropathy associated with MCAS.

Respiratory System

- **Nasal congestion and rhinitis** – Histamine-driven inflammation of nasal passages is often labeled as chronic sinusitis or allergic rhinitis.
- **Asthma-like symptoms** – Can produce airway constriction and excess mucus production in the absence of true asthma or with atypical asthma patterns.
- **Shortness of breath** – Shortness of breath is sometimes triggered by scents, exercise, or emotional stress.
- **Postnasal drip and chronic throat clearing** – This is common and often attributed to acid reflux or allergies.

Musculoskeletal and Connective Tissue

- **Joint pain and swelling** – Mast cell mediators drive synovial inflammation; pain may be migratory and not correlate with imaging findings.
- **Muscle pain and fatigue** – Widespread myalgia is often indistinguishable from fibromyalgia

- **Hypermobility** – A significant proportion of MCAS patients also meet criteria for hypermobile Ehlers-Danlos syndrome (hEDS); the connection between mast cell dysfunction and connective tissue abnormalities is an area of active research.
- **Bone pain** – Tryptase and other mast cell mediators can affect bone metabolism; bone pain without clear structural cause is an underrecognized MCAS symptom.

Genitourinary System

- **Interstitial cystitis-like symptoms** – Pelvic pain, urinary frequency, and bladder irritability without infection can present.
- **Menstrual irregularities and symptom flares** – Many women report significant worsening of MCAS symptoms in the premenstrual phase, driven by estrogen's effect on mast cell sensitivity—explored further in Chapter 10.
- **Sexual dysfunction and pelvic pain** – Mast-cell-mediated neuroinflammation can affect pelvic nerve sensitivity

> **Important Reminder:** *This list is not meant to be alarming—or diagnostic. MCAS looks different in every person, and most individuals have a subset of these symptoms, not all of them. The point is pattern recognition: when symptoms span multiple, seemingly unrelated systems and fluctuate unpredictably, mast cell dysfunction belongs on the differential diagnosis.*

✦ ✦ ✦

The Master of Disguise: Why MCAS Mimics So Many Other Conditions

One of the most frustrating realities of MCAS is that almost every symptom it produces exists as part of some other recognized condition. Hives suggest allergic disease. Gut symptoms suggest IBS. Palpitations suggest cardiac arrhythmia. Anxiety suggests a mental health disorder. Fatigue suggests depression or hypothyroidism. Each specialist sees the part of the elephant in front of them and names it accordingly.

This is not a failure of individual practitioners—it is a structural problem in how medicine organizes itself around single-organ specialties, and it is compounded by how recently MCAS has been formally recognized. The term "mast cell activation syndrome" as a distinct diagnosis only entered mainstream medical literature in the early 2010s, with a consensus definition published in 2011 and refined over subsequent years. Many practitioners trained before that period received no formal education about MCAS and have had little reason to update their framework since.

The conditions most commonly confused with—or genuinely comorbid with—MCAS include:

- **Chronic idiopathic urticaria** – Recurrent hives without identifiable allergic trigger; in many cases, this is MCAS presenting predominantly through skin.
- **Irritable bowel syndrome (IBS)** – The gut is heavily mast-cell-influenced; what is labeled IBS in MCAS patients is often mast-cell-mediated gut inflammation and motility disruption.
- **Fibromyalgia** – Widespread pain, fatigue, and cognitive symptoms overlap substantially; shared neuroinflammatory mechanisms are now recognized.
- **Chronic fatigue syndrome / myalgic encephalomyelitis (ME/CFS)** – Post-viral fatigue, exercise intolerance, and cognitive impairment mirror MCAS post-infectious patterns; significant overlap, particularly in long COVID presentations
- **Anxiety and panic disorder** – The physiological arousal of mast cell mediator release—racing heart, flushing, shortness of breath, sense of doom—is indistinguishable from a panic attack from the patient's subjective experience.
- **POTS (postural orthostatic tachycardia syndrome)** – So frequently comorbid with MCAS that we devote the entire next chapter to this relationship.
- **Lupus and other autoimmune conditions** – Mast cell mediators drive autoimmune pathways; elevated ANA titers and inflammatory markers in MCAS patients can send workups down an autoimmune path that yields no definitive diagnosis.
- **Interstitial cystitis** – Bladder mast cells are directly implicated in the pathology of IC, which may in many cases be a localized MCAS presentation.
- **Eosinophilic esophagitis and gastritis** – Eosinophils and mast cells interact closely; some cases of eosinophilic GI disease have a significant mast cell component.

The tragic consequence of this diagnostic confusion is not merely delay—it is years of treatments aimed at the wrong target. Antidepressants for what is fundamentally a neuroinflammatory process. Proton pump inhibitors for histamine-driven acid excess that doesn't respond because H2 receptors, not proton pumps, are the primary driver. Cognitive behavioral therapy for anxiety that is physiologically mediated. None of these approaches are without value, and many individuals with MCAS benefit from some of them. But without addressing the underlying mast cell dysfunction, they treat symptoms rather than source.

> **Key Insight:** *MCAS doesn't just overlap with other conditions—it can actively cause them. The goal isn't always to replace existing diagnoses but to understand mast cell dysfunction as the thread running beneath them.*

✦ ✦ ✦

Deeper Dive: Diagnostic Challenges and the Evolving Criteria

For the Science-Minded Reader

The diagnosis of MCAS is clinical—meaning it is based primarily on a pattern of symptoms and response to treatment, rather than on a single definitive laboratory test. This is both a challenge and, once understood, a framework for moving forward.

The most widely cited diagnostic criteria, established through expert consensus and refined over the past decade, require three core elements:

1. **Episodic symptoms consistent with mast cell mediator release** – affecting two or more organ systems, occurring in a pattern that suggests mast cell involvement

2. **Evidence of mast cell mediator involvement** – through laboratory markers (elevated levels of serum tryptase, N-methylhistamine, and leukotriene E4) or response to mediator-targeting treatments (such as antihistamines and mast cell stabilizers)

3. **Exclusion of alternative diagnoses** – that might better account for the symptom pattern, including systemic mastocytosis and other clonal mast cell disorders

The laboratory picture in MCAS is where significant confusion arises—and where many people are wrongly told they don't have the condition because their tests came back normal.

The Serum Tryptase Problem

Serum tryptase is the most commonly ordered mast cell marker. In systemic mastocytosis—the clonal mast cell disease—baseline tryptase is typically elevated above 20 ng/mL. In most MCAS patients, baseline tryptase is normal. During acute reactions, tryptase may transiently rise, but this window is narrow: tryptase must be drawn within one to two hours of a suspected reaction to capture the spike, and even then, it may not rise significantly in MCAS because tryptase primarily reflects degranulation of the mucosal mast cell population, which is not always the most activated subset.[22]

This has led to the important clinical principle: a normal tryptase does not rule out MCAS. Other markers are more sensitive in non-clonal disease:

- **24-hour urine histamine and methylhistamine** – Histamine metabolites captured over a full day provide a more reliable picture than a single blood draw.
- **24-hour urine prostaglandin D2 and its metabolite 11β-PGF2α** – A more stable mast cell marker that can be elevated when histamine is not.
- **24-hour urine leukotriene E4** – Another lipid mediator that may be elevated in MCAS.
- **Chromogranin A** – A less specific marker that may be elevated and can help support the picture.
- **Plasma heparin** – It's elevated in some mast cell conditions, though less commonly measured.

The practical challenge is that these tests must often be collected during or shortly after a reaction to have the best sensitivity, which requires the person—and their physician—to be prepared. Routine samples drawn on a routine day when the person feels relatively stable may return normal results even in confirmed MCAS.

Hereditary Alpha-Tryptasemia: A Genetic Modifier

An important genetic factor that can significantly affect both symptom severity and tryptase levels is hereditary alpha-tryptasemia (HαT)—a recently described condition caused by duplications of the TPSAB1 gene.[23] Present in roughly four to seven percent of people of European descent,[24] HαT elevates baseline tryptase levels (usually > 8ng/mL) and increases sensitivity to a wide range of mast cell triggers. People with both HαT and MCAS often have more severe symptoms, a higher burden of comorbidities, and elevated baseline tryptase that may be misread as suggesting systemic mastocytosis.[25] Genetic testing for HαT is now commercially available and is becoming an increasingly important part of the MCAS workup.

The Role of a Therapeutic Trial

Because laboratory confirmation is often elusive, many clinicians experienced in MCAS now rely significantly on a therapeutic trial as part of the diagnostic process. If a patient with a compelling clinical picture experiences meaningful improvement on a combination of H1 and H2 antihistamines, mast cell stabilizers such as cromolyn sodium, and/or mediator-blocking agents like montelukast, this response is considered supportive evidence for the diagnosis. The logic is straightforward: if the symptoms are driven by mast cell mediators, then blocking or stabilizing those mediators should produce clinical benefit.

This approach is not unique to MCAS. Many diagnoses in medicine—migraine, fibromyalgia, autoimmune conditions—are confirmed or supported in part by response to targeted treatment. In MCAS, where the biology is real but the biomarkers are imperfect, therapeutic response is a legitimate and important diagnostic tool.

The Evolving Diagnostic Landscape

It is worth acknowledging an ongoing controversy in the MCAS field. Some researchers and clinicians advocate for stricter diagnostic criteria, concerned that MCAS is being over-diagnosed in people who may have other explanations for their multi-system symptoms. Others—particularly those in functional and integrative medicine who see large numbers of these individuals—argue that strict criteria cause under-diagnosis and leave suffering patients without a useful framework for treatment.

The truth likely lies somewhere between: MCAS is probably more common than traditional allergology has recognized, but it is also a diagnosis that requires careful clinical assessment rather than a simple checklist. What matters most for the person holding this book is not the academic debate—it is whether understanding mast cell dysfunction as a driving mechanism helps explain your experience and opens doors to effective intervention. For the vast majority of people in whom this concept resonates deeply, it does.

> **For Practitioners:** *The most clinically useful approach combines symptom pattern recognition, targeted laboratory testing (ideally during or after a reaction), genetic markers like HaT testing when appropriate, and a structured therapeutic trial. Waiting for a "definitive" biomarker before treating is not supported by current evidence and causes unnecessary delay in care.*

✦ ✦ ✦

What This Means for You: Navigating the Diagnostic Journey

If you have been living with a constellation of unexplained, multi-system symptoms, one of the most powerful things you can do is become a careful observer of your own body. MCAS, more than almost any other condition, rewards self-knowledge. Here is how to approach the diagnostic journey strategically:

Start a symptom and trigger journal. Track what symptoms you experience, when they occur, how severe they are, and what preceded them—foods, activities, environments, emotional states, time of month. Patterns will emerge over time that neither you nor your physician could see without this data. A simple template is provided in the Appendix.

Bring a systems-oriented narrative to your doctor. Instead of presenting each symptom in isolation, offer the full picture: "I have symptoms that involve my skin, gut, heart, and cognition. They fluctuate with identifiable triggers. I've been evaluated for individual conditions in each system, and no single diagnosis has explained all of them." This framing helps direct the conversation toward MCAS.

Ask specifically about mast cell-related testing. Request a serum tryptase, 24-hour urine histamine and methylhistamine, and 24-hour urine prostaglandin D2. Understand that normal results do not definitively rule out MCAS, but abnormal results can powerfully support the diagnosis. Consider timing tests to coincide with a period of higher symptom activity.

Don't wait for a perfect diagnosis to begin reducing your trigger load. The natural interventions described in Parts III and IV of this book—dietary adjustments, nervous system support, gut healing, targeted supplementation—are appropriate and beneficial for anyone with mast cell hyperreactivity, regardless of whether a formal MCAS diagnosis has been attached to the chart. Your biology doesn't require a label to begin healing.

Find physicians familiar with MCAS. This is changing rapidly, but MCAS-literate practitioners are still disproportionately found in functional medicine, integrative medicine, and certain allergy and immunology subspecialties. Patient advocacy organizations and online communities can be valuable sources of practitioner referrals and peer support.

Marcus, whose story opened this chapter, eventually found his way to a physician who recognized the pattern. Within weeks of beginning a systematic approach to reducing his mast cell load—dietary changes, targeted supplements, and nervous system support—he noticed the first real improvement he had experienced in two years. His gut settled. The flushing became less frequent. He slept more deeply. The fog began, slowly, to clear.

He still has work to do. MCAS is rarely resolved in weeks. But he finally had a map. He finally had a name for the storm—and a direction to walk out of it.

✦ ✦ ✦

Chapter 2 at a Glance

What to Remember:

- MCAS is a multi-system condition in which dysregulated mast cells produce symptoms across the skin, gut, cardiovascular system, nervous system, respiratory system, musculoskeletal system, and genitourinary system—often simultaneously and in varying combinations.
- No two MCAS patients look identical. Symptom patterns depend on which mediators are most active, which tissues are most affected, and individual nervous system responses.

- MCAS mimics many common conditions—IBS, fibromyalgia, panic disorder, chronic urticaria, POTS, and others—because mast cell mediators affect the same systems these conditions involve. This leads to chronic misdiagnosis and inappropriate treatment.
- Formal diagnosis requires episodic multi-system symptoms consistent with mediator release, laboratory support (though normal labs don't rule out MCAS), and exclusion of alternative explanations.
- Serum tryptase is often normal in MCAS. More sensitive markers include 24-hour urine histamine, methylhistamine, prostaglandin D2, and leukotriene E4—ideally collected during symptomatic periods.
- A positive therapeutic response to mast cell-targeting treatments (antihistamines, stabilizers, mediator blockers) is considered a valid part of the diagnostic picture when biomarkers are inconclusive.
- Hereditary alpha-tryptasemia (HαT) is a genetic modifier present in a significant minority of MCAS patients and can affect both symptom severity and test interpretation.
- You don't need a perfect diagnosis to begin healing. Reducing the overall mast cell load through natural, evidence-informed interventions is appropriate and beneficial regardless of diagnostic status.

Coming Up in Chapter 3:

One of the most significant and clinically important relationships in MCAS medicine is with postural orthostatic tachycardia syndrome—POTS. For many, these two conditions are inseparable. In Chapter 3, we explore the deep biological links between mast cell dysfunction and cardiovascular autonomic dysregulation, and why treating one often requires understanding the other.

CHAPTER 3

The MCAS-POTS Connection

When the Heart and the Immune System Lose Their Rhythm Together

Standing Up Shouldn't Be This Hard

Priya was twenty-seven when she first fainted in a grocery store. She had felt it coming—the sudden rush of heat, the narrowing of her visual field, the roaring in her ears—and she managed to grip a display shelf before her legs gave out entirely. The store manager called an ambulance. The emergency room found nothing wrong with her heart. She was told she was probably dehydrated and sent home with instructions to drink more water.

Over the following months, fainting gave way to something subtler and in some ways worse: a relentless, disabling dizziness every time she stood up. Her heart would slam against her ribs at rest, then sprint to alarming rates the moment she got vertical. Showering became a tactical challenge—she learned to sit on the shower floor to avoid passing out. Grocery shopping, once unremarkable, now required careful planning: where could she sit if she crashed? How long could she stay upright before the world went gray?

Cardiologists saw a structurally normal heart. A tilt-table test confirmed what her body had been announcing all along: her heart rate shot up more than thirty beats per minute within minutes of being tilted upright. The diagnosis was POTS. She was prescribed salt, fluids, compression stockings, and a beta-blocker to slow her racing heart. It helped, somewhat. But it didn't explain why she also had hives, gut pain, flushing, brain fog so thick she could barely complete sentences, and a body that seemed to react to everything.

It took another two years, two more specialists, and a functional medicine physician who happened to be deeply familiar with both conditions to finally connect the dots. Priya didn't just have POTS. She had MCAS driving her POTS—

a distinction that, once recognized, changed everything about how she was treated and how she healed.

Her story—MCAS and POTS together—is far more common than medicine has traditionally acknowledged. And understanding why they so frequently travel together is one of the most important insights in this entire book.

✦ ✦ ✦

What Is POTS?

Postural orthostatic tachycardia syndrome is a form of dysautonomia—a disorder of the autonomic nervous system, the branch of our nervous system that operates below conscious awareness and regulates the functions we never have to think about: heart rate, blood pressure, digestion, pupil dilation, sweating, breathing rate, and circulation.

In a healthy autonomic nervous system, standing up triggers a cascade of precisely coordinated responses. Gravity pulls blood toward the lower extremities, reducing the amount returning to the heart and brain. Sensors in the blood vessels and heart detect this shift and immediately signal the autonomic nervous system to compensate: blood vessels constrict, heart rate increases slightly, and the body redistributes blood upward to maintain adequate circulation to the brain. The entire process takes seconds. You don't feel it because it works so seamlessly.

In POTS, this compensation fails. Blood pools excessively in the lower body when upright, and the heart—unable to solve the problem through normal vasoconstriction—compensates by racing instead. By definition, POTS is diagnosed when heart rate increases by thirty beats per minute or more within ten minutes of standing (or twenty-five beats per minute in adolescents), in the absence of significant blood pressure drop. This distinguishes it from classical orthostatic hypotension, where blood pressure falls significantly, though the two can coexist.

> **Definition:** *POTS is not a heart condition—it is a circulation and autonomic regulation condition. The heart is racing because it is trying to compensate for a system that isn't managing blood flow properly when upright. Slowing the heart without fixing the underlying problem is like muffling a fire alarm without putting out the fire.*

The experience of POTS is heterogeneous. Some patients faint; others never lose consciousness but live with chronic near-fainting, crushing fatigue, cognitive impairment, and profound exercise intolerance. Many describe the feeling of standing as similar to how a healthy person might feel after running a sprint—heart pounding, light-headed, gasping—except they experience this simply from getting up off the couch. It is exhausting in a way that is difficult to communicate to people who haven't experienced it.

POTS predominantly affects women—estimates suggest roughly four to five times more commonly than men—and frequently first appears or worsens after viral illness, pregnancy, physical trauma, or a period of significant psychological stress.[26] The post-COVID era has generated a surge of POTS diagnoses, with dysautonomia following SARS-CoV-2 infection now recognized as a significant clinical problem.[27] This pattern—triggered by infection, hormonally influenced, and often accompanied by a broader symptom picture—is strikingly similar to MCAS. It is not a coincidence.

✦ ✦ ✦

Two Conditions, One Patient: Shared Symptoms and the Diagnostic Overlap

The symptomatic overlap between MCAS and POTS is so extensive that when a patient presents with one, the other should always be considered. A survey study of patients with MCAS found that more than half also met diagnostic criteria for POTS or reported significant orthostatic symptoms.[28] Conversely, studies of POTS populations have found MCAS in a substantial minority—with some estimates suggesting that fifteen to twenty percent of POTS patients have a significant mast cell component, and many researchers believe the true number is higher when subclinical mast cell dysfunction is included.[29]

The symptoms these conditions share include:

- **Palpitations and tachycardia** – Present in both conditions; in MCAS these occur from mediator release directly affecting cardiac rate and rhythm; in POTS they are the defining cardiovascular compensation—for poor blood flow—mechanism.
- **Orthostatic symptoms** – Dizziness, light-headedness, and near-syncope on standing occur in POTS by definition and are also common in MCAS through histamine-driven vasodilation and volume depletion.
- **Brain fog and cognitive impairment** – Both conditions disrupt cerebral perfusion and neuroinflammation; the cognitive symptoms are often indistinguishable between the two.
- **Fatigue** – Profound and often disproportionate to activity; fatigue is a cardinal feature of both.
- **Exercise intolerance and post-exertional malaise** – POTS patients struggle to exercise because upright exertion dramatically worsens orthostatic stress; MCAS patients may experience exercise as a

mast cell trigger; together, the combination can make even gentle movement feel dangerous.

- **Flushing and temperature dysregulation** – Mast-cell-mediated vasodilation in MCAS; autonomic dysregulation of vascular tone in POTS; in practice, often both.
- **Gastrointestinal symptoms** – Autonomic dysfunction impairs gut motility in POTS; mast cells drive gut inflammation and permeability changes in MCAS; gastroparesis, nausea, bloating, and pain are common in both.
- **Anxiety and hyperarousal** – The physiological experience of a racing heart, flushing, and near-fainting is interpreted by the brain as danger, triggering anxiety that is genuinely physiological rather than primarily psychological.
- **Sleep disruption** – Dysautonomia affects heart rate variability and autonomic tone during sleep; histamine excess disrupts sleep architecture—the structure and pattern of sleep cycles that occur throughout the night, including the different stages of sleep such as non-REM and REM sleep; together, restorative sleep becomes elusive.
- **Hypermobility and joint instability** – Both conditions are strongly associated with hypermobile Ehlers-Danlos syndrome;[30] the triad of MCAS, POTS, and hEDS is now recognized as a clinically significant cluster explored in Chapter 4.

It is worth pausing here to appreciate the clinical consequence of this overlap. When a person with both MCAS and POTS sits across from a cardiologist, she receives a POTS diagnosis and is given medications to manage heart rate and volume. When she visits an allergist, she may receive a partial MCAS workup focused on IgE-mediated allergy. Neither physician sees the full picture, and neither treatment fully works, because each is addressing only part of a shared underlying dysfunction.

> **Clinical Reality:** *MCAS and POTS are not merely comorbid—they are mechanistically linked. In many patients, MCAS is driving POTS, not simply coinciding with it. This distinction has profound implications for treatment; stabilizing mast cells can directly improve orthostatic tolerance and reduce cardiovascular symptoms.*

✦ ✦ ✦

Deeper Dive: How Mast Cells Drive Cardiovascular Dysfunction

For the Science-Minded Reader

The biological mechanisms linking MCAS and POTS are multiple, overlapping, and mutually reinforcing. Understanding them helps explain why these conditions so often appear together, why they amplify each other, and why addressing mast cell dysfunction can produce dramatic improvements in autonomic stability.

1. Histamine and Vascular Tone

Histamine, the most abundant preformed mediator in mast cell granules, is a powerful vasoactive substance. Acting through H1 receptors on vascular smooth muscle, histamine causes vasodilation. This is the same mechanism responsible for the flushing and hypotension that can accompany anaphylaxis. In a patient with chronically elevated mast cell activity, even subclinical histamine release contributes to a persistent state of relative vasodilation. Blood vessels that don't constrict efficiently allow blood to pool in dependent areas when upright, reducing venous return and cardiac output—the very pathophysiology that defines POTS.

Histamine also acts directly on the heart through H1 and H2 receptors located in cardiac tissue. H1 receptor activation slows conduction through the atrioventricular node and can provoke arrhythmia. H2 receptor activation increases heart rate and the force of cardiac contraction. Together, histamine's cardiac effects can produce the tachycardia, palpitations, and irregular rhythms that POTS patients experience even in the absence of the classic orthostatic trigger—simply because mast cells are releasing mediators throughout the day.

2. Blood Volume Depletion

One of POTS's most consistent features is reduced plasma volume—people simply don't have as much circulating blood as they need to maintain adequate perfusion when upright.[31] Mast cell mediators contribute to this through two mechanisms. They often operate with a ten to fifteen percent deficit in plasma volume—a state of 'biological drought' that makes the simple act of standing an exercise in circulatory exhaustion. First, histamine increases vascular permeability: by causing endothelial cells to pull apart slightly, it allows fluid to leak from blood vessels into surrounding tissue. This is what produces the swelling of angioedema and contributes to the "third spacing" of fluid that reduces effective circulating volume. Second, prostaglandins released by mast cells can affect kidney tubular function and influence fluid and sodium retention. The result, in a patient with significant MCAS activity, is a tendency toward relative hypovolemia that compounds the postural challenge of POTS.

3. Mast Cells and the Autonomic Nervous System

The relationship between mast cells and the autonomic nervous system is bidirectional and deeply intimate. Mast cells are anatomically positioned in close proximity to autonomic nerve fibers throughout the body—in the gut, the skin, and in perivascular spaces. This proximity is not incidental; mast cells and autonomic nerves communicate directly through chemical signals.

The sympathetic nervous system—the "fight-or-flight" branch of the autonomic system—releases norepinephrine, which can directly activate mast cells through adrenergic receptors. When POTS patients experience the orthostatic surge of sympathetic activity that is the hallmark of their condition, this sympathetic activation can trigger mast cell degranulation. The mast cells then release histamine and other mediators that further perturb vascular tone and autonomic signaling—a vicious cycle in which POTS triggers MCAS activation, which worsens POTS.

Conversely, the parasympathetic nervous system—the "rest-and-digest" branch, mediated largely through the vagus nerve—has a suppressive effect on mast cell activity. Acetylcholine, the primary parasympathetic neurotransmitter, acts through muscarinic receptors to dampen mast cell degranulation. In patients with dysautonomia, parasympathetic tone is often reduced relative to sympathetic activity. This autonomic imbalance means the natural brake on mast cell activation is chronically underperforming, leaving mast cells more reactive and the threshold for degranulation lower.

> **Key Mechanism:** *Sympathetic overdrive activates mast cells. Reduced parasympathetic tone removes the brakes on mast cell activity. The autonomic imbalance of POTS creates precisely the neurochemical environment in which MCAS thrives—and MCAS mediators, in turn, perpetuate the autonomic imbalance. This is the bidirectional engine at the heart of their co-occurrence.*

4. Corticotropin-Releasing Hormone and the Stress Axis

Corticotropin-releasing hormone (CRH), the primary orchestrator of the body's stress response, is a potent mast cell activator. CRH binds to receptors on mast cells and triggers degranulation through a non-IgE pathway—meaning it doesn't require prior sensitization and operates independently of allergy. In people with POTS, the chronic physical stress of orthostatic intolerance, the psychological burden of a disabling condition, and the sleep deprivation that accompanies both create a state of persistently elevated CRH output. This hormonal environment keeps mast cells primed and reactive.

At the same time, mast cells release their own CRH-like peptides and directly stimulate the hypothalamic-pituitary-adrenal (HPA) axis—the central control system for the stress response. This bidirectional cross-talk between the mast cell population and the HPA axis creates another reinforcing loop: stress activates mast cells, activated mast cells amplify the stress response, and the combined effect perpetuates both the autonomic dysfunction of POTS and the mediator excess of MCAS.

5. Neuropeptides and Small-Fiber Neuropathy

Substance P, calcitonin gene-related peptide (CGRP), and other neuropeptides released from sensory nerve fibers are powerful mast cell activators that also directly influence vascular tone. In MCAS, the sustained neuro-immune cross-talk between sensitized sensory nerves and reactive mast cells creates a local inflammatory environment that, over time, can damage the small unmyelinated nerve fibers that regulate vascular response and autonomic function. This small-fiber neuropathy—detectable through skin biopsy in a meaningful proportion of POTS and MCAS patients—contributes directly to the impaired vascular compensation that defines orthostatic intolerance.

Conversely, the neuropeptide-mast cell interaction helps explain why MCAS flares so frequently accompany emotional stress, physical trauma, or environmental triggers that activate the sensory nervous system. The nerves speak; the mast cells listen—and in a sensitized system, the response is amplified far beyond what the original signal warranted.

6. Renin-Angiotensin-Aldosterone System Interactions

Some POTS subtypes involve abnormalities in the renin-angiotensin-aldosterone system (RAAS), which regulates blood volume and vascular resistance. Mast cell mediators—particularly heparin, tryptase, and certain prostaglandins—interact with components of the RAAS in ways that can impair sodium retention and vascular responsiveness. Tryptase, for instance, can activate protease-activated receptors (PARs) on endothelial cells and vascular smooth muscle in ways that alter vasomotor tone. These interactions are not fully characterized but represent an active area of research into why MCAS and POTS so frequently co-occur and why addressing mast cell activity can improve blood pressure regulation.

✦ ✦ ✦

What This Means for You: A Unified Approach to MCAS and POTS

If you have been diagnosed with POTS and suspect you may also have MCAS—or if you have been diagnosed with MCAS and recognize the orthostatic symptoms described in this chapter—the most important thing to understand is this: these conditions are not separate problems requiring separate solutions. They are two expressions of a shared underlying dysfunction in the communication between your immune system, your nervous system, and your cardiovascular system. Treating them in concert is far more effective than treating each in isolation.

Here are the foundational principles of a unified approach:

Mast cell stabilization improves orthostatic tolerance. For individuals with POTS with a significant MCAS component, reducing mast cell reactivity through dietary changes, targeted supplementation, and nervous system support can improve vascular tone and reduce the pathological vasodilation that worsens postural symptoms. Many people report that their POTS becomes significantly more manageable once MCAS is addressed—even before conventional POTS medications are adjusted.

Standard POTS interventions remain important. Increased salt and fluid intake, compression garments, and graduated reconditioning exercises are the foundation of conventional POTS management, and they remain relevant and helpful in the person with comorbid MCAS-POTS. The goal is not to replace these strategies but to add the mast cell dimension to the treatment picture. Natural approaches to POTS are explored in detail later in this book.

The nervous system is the shared terrain. Because autonomic dysfunction underlies both conditions, interventions that support nervous system regulation—vagus nerve exercises, breathwork, somatic practices, and sleep optimization—address both MCAS reactivity and orthostatic instability simultaneously. This is not coincidental; it reflects the biology we've just explored. The vagus nerve, through the cholinergic anti-inflammatory pathway, suppresses mast cell activation. Strengthening vagal tone is one of the most powerful dual interventions available in natural MCAS-POTS management. Chapter 14 is devoted to these practices.

Exercise requires a thoughtful strategy. Exercise is genuinely therapeutic for POTS—it increases plasma volume, improves vascular tone, and reconditions the cardiovascular system. But exercise can also be a mast cell trigger, and the post-exertional malaise pattern seen in many MCAS-POTS patients can make standard reconditioning advice dangerous if applied without nuance. The recumbent exercise protocols, pacing strategies, and gradual reconditioning approaches outlined in Chapter 23 are designed specifically for this population.

Histamine management has direct cardiovascular benefits. Reducing dietary histamine load, supporting DAO enzyme activity, and using natural mast cell stabilizers doesn't just help with skin and gut symptoms—it directly reduces the vasodilatory and tachycardic effects of histamine on the cardiovascular system. For many, this is the most immediate and surprising benefit of a low-histamine approach: their heart rate becomes more stable and their orthostatic tolerance improves within days to weeks.

Track both sets of symptoms together. Using the symptom tracker in the Appendix, note your orthostatic symptoms alongside your classic MCAS symptoms. You will likely find that the same triggers that worsen your hives or gut pain also worsen your heart rate and dizziness. This convergence is the clearest evidence that mast cells are driving your cardiovascular symptoms—and it points directly toward the most effective interventions.

Priya's recovery was not linear. It never is. But once her treatment team began addressing her MCAS alongside her POTS—introducing a low-histamine protocol, supporting her vagus nerve, and using targeted mast cell stabilizers—the two conditions began to quiet together. Her resting heart rate normalized. The dizziness on standing became manageable. The hives that had seemed unrelated to her cardiovascular symptoms faded alongside them. Her body was not running two separate fires. It was running one, and they had finally found the right extinguisher.

✧ ✧ ✧

Chapter 3 at a Glance

What to Remember:

- POTS is a form of dysautonomia characterized by a heart rate increase of thirty or more beats per minute upon standing, caused by impaired autonomic compensation for gravity's effect on blood distribution.
- MCAS and POTS co-occur at rates far above chance. In many people, MCAS is not merely comorbid with POTS—it is actively driving it through direct effects on vascular tone, blood volume, and autonomic signaling.
- Histamine causes vasodilation and directly affects cardiac rate and rhythm through H1 and H2 receptors in cardiac tissue—mechanisms that directly worsen the orthostatic instability of POTS.
- Mast cell mediators reduce effective circulating blood volume by increasing vascular permeability, compounding the postural challenge of POTS.
- The autonomic nervous system and mast cells communicate bidirectionally: sympathetic overdrive activates mast cells, while reduced parasympathetic (vagal) tone removes the natural brake on mast cell reactivity. POTS creates the neurochemical environment in which MCAS thrives, and MCAS perpetuates autonomic dysfunction.
- Corticotropin-releasing hormone (CRH), released during physical and emotional stress, is a potent non-IgE mast cell activator—linking the chronic stress of living with POTS to ongoing mast cell priming.
- Small-fiber neuropathy, driven by the sustained neuro-immune cross-talk of MCAS, can directly damage the nerve fibers that regulate vascular response, contributing structurally to orthostatic intolerance.

- Treating MCAS and POTS in concert is more effective than treating each in isolation. Mast cell stabilization, vagus nerve support, histamine reduction, and recumbent exercise protocols address both conditions simultaneously through shared biological mechanisms.

Coming Up in Chapter 4:

MCAS and POTS do not travel alone. For a significant number of people, a third companion joins the picture: hypermobile Ehlers-Danlos syndrome, a connective tissue disorder that shares biological terrain with both. In Chapter 4, we explore the emerging science behind the MCAS–POTS–hEDS triad, its connections to chronic fatigue, long COVID, and autoimmune disease, and why these conditions so reliably cluster together in the same bodies.

CHAPTER 4

The Bigger Picture

MCAS, hEDS, Dysautonomia, Long COVID, and Why These Conditions Find Each Other

The Patient That Medicine Keeps Missing

She has been told she is complicated. That is the word doctors use—sometimes gently, sometimes with barely concealed frustration—when a patient's chart spans multiple specialties, when the diagnoses don't quite cohere, and when the treatments for each individual problem don't seem to add up to a person who is getting better.

Her name is Sofia. She is thirty-nine. Since her early twenties she has been hypermobile—her joints bend further than they should, she sprains her ankles on flat ground, and she has learned to be careful about how she sits and stands. Her physical therapist mentioned Ehlers-Danlos syndrome once, but her rheumatologist said she didn't quite meet the criteria and left it at that. In her late twenties, after a bout of mononucleosis (Epstein-Barr virus infection), she developed the racing heart and dizziness of POTS. She has been managing that for over a decade with salt, fluids, and compression. The hives, gut pain, and brain fog arrived gradually in her mid-thirties, worsening after a difficult pregnancy. No single physician has ever looked at all three problems together.

Sofia isn't three people who happen to share a body. She is one person, with one underlying biological disruption expressing itself in three interconnected ways. The triad of MCAS, POTS, and hypermobile Ehlers-Danlos syndrome (hEDS) is now one of the most recognized patterns in complex chronic illness medicine, even as mainstream medicine continues to treat each component separately.

This chapter is about the bigger picture: why these three conditions cluster, how they share biological terrain with chronic fatigue syndrome, long COVID, and autoimmune disease, and what understanding these connections means for the path toward healing.

✦ ✦ ✦

The Triad: MCAS, POTS, and Hypermobile Ehlers-Danlos Syndrome

Ehlers-Danlos syndrome (EDS) is a group of heritable connective tissue disorders characterized by defects in collagen—the structural protein that gives skin its elasticity, joints their stability, and blood vessels their integrity. There are thirteen recognized subtypes, distinguished by their genetic cause and clinical features. The most common by far—and the one most relevant to this discussion—is hEDS, which accounts for the vast majority of EDS diagnoses and is characterized primarily by joint hypermobility, chronic pain, and connective tissue fragility throughout the body.

The formal diagnosis of hEDS remains clinical—there is currently no confirmatory genetic test, which itself speaks to the complexity of connective tissue biology. Diagnosis relies on a structured assessment of joint mobility (typically using the Beighton score), the presence of characteristic musculoskeletal features, and the exclusion of other connective tissue disorders. A related condition, hypermobility spectrum disorder (HSD), describes patients who have significant hypermobility and its consequences without meeting the full hEDS criteria. For practical purposes in this discussion, hEDS and HSD share most of the same clinical territory.

> **Key Context:** *Hypermobility is far more common than most people realize. Estimates suggest that as many as one in five hundred to one in five thousand people meet criteria for hEDS, and hypermobility spectrum disorder is considerably more prevalent.*[32,33] *Many people with hypermobility have been told their whole lives that they are simply 'flexible' or 'double-jointed'—a benign description that dramatically underestimates the systemic consequences of defective connective tissue.*

The co-occurrence of MCAS, POTS, and hEDS is not a statistical coincidence. Clinical observations from centers specializing in these conditions consistently find that patients with one of the three have dramatically elevated rates of the other two.[34] Surveys of hEDS patient populations have found POTS in thirty to fifty percent and MCAS-consistent symptom patterns in a substantial majority.[35,36] The correlation between these three conditions is so strong that the view has shifted from viewing these as three separate conditions to a single multisystemic phenotype.[37,38] The question has shifted from whether these conditions cluster to why—and the answers emerging from research are illuminating.

Connective Tissue, Mast Cells, and a Shared Root

Collagen is not merely structural scaffolding. It is the medium in which mast cells live, migrate, and communicate with their neighbors—nerve fibers, blood vessels, and immune cells. When collagen is structurally abnormal, as in hEDS, it changes the physical and chemical environment in which mast cells operate. Connective tissue laxity (a condition where connective tissues are overly flexible or loose) alters the mechanical forces that mast cells experience. Research has shown that physical forces—pressure, stretch, vibration—can directly activate mast cells through mechanosensitive receptors including MRGPRX2.[39,40,41] In a body where connective tissue doesn't provide normal structural containment and resistance, mast cells may be chronically exposed to the kinds of mechanical stimulation that trigger their activation.

Beyond this mechanical hypothesis, there is emerging evidence that the genetic and epigenetic landscape of hEDS—poorly characterized as it remains—may directly predispose to mast cell dysfunction.[42,43] Dr. Lawrence Afrin and colleagues have theorized that the somatic mutations underlying MCAS and the germline or epigenetic defects contributing to hEDS may be linked at a deeper level: that the same impairment in cellular regulatory machinery that allows mast cell mutations to accumulate may also permit the expression of connective tissue fragility.[44,45,46] This hypothesis is not yet proven, but it is consistent with the clinical reality that these conditions cluster in families and that they tend to share not just symptoms but a similar natural history and progression.

The connective tissue laxity of hEDS also directly worsens POTS. Normally, blood vessel walls maintain tone partly through the structural integrity of the collagen surrounding them. In hEDS, vascular walls are more compliant—they stretch more readily—which means blood pools more aggressively in dependent vessels when upright. This is one of the clearest mechanical explanations for why hEDS patients have such elevated rates of orthostatic intolerance: their blood vessels, like their joints, lack the structural stiffness to maintain normal function under the ordinary physical stress of gravity.

The Neurological Thread: Dysautonomia in hEDS

Autonomic dysfunction in hEDS extends beyond the postural intolerance of POTS. Many hEDS patients experience a broader dysautonomic picture: impaired temperature regulation, abnormal sweating, gut dysmotility (slow or unpredictable gut movement), bladder dysfunction, and widespread abnormalities in how pain is processed and amplified.[47,48,49] This connects to the small-fiber neuropathy discussed in Chapter 3—the progressive damage to unmyelinated nerve fibers that regulate autonomic and sensory function—which is now documented in meaningful proportions of people with hEDS and appears to worsen with MCAS activity.

There is also the question of central sensitization: a state in which the central nervous system becomes persistently primed to amplify incoming signals, lowering the threshold at which pain, sensory input, and other stimuli are perceived as threatening. Central sensitization is well-documented in hEDS and fibromyalgia,[50,51] and there is mounting evidence that mast cell mediators—particularly those that cross the blood-brain barrier or activate meningeal mast cells—contribute directly to the neuroinflammatory processes that drive central sensitization.[52] In this model, MCAS does not merely accompany the pain and neurological symptoms of hEDS; it actively maintains and amplifies them.

> **Clinical Implication:** *For people with the full MCAS–POTS–hEDS triad, the nervous system is not merely a passive victim of these conditions. It is an active participant, maintained in a state of sensitization by chronic mast cell mediator exposure. Addressing mast cell dysfunction is therefore essential not just for immune and cardiovascular symptoms, but for the central nervous system dimensions of this triad—chronic pain, sensory hypersensitivity, and autonomic dysregulation.*

✦ ✦ ✦

Beyond the Triad: Chronic Fatigue, Long COVID, and Autoimmune Links

The MCAS–POTS–hEDS cluster does not exist in isolation. It overlaps substantially with a broader family of complex chronic conditions that share features of immune dysregulation, autonomic dysfunction, metabolic disruption, and a characteristic tendency to be triggered or worsened by infections, physical stress, or major physiological transitions.

Chronic Fatigue Syndrome and Myalgic Encephalomyelitis (ME/CFS)

Myalgic encephalomyelitis, commonly called chronic fatigue syndrome or ME/CFS, is characterized by profound fatigue that is not relieved by rest, post-exertional malaise (a worsening of symptoms following physical or cognitive effort that can last days to weeks), cognitive impairment, orthostatic intolerance, and unrefreshing sleep. It frequently follows viral or bacterial infection[53] and shares a demographic profile—predominantly affecting women, often onset in young adulthood—that overlaps substantially with MCAS and POTS.

There is increasing evidence of overlapping neuroimmune and inflammatory mechanisms between ME/CFS and mast cell activation disorders, suggesting a potential pathophysiologic connection, although definitive mechanistic links remain under investigation.[54,55] Elevated mast cell mediators have been measured in ME/CFS cohorts. The post-exertional malaise of ME/CFS—arguably its most defining and disabling feature—may in part reflect mast cell activation triggered by physical exertion, a pattern well recognized in MCAS. The immune dysregulation documented in ME/CFS, including natural killer cell dysfunction, elevated pro-inflammatory cytokines, and altered T-cell populations, overlaps with the immunological consequences of chronic mast cell mediator excess. And the small-fiber neuropathy, autonomic dysfunction, and neuroinflammation increasingly documented in ME/CFS are identical in character to what we see in the MCAS–POTS–hEDS triad.

Many researchers now believe that ME/CFS is not a single disease but a clinical phenotype—a common endpoint reached by different underlying disruptions in different people, with mast cell dysfunction being a significant contributor in a meaningful subset.[56] For people with both ME/CFS and MCAS features, natural approaches that address mast cell reactivity, support the autonomic nervous system, and reduce overall inflammatory burden have shown promise in improving both symptom clusters simultaneously.

Long COVID: A Modern Convergence

Perhaps no development in recent medicine has illuminated the MCAS–POTS–chronic illness connection more vividly than the emergence of long COVID. Post-acute sequelae of SARS-CoV-2 infection (PASC)—colloquially known as long COVID—describes a syndrome of persistent symptoms following COVID-19 infection that affects an estimated ten to thirty percent of those infected, regardless of acute illness severity.[57,58] Its hallmark features are exhaustingly familiar: profound fatigue, cognitive impairment, orthostatic intolerance, palpitations, gut dysfunction, sleep disruption, and a diverse array of inflammatory symptoms that vary considerably between individuals.

The parallels to MCAS are not superficial. Research published from 2021 onward has documented elevated mast cell mediators—histamine, tryptase, prostaglandins—in long COVID patients.[59,60] Studies have identified mast cell activation in multiple tissues of long COVID patients at autopsy and in living tissue samples.[61,62] The clinical picture of long COVID in many individuals is indistinguishable from MCAS: multi-system symptoms with no clear structural cause, fluctuating reactivity to foods and environmental triggers, and a pronounced sensitivity to exertion. And the treatment approaches that have shown the most benefit in long COVID clinics—low-histamine diets, H1 and H2 antihistamines, mast cell stabilizers, and autonomic rehabilitation—are precisely the approaches used to manage MCAS.

The SARS-CoV-2 virus appears to interact with mast cells directly through multiple pathways. The spike protein has been shown to activate mast cells through both ACE2 receptor binding and through pattern-recognition receptors that respond to viral components.[63] Viral RNA fragments that persist in tissue reservoirs in some long COVID patients may represent an ongoing source of mast cell activation. And the neurological effects of SARS-CoV-2—including its documented disruption of autonomic function and its capacity to trigger small-fiber neuropathy—may both reflect and perpetuate mast cell-driven neuroinflammation.

> **For Long COVID Patients:** *If you developed long COVID and recognize yourself in the descriptions of MCAS and POTS in this book, that recognition is clinically meaningful. Your symptoms are not imaginary, not purely psychological, and not simply 'post-viral fatigue' in the trivializing sense that phrase is sometimes used. They reflect a genuine biological disruption of mast cell regulation and autonomic function—and the natural approaches in this book are directly relevant to your recovery.*

Autoimmune Connections: Inflammation Without an Off Switch

The relationship between MCAS and autoimmune disease is bidirectional and complex. On one hand, mast cell mediators—particularly cytokines like TNF-alpha, IL-6, and IL-33—actively promote autoimmune inflammation by stimulating dendritic cell maturation, promoting Th2 immune skewing, and directly activating autoreactive lymphocytes.[64] Chronic mast cell activation can, over time, push the immune system toward sustained self-directed inflammation. On the other hand, many autoimmune conditions directly activate mast cells: autoantibodies can cross-link IgE receptors on mast cells, complement activation can trigger mast cell degranulation, and the inflammatory cytokine environment of active autoimmune disease provides a potent stimulus for mast cell priming.[65]

This bidirectional relationship explains several patterns frequently observed in complex chronic illness patients. Mildly elevated antinuclear antibody (ANA) titers—a common feature of systemic lupus erythematosus and other autoimmune conditions—appear in a proportion of MCAS patients without full autoimmune disease,[66] possibly reflecting mast-cell-driven immune dysregulation that hasn't yet crossed the threshold of clinical autoimmunity. Sjögren's-like symptoms (dry eyes, dry mouth, fatigue), thyroid autoimmunity, and autoimmune skin conditions all appear with elevated frequency in MCAS populations.[67] And conversely, patients with established autoimmune diagnoses who also have MCAS often find that their autoimmune symptoms are more severe, more reactive, and harder to control—because mast cells are amplifying their underlying immune dysfunction.

It is also worth noting that some autoimmune medications directly affect mast cells. Hydroxychloroquine, commonly used in lupus and Sjögren's, has mast cell-stabilizing properties. Low-dose naltrexone, increasingly used off-label in autoimmune and chronic inflammatory conditions, influences mast cell activity through opioid receptor pathways. The therapeutic overlap is not coincidental—it reflects shared biological terrain.

✦ ✦ ✦

Deeper Dive: Why Do These Conditions Cluster?

For the Science-Minded Reader

The clustering of MCAS, POTS, hEDS, ME/CFS, long COVID, and related conditions in the same individuals and families is not adequately explained by coincidence or by simple shared genetic risk for each condition independently. Something deeper is operating—a shared biological vulnerability that makes the entire system more susceptible to a family of interconnected dysfunctions. Several overlapping explanations have emerged from recent research.

The Connective Tissue Matrix as a Shared Vulnerability

Collagen is not only the structural backbone of joints, skin, and blood vessels—it is also the scaffolding within which most organ systems are embedded and through which chemical signals diffuse. When collagen is structurally abnormal, as in hEDS, the mechanical and chemical signaling environment throughout the body is altered.[68] This affects mast cell behavior (as discussed above), vascular integrity (worsening POTS), and the mechanical properties of nerves (potentially contributing to peripheral neuropathy and autonomic dysfunction). The extracellular matrix—the broader mesh of collagen, elastin, glycoproteins, and proteoglycans that surrounds cells—is increasingly recognized as an active signaling environment, not passive scaffolding.[69] Disruptions in its composition and mechanics may represent a unifying vulnerability underlying this cluster of conditions.

Shared Genetic and Epigenetic Architecture

Genome-wide association studies and emerging epigenomic research are beginning to identify shared genetic loci that influence susceptibility to multiple conditions in this cluster.[70,71,72] Variants affecting mast cell receptor signaling, connective tissue gene expression, autonomic nervous system development, and immune regulation appear in overlapping patterns across MCAS, hEDS, and dysautonomia populations. More intriguing still is the epigenetic dimension: the regulation of gene expression through methylation, acetylation, and other modifications that can be influenced by environmental exposures, chronic stress, infections, and developmental experiences.

Dr. Lawrence Afrin's hypothesis of impaired DNA repair machinery as the root driver of somatic mast cell mutations—described in Chapter 11—suggests that the same epigenetic dysregulation that allows mast cell mutations to accumulate may also underlie the connective tissue and autonomic vulnerabilities of this population. This is speculative but mechanistically coherent: a system that fails to maintain cellular integrity precisely would be expected to produce multiple expressions of that failure across different cell types and tissues, explaining why the same people who develop MCAS also develop hEDS-like connective tissue changes and dysautonomia.

The Role of Infectious Triggers

The frequency with which MCAS, POTS, hEDS symptom amplification, ME/CFS, and long COVID are triggered or dramatically worsened by infection is one of the most consistent features of this population and one of the strongest arguments for a shared underlying mechanism. Infections—particularly viral infections—activate mast cells directly through toll-like receptors and other pattern-recognition pathways.[73] They trigger massive cytokine release that can prime the immune system in a persistently dysregulated state. They can damage autonomic nerve fibers through direct neurotropic effects or through immune-mediated injury. And in genetically or epigenetically vulnerable individuals, a single significant infection can tip a previously compensated system into overt, disabling disease. Even after partial stabilization, subsequent infections may again disrupt this fragile equilibrium, leading to renewed or even more severe symptom exacerbations.

The pathogens most frequently identified as triggers in this cluster—Epstein-Barr virus (EBV), *Borrelia burgdorferi* (Lyme disease), enteroviruses, and most recently SARS-CoV-2—all share characteristics relevant to mast cell biology; they are capable of persistent infection or latency, they interact directly with immune receptors present on mast cells, and they provoke chronic or recurrent immune activation. We explore these infectious triggers in detail in Chapter 7.

Trauma, the Nervous System, and Biological Embedding

One of the most important—and most frequently overlooked—contributors to the clustering of these conditions is the role of adverse early experiences, chronic stress, and psychological trauma in shaping the immune and autonomic systems in ways that increase lifelong vulnerability.[74] This is not a psychological explanation for physical illness. It is a biological one.

The developing autonomic nervous system and immune system are exquisitely sensitive to early environmental signals. Adverse childhood experiences (ACEs)—abuse, neglect, family instability, chronic illness in the household—alter the set point of the HPA axis stress response, shape autonomic nervous system baseline tone, and influence the regulation of inflammatory pathways including mast cell reactivity.[75,76,77,78] These changes are encoded epigenetically and persist into adulthood. Adults with histories of significant adverse experiences show measurably higher baseline inflammatory markers, greater sympathetic nervous system reactivity, reduced vagal tone, and in multiple studies, elevated rates of conditions including fibromyalgia, IBS, chronic pelvic pain, and—increasingly evident—MCAS and dysautonomia.

This does not mean that MCAS or hEDS or POTS is caused by trauma in any simple or reductive sense. Many individuals with this triad have no identifiable adverse history and many people with significant trauma histories do not develop these conditions. But it does mean that for a meaningful proportion of people, the biological soil in which these conditions take root has been shaped by experiences that medicine has historically dismissed as irrelevant to physical disease. Understanding this connection opens important therapeutic doors—somatic therapies, nervous system regulation, and trauma-informed approaches to healing—that purely biomedical frameworks miss entirely. Chapter 14 addresses these approaches in depth.

> **Important Note:** *Recognizing the role of stress and trauma in biological vulnerability is not the same as saying symptoms are 'in your head.' The biological pathways are real, measurable, and treatable. This understanding should empower treatment options, not diminish the reality of your suffering.*

✦ ✦ ✦

What This Means for You: Thinking Systemically About Your Health

Understanding the bigger picture changes how you approach your own healing in several important ways. When your conditions are interconnected, isolated treatments—managing POTS without addressing mast cells, treating gut symptoms without considering connective tissue and nervous system dysfunction—inevitably fall short. The good news is that the shared biological terrain of these conditions means that interventions that address the underlying dysfunction can improve multiple symptom clusters simultaneously.

Seek a unified framework, not a specialist for each symptom. The most effective care for individuals in this cluster comes from physicians and practitioners who understand the interconnections—functional medicine doctors, integrative practitioners, and a growing number of specialists in MCAS, hEDS, and dysautonomia who are trained to see the whole picture. When building your care team, look for someone willing to hold the whole map, not just their corner of it.

Recognize that your history matters. If you have experienced significant infections, adverse experiences, or major physiological transitions (pregnancies, surgeries, periods of extreme stress) that preceded or dramatically worsened your symptoms, this history is clinically relevant. Share it with your practitioners. It is not background noise—it is signal.

Prioritize foundational interventions that work across the triad. Several natural interventions benefit all three conditions simultaneously; nervous system regulation (vagus nerve support, breathwork, somatic practices) improves mast cell reactivity, orthostatic tolerance, and connective tissue pain simultaneously. Low-histamine dietary approaches reduce mediator load, reduce neuroinflammation, and improve gut-driven autonomic signals. Anti-inflammatory supplementation addresses the shared inflammatory terrain of all three conditions. These are not fragmented symptom treatments—they are systemic interventions for a systemic problem.

Understand why long COVID and ME/CFS belong in your vocabulary. If you experience post-exertional malaise—a worsening of symptoms after physical or cognitive effort that lasts hours to days—this pattern deserves specific attention. Post-exertional malaise is the clinical signal of a system that cannot adequately recover from physiological demand, and it requires a pacing strategy fundamentally different from conventional exercise advice. Chapter 23 addresses this in detail.

Be patient with the complexity. The MCAS–POTS–hEDS cluster is among the most complex presentations in chronic illness medicine. Healing is rarely linear, and interventions that work powerfully for one person may need significant adjustment for another. The personalized protocol framework found later in this book is designed specifically for this complexity—to help you identify your own dominant drivers, your own most effective interventions, and your own sustainable path forward.

Sofia—whose story opened this chapter—is still navigating her recovery. She has good weeks and harder ones. But she is no longer confused about the terrain. She understands that her hypermobility, her POTS, and her mast cell symptoms are not three separate problems competing for her attention. They are three windows into the same underlying landscape. And knowing the landscape, she knows which direction to walk.

✦ ✦ ✦

Chapter 4 at a Glance

What to Remember:

- The triad of MCAS, POTS, and hypermobile Ehlers-Danlos syndrome (hEDS) is one of the most recognized patterns in complex chronic illness. These three conditions co-occur at rates far above chance and are mechanistically interconnected, not merely coincidentally comorbid.

- hEDS involves defective collagen and connective tissue throughout the body. Connective tissue laxity directly worsens POTS by reducing vascular wall integrity, and may prime mast cell activation through altered mechanical signaling in the extracellular matrix.
- Dysautonomia in hEDS extends beyond POTS to include broad autonomic dysfunction, small-fiber neuropathy, and central sensitization—all of which are amplified and maintained by chronic mast cell mediator exposure.
- ME/CFS and MCAS share overlapping mechanisms including elevated mast cell mediators, post-exertional immune activation, small-fiber neuropathy, and autonomic dysfunction. In many ME/CFS patients, mast cell dysfunction is a significant contributor to the clinical picture.
- Long COVID represents a modern, large-scale example of post-infectious mast cell activation and autonomic dysregulation. Mast cell mediators are elevated in long COVID patients, and the clinical pattern—multi-system, reactive, exertion-sensitive—maps closely onto MCAS.
- MCAS and autoimmune disease interact bidirectionally: mast cell mediators promote autoimmune inflammation, while autoimmune processes activate mast cells. Mildly elevated ANA titers and Sjögren's-like features are common in MCAS without constituting full autoimmune disease.
- These conditions cluster due to overlapping biological vulnerabilities: shared connective tissue matrix disruption, shared genetic and epigenetic architecture, infectious triggers that activate common pathways, and the biological embedding of stress and adverse experience in immune and autonomic regulation.
- Foundational interventions—nervous system regulation, low-histamine dietary approaches, anti-inflammatory supplementation—address the shared biological terrain of the entire cluster simultaneously, making them especially powerful in complex multi-condition patients.

Coming Up in the Next Chapters:

With a clear picture of what MCAS is, how it presents, and why it so frequently travels with POTS, hEDS, and related conditions, we are ready to go deeper—into the root causes and triggers that drive mast cell dysfunction in the first place. The next chapter opens with one of the most useful conceptual frameworks in all of MCAS medicine: the bucket theory of triggers. Understanding why your symptoms fluctuate, why the same food bothers you one day and not the next, and how cumulative load shapes your mast cell threshold is the foundation of everything that follows.

Why the Barrier Model Explains Key MCAS Patterns

The epithelial barrier model suggests that MCAS is caused by a "leaky" protective lining in the body that lets in irritants, which then constantly overstimulate the immune cells waiting just underneath. This model clarifies several clinical observations that are otherwise difficult to explain—patterns practitioners have long recognized but struggled to connect with a unifying mechanism.

The EDS, IBS, and MCAS Triad

Ehlers-Danlos Syndrome (hEDS) involves abnormal connective tissue throughout the body—including the connective tissue scaffold that supports epithelial barriers. Individuals with hEDS have documented higher rates of gut permeability, and this structural vulnerability offers a compelling explanation for why EDS, IBS, and MCAS so consistently co-occur. The triad is not coincidence—it may reflect a shared upstream defect in barrier architecture that predisposes all three conditions simultaneously.

Microbiome Restoration and Systemic Improvement

If the gut microbiome is one of the primary regulators of epithelial integrity—which the evidence strongly supports—then interventions that restore microbiome health (probiotics, prebiotics, dietary fiber, dysbiosis treatment) would be expected to improve MCAS symptoms indirectly, by rebuilding barrier function and reducing the chronic antigen load reaching subepithelial mast cells. This is precisely what is observed clinically: microbiome-focused interventions producing systemic MCAS improvement that cannot be explained by direct mast cell effect alone.

Environmental Sensitivity and Geographic Symptom Variation

Many individuals with MCAS notice their symptoms worsen dramatically in specific environments—moldy buildings, high-pollution areas, or during high-pollen seasons. The respiratory epithelium is continuously stressed by these environments, releasing alarm signals that lower the systemic mast cell threshold. This explains why the symptom burden often increases far beyond what the specific trigger alone would produce: the respiratory barrier is actively amplifying the total mast cell load, even when the gut and skin appear stable.

Key Insight: *These three patterns share a common thread—the epithelial barrier as a systemic amplifier. Addressing barrier health across all three surfaces, not simply managing individual triggers, is where lasting improvement becomes possible. The strategies in this book act like act like a "universal repair kit" that strengthens the cellular glue holding epithelial linings together. By sealing the gaps in your gut, skin, and airways, they prevent irritants from leaking through and causing the immune system to overreact.*

CHAPTER 5

The Bucket Theory of Triggers

Why Your Body Overflows—and How to Start Emptying the Bucket

The Day the Strawberries Became the Enemy

For most of her adult life, Rachel ate strawberries without a second thought. She put them in smoothies, tossed them into salads, and looked forward to them every summer. They were, as far as she was concerned, one of life's uncomplicated pleasures.

Then, at thirty-six, she ate a handful of strawberries on a Tuesday afternoon and broke out in hives from her collarbone to her waist.

Her doctor tested her for a strawberry allergy. The test came back negative. She was told to avoid strawberries anyway, just to be safe. She did. And for several weeks, nothing happened. Then, on a particularly stressful Wednesday—the day her mother was admitted to hospital, the day she'd barely slept, the day she'd pushed through a gym class she probably shouldn't have—she ate a piece of leftover birthday cake. Hives again. Not as bad as the strawberries had triggered, but unmistakable.

The cake didn't have strawberries in it. It was vanilla.

What was happening? If the strawberries were the problem, why did vanilla cake cause hives? And if strawberries were fine before, why were they suddenly a problem at all?

The answer lies in one of the most important concepts in all of MCAS medicine—and one of the most immediately practical. Once Rachel understood it, her symptoms began to make sense for the first time. More importantly, she discovered she had far more control over her situation than she had believed.

The concept is called the bucket theory of triggers. And it changes everything about how you understand your reactions.

✦ ✦ ✦

The Bucket: A Simple Model for a Complex Reality

Imagine your body's tolerance for triggers as a bucket. Every day, various things fill that bucket—foods that are high in histamine, stress, poor sleep, environmental exposures, hormonal fluctuations, infections, physical exertion, emotional strain. Some of these things add a large amount to the bucket. Others add just a small splash. As long as the water stays below the rim, you feel reasonably okay. Your mast cells are activated to some degree—they're always doing their job—but the response stays within manageable bounds.

When the bucket overflows, symptoms appear.

This is the core insight: it's not always the last thing you added to the bucket that causes the overflow. It's the total volume—the cumulative load of everything that has been building up. The strawberries weren't the villain in Rachel's story. They were simply the thing that pushed an already-very-full bucket over the rim. On a calm day with good sleep, manageable stress, and a light trigger load, she might have eaten those same strawberries without a single hive. But on the day her bucket was nearly full, even a small addition was enough.

> **The Bucket Principle:** *Your symptoms aren't caused by triggers in isolation—they're caused by triggers in context. The same food, the same environment, the same stressor can produce very different reactions on different days, depending on how full your bucket already is.*

This explains one of the most maddeningly inconsistent features of MCAS: the fact that the same thing bothers you one day and not the next. It explains why your reactions seem random when they aren't. It explains why you can eat a food a dozen times without issue and then react violently the thirteenth time—because the thirteenth time, the rest of your bucket happened to be fuller. And it explains why, counterintuitively, addressing what seems like a small contributor—getting a better night's sleep, reducing a stressful relationship, fixing a gut problem—can have a dramatic effect on your overall reactivity, even without changing anything about the specific triggers that seem most obvious.

The bucket model also helps explain the phenomenon many people with MCAS describe as "sensitization over time"—the gradual expansion of the list of things they react to. When the bucket is consistently full or overflowing, the threshold for mast cell activation gets lower. Repeated overflow events can prime mast cells to be even more reactive, and the immune system learns, incorrectly, that a growing number of stimuli are threats. The bucket doesn't just overflow; over time, if it's never properly emptied, it seems to get smaller.

The good news—and this is critical—is that the relationship works in both directions. Just as adding to the bucket causes overflow, emptying the bucket reduces reactivity. Every trigger you reduce or eliminate lowers the water level. Every foundational intervention—better sleep, reduced stress, dietary adjustment, gut healing, nervous system support—creates more room. More room means a higher threshold before you react. A higher threshold means foods and environments that once triggered you consistently may become manageable again. The bucket gets bigger. Or rather, the water level drops low enough that the bucket's size stops mattering.

> **A Word of Hope:** *Individuals who understand the bucket theory often report a turning point in their relationship with their illness. They stop feeling at the mercy of an unpredictable, hostile body and start seeing their condition as something they can actively influence. That shift in perspective is not small. It is, for many, the beginning of genuine healing.*

✦ ✦ ✦

What Goes Into the Bucket? A Guide to Trigger Categories

Triggers fall into several broad categories, and understanding them helps you make strategic decisions about where to focus your energy. Not all triggers are equally significant for every person—part of the work ahead is identifying which categories fill your bucket most rapidly. But knowing the full landscape is the first step.

Food and Drink Triggers

Food is one of the most visible trigger categories for most individuals with MCAS, because dietary reactions are relatively easy to observe and track. But food triggers in MCAS are not the same as food allergies. In a classic food allergy, a specific food triggers an IgE-mediated immune response that is consistent, immediate, and usually dose-dependent. With MCAS, food reactions are more variable—the same food may be tolerable in small amounts, catastrophic in larger amounts, fine on a low-trigger day, and problematic on a high-trigger day.

The most significant food-related triggers include:

- **High-histamine foods – These include** aged cheeses, fermented foods, cured and processed meats, alcohol (especially red wine and beer), vinegar, certain fish (particularly canned or smoked), tomatoes, spinach, eggplant, avocado, and leftovers (histamine content rises with storage time as bacteria react with histidine).[79] These foods don't trigger mast cell degranulation directly—they add histamine to the system directly, reducing the margin before symptoms appear.

- **Histamine-liberating foods** – Some foods don't contain high histamine themselves but prompt the body to release histamine from existing stores. Strawberries, citrus fruits, pineapple, papaya, tomatoes, chocolate, alcohol, and certain food additives fall into this category—which explains why Rachel's strawberries were a problem even without testing positive for a strawberry allergy.[80] These foods naturally contain certain proteins or chemical triggers that act directly on mast cells, signaling them to degranulate; or in the case of alcohol block the enzyme—diamine oxidase (DAO)—that breaks down histamine in food.
- **DAO-blocking foods and substances** –DAO is the primary enzyme responsible for breaking down histamine in the gut. Alcohol, black tea, energy drinks, and certain medications block DAO activity,[81] allowing histamine to accumulate rather than be cleared efficiently. A DAO-blocking food adds to the bucket not by adding histamine but by reducing the drain.
- **Foods that directly activate mast cells** – Some compounds in food can trigger mast cell degranulation through non-histamine pathways. Alcohol, certain food dyes and preservatives (particularly sulfites and benzoates), lectins in high amounts, and gluten (in some people) may directly stimulate mast cells or amplify their reactivity.[82,83,84,85,86]
- **Glyphosate residues on foods** – Widely used in modern agriculture, glyphosate residues have been detected on a range of foods. Glyphosate can directly stimulate mast cell degranulation and is known to affect intestinal barrier function.[87,88] When these tight junctions are compromised (leaky gut), larger proteins and environmental toxins can enter the bloodstream triggering a chronic, low-grade mast cell activation and histamine release.
- **Oxalates and salicylates** – These naturally occurring compounds in many healthy foods can trigger reactions in a subset of MCAS patients,[89] adding another layer of complexity to dietary management. Salicylate sensitivity is often unrecognized and can masquerade as reactions to seemingly unrelated foods.

It is important to note that a low-histamine diet is not meant to be a permanent, maximally restrictive state. It is a tool for lowering the water level in your bucket while your mast cells stabilize and your gut—the primary site of histamine clearance—heals. As you recover, many people find they can reintroduce previously reactive foods without issue. Chapter 13 covers the practical details of the low-histamine lifestyle, and Chapter 15 explores the foods that actively support mast cell stabilization.

Stress and Emotional Triggers

Stress is not a soft trigger. It is one of the most potent mast cell activators in the human body, operating through multiple direct biological pathways.[90]

When you experience stress—whether from a difficult conversation, a looming deadline, a frightening medical appointment, or simply the accumulated weight of a difficult life—your brain releases corticotropin-releasing hormone (CRH), which directly activates mast cells through specific surface receptors. At the same time, your sympathetic nervous system surges, releasing norepinephrine that also stimulates mast cell degranulation. These are not metaphorical effects. Stress physically triggers your mast cells within minutes, adding a substantial volume to your bucket regardless of what you've eaten or how well you've slept.

Emotional stress is often the hidden variable that explains why your symptoms fluctuate so dramatically. A week of unusually good eating may be undermined by a period of unusual stress, leaving you scratching your head at reactions that seem to have no dietary explanation. Conversely, individuals who make significant progress on stress reduction and nervous system regulation often find their dietary tolerance improving dramatically—not because they changed what they ate, but because they lowered the non-dietary contributions to their bucket.

This does not mean you need to achieve perfect serenity to recover—an unrealistic and somewhat unkind standard. It means that nervous system support is as genuinely medical as any dietary protocol, and deserves to be treated with the same seriousness. Chapter 14 provides concrete, practical tools for this work.

Sleep and Circadian Disruption

Sleep is when your body performs its most critical repair and regulatory work. The glymphatic system—your brain's waste-clearance mechanism—runs primarily during deep sleep, flushing out inflammatory debris including the byproducts of mast cell mediator activity. Histamine itself is a wakefulness-promoting neurotransmitter, so excess histamine disrupts sleep, and poor sleep leads to higher histamine levels the following day: a vicious cycle familiar to many people with MCAS.

Even a single night of significantly disrupted sleep elevates inflammatory markers, reduces immune regulation, and lowers the threshold for mast cell reactivity the following day.[91] Chronically poor sleep—which is nearly universal in individuals with MCAS—is one of the most consistent and underappreciated bucket-fillers, because it affects every other trigger simultaneously: food reactions worsen, stress tolerance drops, pain amplifies, and cognitive function deteriorates.

Sleep optimization is therefore not optional in MCAS management—it is foundational. Chapter 14 addresses sleep support strategies in depth, including approaches tailored specifically to the histamine-disrupted sleep architecture common in this population.

Environmental and Chemical Triggers

Mast cells in the skin, respiratory tract, and tissues respond to a wide range of environmental stimuli that most people encounter without incident. For someone with sensitized mast cells and a frequently full bucket, these same stimuli become significant contributors:

- **Fragrances and synthetic chemicals** – Perfumes, scented cleaning products, fabric softeners, air fresheners, and personal care products containing synthetic fragrance compounds are among the most common environmental triggers.[92] Even brief exposure in a shared space can add enough to the bucket to push a sensitized person over threshold.
- **Mold and mycotoxins** – Mold exposure is explored in detail in Chapter 8, but it deserves mention here as a powerful and often unrecognized bucket-filler. Mast cells in the respiratory and mucosal tissues respond strongly to mold spores and the mycotoxins they produce, and living or working in a water-damaged building can keep the bucket perpetually full regardless of what else is being done to lower it.[93]
- **Temperature extremes** – Both heat and cold can directly trigger mast cell degranulation.[94,95] Many people with MCAS notice significant worsening with sudden temperature changes—stepping from air conditioning into summer heat, or from a warm room into cold air. Exercise-induced overheating is a related trigger for some.
- **Electromagnetic fields and vibration** – While the evidence is limited and this remains an area of debate, some MCAS patients report sensitivity to electromagnetic fields and vibration.[96] This may relate to MRGPRX2 receptor activation by physical forces, as discussed in Chapter 1.
- **Air quality and pollution** – Particulate matter, diesel exhaust, and other air pollutants directly activate mast cells in the respiratory mucosa.[97] Urban environments, high-traffic areas, and wildfire smoke can produce measurable increases in mast cell reactivity.

Hormonal Fluctuations

Hormones, particularly estrogen, have direct effects on mast cell sensitivity and activity.[98] Estrogen upregulates the expression of mast cell surface receptors and enhances their responsiveness to both IgE-mediated and non-IgE triggers. This estrogen-histamine interaction—explored fully in Chapter 10—explains why many women with MCAS experience dramatic symptom fluctuation across the menstrual cycle, with significant worsening in the premenstrual phase when estrogen dominates and progesterone is falling.

Hormonal transitions more broadly—puberty, pregnancy, postpartum, perimenopause—are frequently reported as trigger points for the onset or significant worsening of MCAS. Thyroid dysfunction and adrenal imbalance also influence mast cell reactivity and overall inflammatory threshold.[99] For people whose bucket seems to refill rapidly despite addressing other triggers, hormonal assessment is a critical piece of the diagnostic picture.

Infections and Immune Challenges

Any active infection—viral, bacterial, or fungal—significantly fills the bucket. The immune activation involved in fighting an infection directly primes and activates mast cells, which is part of their normal role in immune defense. For individuals with MCAS, even relatively minor illnesses that a healthy person would shake off in a few days can trigger prolonged flares that last weeks to months.

Chronic or latent infections—the Epstein-Barr virus sitting dormant, low-grade Lyme disease, small intestinal bacterial overgrowth (SIBO), or chronic fungal overgrowth—are persistent contributors to bucket loads that often go unidentified. These are explored in Chapters 6 and 7. Vaccination, surgical procedures, dental work, and other medical interventions that acutely challenge the immune system can also temporarily fill the bucket, sometimes triggering prolonged flares that leave both patient and physician confused about what went wrong.

Physical Factors

Physical forces—exertion, mechanical pressure, vibration, and even touch—can directly activate mast cells through mechanosensitive pathways. This helps explain why some people with MCAS react to tight clothing, firm massage, or prolonged sitting in ways that seem entirely disconnected from the conventional understanding of allergy.

Exercise is a complex trigger. At moderate levels it can be anti-inflammatory and genuinely therapeutic—but pushed too hard, it triggers significant mast cell activation through both thermal (overheating) and mechanical pathways, plus the sympathetic surge that accompanies intense effort. Finding the therapeutic window for movement—enough to support cardiovascular health and nervous system regulation, not so much as to trigger flares—is one of the practical arts of MCAS management. Chapter 23 is devoted entirely to this question.

✦ ✦ ✦

Deeper Dive: The Biology of Cumulative Load and Threshold

For the Science-Minded Reader

The bucket theory is a conceptual model, but it maps onto real and measurable biology. Understanding the mechanisms behind threshold and cumulative load helps explain why this model is so clinically accurate—and why the interventions it suggests work.

Mast Cell Priming and the Lowered Threshold

Mast cells exist on a spectrum of activation states. At baseline, they are in a resting or "surveying" state—monitoring the environment but not releasing mediators. When exposed to a sensitizing signal, they become primed: their surface receptors are upregulated, their granules are positioned closer to the cell membrane, and the threshold signal required to trigger degranulation is significantly lower. A primed mast cell responds to stimuli that a resting mast cell would ignore entirely.

What primes mast cells? Essentially, the very triggers described above—sustained stress, chronic infection, environmental exposures, sleep deprivation, and hormonal shifts. Each of these priming signals doesn't just add to the bucket in the moment; it lowers the bucket's rim, making future overflow easier. This is the biological basis for sensitization over time: every period of high trigger load leaves the mast cell population slightly more reactive than it was before, until what once seemed like a high threshold becomes vanishingly low.

The reverse is also true. Interventions that reduce trigger load—consistently, over weeks to months—allow mast cells to return toward a more rested, less primed state. Surface receptor expression normalizes. The threshold rises. The bucket, in the biological sense, gets deeper.

Mediator Load and the Saturation of Clearance Systems

The body has several systems for clearing histamine and other mast cell mediators once they've been released. Diamine oxidase (DAO) in the gut lining breaks down histamine from food before it enters the bloodstream. Histamine N-methyltransferase (HNMT) within cells converts histamine into an inactive metabolite. The liver processes and conjugates a wide range of inflammatory mediators for excretion. When trigger load is low, these clearance systems keep pace and mediator levels stay manageable.

When trigger load is high—when the mast cells are releasing mediators faster than clearance systems can process them—mediators accumulate. This is the biochemical reality of a full bucket: not just mast cells firing, but their products building up in tissues and circulation because the drain can't keep up with the inflow. Interventions that support DAO activity (supplemental DAO enzymes, certain probiotics, B6 and copper), optimize liver detoxification, and reduce the rate of mediator release all work partly by improving the drainage side of the bucket equation.

Individual Variation in Threshold

Why do some people's buckets seem much smaller than others? Several factors determine individual mast cell threshold:

- **Genetics** – Variants in genes encoding mast cell receptors, histamine-metabolizing enzymes, and inflammatory signaling pathways influence baseline reactivity. Hereditary alpha-tryptasemia (HαT), discussed in Chapter 2, is one example of a genetic factor that demonstrably lowers the threshold.
- **Epigenetic programming** – As discussed in Chapter 4, early life experiences and chronic stress alter the epigenetic regulation of immune and autonomic function in ways that affect mast cell behavior throughout life.
- **Gut microbiome** – The gut microbiome profoundly influences histamine metabolism, immune regulation, and the integrity of the intestinal barrier through which dietary histamine is absorbed. A dysbiotic microbiome—one that is out of balance—can significantly reduce the body's capacity to clear histamine and regulate mast cell activity.[100,101] Chapter 6 explores this in depth.
- **Hormonal status** – Estrogen's mast-cell-sensitizing effects mean that hormonal phase, hormonal health, and hormonal history significantly affect individual threshold.
- **Body burden of toxins** – Accumulation of heavy metals, mycotoxins, and chemical exposures impairs cellular function including the regulatory pathways that keep mast cells from overreacting. Chapter 8 explores the role of environmental toxins as a persistent bucket contributor.

> **The Practical Implication:** *Because individual threshold is determined by multiple factors—many of which are modifiable—there is genuine room to raise your threshold over time. This is not wishful thinking; it is the mechanism by which patients recover. Raising the threshold is not about eliminating every trigger. It is about systematically reducing the factors that keep your threshold low.*

Identifying Your Personal Thresholds

One of the most valuable skills you can develop is learning to recognize the early warning signs that your bucket is getting full—before it overflows. Most individuals with MCAS, once they start paying careful attention, can identify a pattern—a set of subtle signals that precede a full reaction by hours or even days. These might include:

- Increased skin sensitivity or mild itching without visible hives
- A heightened sense of smell or increased irritation from odors
- Mild digestive discomfort or bloating that feels different from usual
- A low-grade feeling of unease or heightened anxiety
- Sleep that is slightly more disrupted than normal
- A subtle increase in heart rate variability or palpitations
- A feeling some people describe as "wired but tired" or "on edge"

These are your early warning system—your body's way of telling you the bucket is filling. Learning to recognize them and respond proactively—resting, reducing triggers, adding a stabilizing supplement, prioritizing sleep—can interrupt the cascade before it reaches overflow. This early intervention skill, more than almost anything else, gives patients a genuine sense of agency over their condition.

✦ ✦ ✦

What This Means for You: Finding Your Personal Trigger Pattern

The bucket theory is only useful if you put it to work. Here is how to translate the concept into practical, daily self-knowledge.

Start tracking—but track smartly. A symptom journal is the single most important tool in the early stages of MCAS management. But tracking everything at once can become overwhelming and counterproductive. Start with three columns: symptoms (what happened, severity on a 1–10 scale), likely contributors (what you ate, your sleep quality, stress level, any unusual exposures), and bucket assessment (on a scale of 1–10, how full did your bucket feel that day overall?). Over two to four weeks, patterns will emerge that no amount of specialist testing has been able to reveal. The Appendix contains a structured symptom tracker designed specifically for this purpose.

Look for the patterns behind the patterns. When you review your tracking data, resist the urge to identify single causes. Instead, ask: On the days I reacted, what else was happening? Was sleep worse? Was stress higher? Had I been exposed to more environmental triggers? Often the most illuminating insight is not which food triggered you, but which combination of circumstances—a full bucket plus a trigger—reliably produces symptoms.

Rank your triggers by bucket contribution. Once you have a reasonable picture of your trigger landscape, try to rank your triggers roughly by how much they fill your bucket. Some triggers are major contributors—a poor night's sleep, a period of high stress, significant mold exposure, a gut infection. Others are minor contributors that only matter when the bucket is already full. Focusing your early energy on reducing the major contributors produces the most significant and fastest improvement in overall reactivity.

Understand the difference between elimination and management. The bucket theory does not require you to eliminate every trigger permanently. It requires you to understand your threshold and manage your total load. Many individuals discover that once their bucket is consistently lower—through gut healing, nervous system regulation, and foundational dietary adjustments—they can tolerate occasional exposures to moderate triggers without reacting. Recovery is not about achieving a pristine, zero-trigger life. It is about raising your threshold high enough that ordinary life becomes livable.

Be strategic about timing. Because your bucket level fluctuates, strategic timing of activities can make a significant difference. Save higher-trigger events—restaurants with less dietary control, social situations that are stressful, higher-intensity exercise—for days when your bucket has been consistently lower. Use known high-bucket periods—the premenstrual week, high-stress periods at work, the first days of a new season—as times to be especially diligent with supportive practices.

Celebrate the small empties. Every intervention that reduces your trigger load—every good night's sleep, every low-histamine meal, every stress-management practice, every reduction in environmental chemical exposure—is emptying the bucket. The effects may not be dramatically visible day to day, but they accumulate. Individuals who feel discouraged because a single change didn't transform their symptoms often don't appreciate how many small empties are needed before the bucket drops to a consistently safe level. Progress in MCAS management tends to be gradual, then suddenly noticeable.

Rachel, whose strawberry story opened this chapter, eventually understood what had been happening. Her bucket on that Tuesday afternoon had been nearly full before she ate a single berry: She'd been sleeping poorly for a week, her mother's health was worrying her, she'd skipped meals and eaten more leftovers than usual, and she'd been pushing herself through workouts she didn't have the energy for. The strawberries weren't the cause. They were the final drop.

Once she understood that, she stopped being afraid of strawberries. She started paying attention to the bucket instead. And slowly, with fewer overflows and more intentional management, her body began to find a kind of steadiness it hadn't known in years.

✦ ✦ ✦

Chapter 5 at a Glance

What to Remember:

- The bucket theory of triggers explains why MCAS symptoms fluctuate unpredictably: your body has a tolerance threshold for mast cell activation, and symptoms occur when the cumulative load of all triggers—not any single trigger—exceeds that threshold.
- The same food, environment, or stressor can cause a reaction one day and be tolerated another day, depending entirely on how much else has been added to the bucket.
- Trigger categories include: food and drink (high-histamine foods, histamine liberators, DAO-blocking substances), stress and emotional load, sleep quality and circadian rhythm, environmental and chemical exposures, hormonal fluctuations, active and chronic infections, and physical factors including exercise and temperature.
- Repeated overflow events can prime mast cells to be more reactive over time, effectively making the bucket smaller. Consistent reduction of trigger load allows mast cells to return toward a less primed state, raising the threshold and making the bucket deeper.
- Clearance systems—including DAO in the gut, HNMT within cells, and liver detoxification—represent the drain of the bucket. Supporting these systems is as important as reducing what goes in.
- Individual threshold varies based on genetics, epigenetic programming, gut microbiome health, hormonal status, and accumulated toxin burden—many of which are modifiable over time.
- Learning your personal early warning signs—the subtle signals that your bucket is filling—gives you the ability to intervene before overflow and develop genuine agency over your condition.
- Recovery does not require eliminating every trigger. It requires raising your threshold high enough, through consistent foundational interventions, that ordinary life becomes tolerable and progressively more comfortable.

Coming Up in Chapter 6:

Of all the root causes and trigger amplifiers explored in this book, few are more foundational—or more correctable—than the state of the gut. The gastrointestinal tract is the site of histamine production, histamine clearance, immune education, and the first line of defense against a world full of potential triggers. In Chapter 6, we explore how gut dysfunction and an imbalanced microbiome feed directly into MCAS, why leaky gut and SIBO are so common in this population, and what you can do to begin healing from the inside out.

CHAPTER 6

Gut Dysfunction and the Microbiome

How the State of Your Gut Shapes the Reactivity of Your Entire Body

The Gut That Started Everything

Daniel had always had a sensitive stomach. As a child, he'd been prone to what his parents called "tummy trouble"—episodes of cramping and loose stools that came and went without obvious cause. By his twenties, he'd been given a diagnosis of irritable bowel syndrome, handed a pamphlet about dietary fiber and stress management, and largely left to make peace with the fact that his gut was simply unreliable.

What nobody told Daniel was that his gut wasn't just causing discomfort. It was shaping his immune system.

By his mid-thirties, Daniel had developed what he could only describe as a body that had "gone haywire." Foods he'd eaten for years without issue were now triggering hives, flushing, and a terrifying pounding in his chest. His brain fog had become so thick that he'd had to reduce his hours at work. He was exhausted in ways that sleep didn't fix. His skin itched constantly. His gastroenterologist said his IBS was "unchanged" based on his colonoscopy. His allergist found no IgE-mediated allergies. Nobody made the connection between his lifelong gut dysfunction and his new systemic reactivity—because in conventional medicine, the gut and the immune system are still treated as mostly separate stories.

They are not separate stories. They are the same story, told from different angles.

The gut is not simply a food-processing tube. It is the site of seventy percent of the body's immune tissue, home to trillions of microorganisms that directly regulate inflammation and immune tolerance, and—critically for MCAS patients—both the primary site of histamine production and the primary site of histamine clearance.

When the gut is dysfunctional, the consequences ripple outward into virtually every system in the body, including—and especially—the mast cell network.

This chapter is about that connection: why gut health is not peripheral to MCAS management but central to it, and what you can do to begin healing it.

✦ ✦ ✦

Your Gut: The Immune System's Headquarters

To understand why gut dysfunction matters so profoundly in MCAS, it helps to appreciate just how much immunological work the gut does every single day.

The gut lining—the mucosal surface of the intestines—faces an extraordinary challenge. Its job is to allow nutrients to pass into the bloodstream while keeping everything else out: bacteria, undigested food particles, toxins, and pathogens. This is a feat of remarkable discrimination, performed across a surface area roughly the size of a tennis court, by a barrier that is, in most places, only a single cell thick.

To manage this challenge, the gut houses an enormous and sophisticated immune apparatus. Peyer's patches and mesenteric lymph nodes process a constant stream of antigens, training immune cells to distinguish between harmless food proteins and genuine threats. Secretory IgA—an antibody produced in vast quantities in the gut lining—forms a first line of defense, coating pathogens and preventing them from breaching the barrier. Regulatory T cells cultivated in the gut mucosa travel throughout the body helping to maintain immune tolerance—the ability to not overreact to the environment.

And mast cells. The gut wall is one of the most mast-cell-dense environments in the body.[102] These tissue-resident immune cells are positioned directly beneath the gut epithelium, ideally situated to respond to anything that breaches or threatens the barrier—and, as we've seen, to respond excessively when their threshold is chronically lowered.

> **The Key Insight:** *The gut doesn't just react to MCAS—it drives it. A gut that is inflamed, poorly sealed, or populated by the wrong microbial community, is a gut that is continuously filling the mast cell bucket, day after day, whether or not any obvious dietary trigger is present.*

Three distinct but overlapping mechanisms connect gut health to MCAS: intestinal permeability ("leaky gut"), microbiome composition (the balance of histamine-producing versus histamine-degrading bacteria), and specific gut conditions including IBS, small intestinal bacterial overgrowth (SIBO), and candida overgrowth. Let's explore each in turn.

✦ ✦ ✦

Leaky Gut and Mast Cell Activation

"Leaky gut" is a colloquial term that has attracted both popular enthusiasm and clinical skepticism. The skepticism is understandable—the term has been used loosely and sometimes associated with exaggerated health claims. But the underlying phenomenon is real, measurable, and increasingly well-documented in peer-reviewed literature.[103,104,105] Its proper name is increased intestinal permeability, and its relevance to MCAS is difficult to overstate.

The cells lining the intestinal wall—enterocytes—are joined together by protein structures called tight junctions. When functioning properly, tight junctions act like the grout between bathroom tiles: they seal the gaps between cells, preventing large molecules from slipping through. When tight junctions are disrupted—by inflammation, by certain foods, by microbial toxins, by stress, by certain medications including non-steroidal anti-inflammatory drugs (NSAIDs) and proton pump inhibitors—the gaps widen. Substances that should stay in the gut lumen pass into the underlying tissue and, from there, into the bloodstream.

These substances include partially digested food proteins, bacterial fragments called lipopolysaccharides (LPS), bacterial toxins, and other immune-activating compounds. When they breach the gut barrier, they encounter the dense population of mast cells just beneath the epithelium—and they activate them.

Here is the vicious cycle that results: intestinal permeability activates subepithelial mast cells, which release mediators that further damage the gut lining, which worsens permeability, which activates more mast cells. Activated gut mast cells also release mediators that drive systemic inflammation, further priming mast cells throughout the body. The gut, in this model, is not just experiencing the consequences of MCAS—it is perpetuating it.

What Causes Increased Intestinal Permeability?

The factors that disrupt tight junction integrity overlap substantially with the trigger categories described in Chapter 5. They include:

- **Chronic psychological stress** – Cortisol and CRH directly disrupt tight junction proteins,[106] one of the clearest demonstrations that stress has a literal structural effect on the gut barrier.
- **Dysbiosis** – An imbalanced gut microbiome produces less of the short-chain fatty acids (particularly butyrate) that nourish enterocytes and maintain tight junction integrity, and more of the inflammatory metabolites that damage it.[107,108]

- **Dietary factors** – Ultra-processed foods, excessive sugar, gluten (particularly in genetically susceptible individuals), and certain food additives including emulsifiers and surfactants have been shown to disrupt tight junctions in laboratory and clinical studies.[109,110]
- **Alcohol – Alcohol is** directly toxic to the gut epithelium and a potent disruptor of tight junction proteins,[111,112] explaining in part why even small amounts of alcohol are so problematic for many MCAS patients.
- **NSAIDs and certain medications** – Ibuprofen, naproxen, and aspirin increase intestinal permeability even at standard doses;[113,114] proton pump inhibitors alter gut pH in ways that promote dysbiosis and may secondarily affect barrier function.[115,116]
- **Infections and microbial imbalance** – Bacterial toxins, fungal metabolites, and parasitic infections all damage the gut epithelium and disrupt tight junctions.[117,118,119]
- **Mast cell mediators themselves** – Histamine, tryptase, and certain prostaglandins released by activated gut mast cells increase intestinal permeability directly,[120,121,122] closing the loop of the vicious cycle.

Testing for intestinal permeability is possible but imperfect. The lactulose-mannitol test measures the ratio of these two sugars in urine after oral administration—a higher ratio suggests increased permeability.[123] Serum zonulin (a protein that regulates tight junction opening) is available through some functional medicine laboratories, though its sensitivity and specificity remain subjects of debate.[124,125,126] Elevated serum LPS-binding protein provides indirect evidence of bacterial translocation.[127,128,129] For most patients, the combination of clinical picture and therapeutic response—improvement in systemic symptoms when gut healing protocols are implemented—is the most practical evidence for intestinal permeability as a contributing factor.

✦ ✦ ✦

The Microbiome: Your Inner Ecosystem and Histamine Balance

Living in your gut right now are somewhere between thirty-eight trillion microorganisms—bacteria, archaea, fungi, and viruses—collectively called the gut microbiome.[130] These organisms are not passive passengers. They digest dietary fibers you cannot process yourself, produce vitamins including K2 and several B vitamins, train and regulate your immune system, communicate with your nervous system through the gut-brain axis, and directly influence your body's histamine levels.

That last point is the one most immediately relevant to MCAS.

Histamine-Producing Bacteria: The Microbiome's Contribution to Your Bucket

Certain bacteria in the gut produce histamine as a metabolic byproduct, using an enzyme called histidine decarboxylase to convert the amino acid histidine—found in many protein-containing foods—into histamine.[131] This is entirely normal in a balanced microbiome, where histamine-producing bacteria are present in modest numbers and histamine-degrading counterparts keep the balance in check. But in a dysbiotic gut—one where this balance has been disrupted—histamine-producing bacteria can dominate, generating a continuous internal source of histamine that fills the bucket from the inside regardless of what is being eaten.

The most significant histamine-producing bacteria include:

- ***Lactobacillus reuteri*, *Lactobacillus casei*, and *Lactobacillus bulgaricus*** – These are commonly found in fermented foods and many commercial probiotic products—a critical point for MCAS patients, who may inadvertently worsen their histamine load by consuming fermented foods or the wrong probiotics in an attempt to support gut health.[132,133,134]
- ***Morganella morganii*, *Klebsiella pneumoniae*, and *Hafnia alvei*** – These are opportunistic bacteria that can overgrow during dysbiosis and are among the most prolific histamine producers in the gut.[135,136]
- ***Enterococcus faecalis* and *Enterococcus faecium*** – Present in many healthy guts but capable of significant histamine production when in excessive numbers;[137] however, this production is contingent on the presence of histidine decarboxylase genes and appropriate environmental conditions.

> **Critical Note for People with MCAS:** *Not all probiotics are appropriate for MCAS. Several commonly recommended strains—including Lactobacillus casei, Lactobacillus reuteri, and Lactobacillus bulgaricus—are histamine producers and may worsen symptoms. Strain selection matters enormously. Chapter 19 covers probiotic guidance in detail, including which strains are appropriate and which to avoid.*

Histamine-Degrading Bacteria: The Microbiome's Natural Drain

Just as some bacteria produce histamine, others help break it down or prevent its accumulation. A healthy, diverse microbiome contains substantial populations of these beneficial organisms, providing a natural biological drain for the histamine bucket.

The most clinically relevant histamine-degrading and histamine-neutral strains include:

- ***Lactobacillus rhamnosus*** – One of the best-studied strains for histamine intolerance and mast cell reactivity, it is believed to upregulate DAO enzyme production in the gut and reduce histamine-mediated intestinal inflammation.[138,139,140]
- ***Lactobacillus plantarum*** – It does not produce histamine and has anti-inflammatory effects in the gut mucosa;[141,142] it also demonstrates a capacity to degrade biogenic amines including histamine.[143]
- ***Bifidobacterium longum*** **and** ***Bifidobacterium infantis*** **– They are** important butyrate producers and immune modulators that support barrier integrity and reduce inflammatory signaling in gut mast cells.[144]
- ***Lactobacillus salivarius*** – This is histamine-neutral and demonstrated to have mast cell-stabilizing effects in some research models.[145]

The practical implication is straightforward but often counterintuitive to patients who have been told to "eat more fermented foods" for gut health. In MCAS, the value of any probiotic or fermented food depends entirely on which bacteria it contains. Sauerkraut, kimchi, kefir, aged cheeses, and most commercial yogurts—standard recommendations for general gut health—are among the highest-histamine foods available and among the most significant bucket-fillers for MCAS patients. Fermented foods are not universally beneficial. For someone with significant mast cell dysfunction, they can be profoundly destabilizing until the gut has healed sufficiently to handle the histamine load they introduce.

The Microbiome Beyond Histamine

The gut microbiome's influence on MCAS extends well beyond histamine metabolism. Several additional mechanisms deserve attention:

- **Short-chain fatty acid production** – Beneficial bacteria ferment dietary fiber to produce short-chain fatty acids, particularly butyrate, propionate, and acetate. Butyrate is the primary energy source for colonocytes (the cells lining the colon) and is essential for maintaining tight junction integrity and a healthy gut barrier.[146] A fiber-poor diet or a depleted microbiome means less butyrate, which means a weaker gut barrier—and more mast cell activation.
- **Immune system education** – The microbiome plays a critical role in training regulatory T cells and educating the immune system to distinguish friend from foe.[147] Dysbiosis impairs this training, contributing to the immune dysregulation and loss of tolerance that characterizes MCAS.
- **Gut-brain axis communication** – Gut bacteria produce and modulate neurotransmitters, including serotonin, GABA, and dopamine, and communicate with the nervous system through the vagus nerve.[148] A

disrupted microbiome disrupts these signals, potentially contributing to the anxiety, depression, and autonomic dysregulation seen in MCAS patients.

- **Tryptophan metabolism** – The microbiome is central to how tryptophan—an essential amino acid—is metabolized.[149] In a healthy gut, tryptophan is directed toward serotonin production and anti-inflammatory indole metabolites. In dysbiosis, it may be shunted toward inflammatory kynurenine pathways that contribute to neuroinflammation and mood disruption.

✦ ✦ ✦

IBS, SIBO, Candida, and Dysbiosis: The Gut Conditions Behind the Reactivity

For many individuals living with MCAS, gut dysfunction isn't just a general imbalance; it takes the form of specific, identifiable conditions that deserve targeted attention. The three most commonly encountered in this population are irritable bowel syndrome (IBS), small intestinal bacterial overgrowth (SIBO), and candida overgrowth.

Irritable Bowel Syndrome: The Mast Cell Connection

IBS is the most common gastrointestinal diagnosis in the developed world, affecting an estimated ten to fifteen percent of the population.[150] It is characterized by chronic abdominal pain, bloating, and altered bowel habits—diarrhea, constipation, or both—in the absence of structural disease detectable by standard testing. For decades it was considered primarily a disorder of gut motility and hypersensitivity, with the gut-brain axis playing a central role.

What has become increasingly clear over the past two decades is that mast cells are a central player in the pathophysiology of IBS—not just a bystander.[151] Studies consistently find elevated mast cell numbers in the gut mucosa of people with IBS, increased proximity of mast cells to enteric nerve fibers, and elevated mast cell mediator release in intestinal biopsies.[152,153] Tryptase released by activated gut mast cells directly sensitizes the enteric nervous system, lowering the pain threshold and driving the visceral hypersensitivity that is IBS's defining feature. Histamine, released by gut mast cells, alters gut motility and secretion in both directions—driving diarrhea through increased motility and secretion, or constipation through smooth muscle spasm.

This means that what most individuals living with IBS have been given as a diagnosis—a label for a pattern of gut symptoms—is in many cases a description of chronic gut mast cell activation looking for its underlying cause. For people with MCAS and IBS, the gut symptoms are not a separate condition to manage alongside MCAS; they are MCAS expressing itself in the gut. Treating the mast cell dysfunction addresses the IBS.

> **Reframing IBS:** *If you have been diagnosed with IBS and are now reading this book, consider the possibility that your gut symptoms and your systemic reactivity—the skin reactions, the palpitations, the brain fog—are the same condition wearing different clothes. Treating them as one unified problem, rather than two parallel problems, is typically far more effective.*

Small Intestinal Bacterial Overgrowth (SIBO)

The small intestine is not supposed to house large populations of bacteria. The vast majority of the gut's microbial community lives in the colon, where it performs its fermentation and immune functions at a safe distance from the nutrient-absorbing small intestine. When bacteria migrate upstream into the small intestine and establish significant colonies there—a condition called small intestinal bacterial overgrowth—the consequences are substantial.

SIBO produces symptoms that overlap heavily with both IBS and MCAS: bloating, abdominal pain, altered bowel habits, nausea, and fatigue. But it also does something more relevant to mast cell health: it dramatically increases the production of histamine and other biogenic amines in the small intestine, right where absorption is most efficient. SIBO-derived histamine is absorbed directly into the portal circulation, flooding the liver with a histamine load that may exceed its clearance capacity, particularly if DAO enzyme activity is reduced—which it frequently is in the inflamed small intestinal mucosa of individuals with SIBO.

The result is a gut that is functioning as a histamine factory, continuously producing histamine internally regardless of dietary choices. This explains why some people with MCAS find that even the most rigorous low-histamine diet produces only modest improvement—they are addressing the intake side of the equation while ignoring the internal production side.

SIBO is diagnosed through breath testing—hydrogen and methane breath tests detect the fermentation gases produced by bacterial overgrowth in the small intestine. It is found at elevated rates in people with IBS, in those with gut motility disorders, in individuals with a history of food poisoning or gastroenteritis, and increasingly in people with MCAS. It can be driven by proton pump inhibitor use (which reduces the acid that normally limits bacterial colonization of the upper gut), by slow gut motility (common in dysautonomia), by structural abnormalities, and by immune dysfunction that allows gut bacteria to migrate where they shouldn't.

Treatment of SIBO typically involves a combination of antimicrobial therapy (either pharmaceutical or herbal), prokinetic agents to improve gut motility and prevent recurrence, and dietary strategies to limit fermentable carbohydrates during treatment. Chapter 19 addresses gut healing protocols, including SIBO management, in practical detail.

Candida Overgrowth and Fungal Dysbiosis

Candida albicans is a yeast that lives in small amounts in most human guts without causing problems. In the right conditions—particularly after antibiotic use, in the context of a high-sugar diet, with impaired immune function, or with prolonged use of corticosteroids or oral contraceptives—*Candida* can shift from a harmless commensal organism to a problematic overgrowth.[154,155] In its hyphal (thread-like) form, Candida can physically penetrate the intestinal epithelium, directly increasing intestinal permeability.[156] It also produces a range of metabolites, including acetaldehyde (a toxic alcohol breakdown product) that impairs immune function and further damages the gut barrier.[157,158]

Candida and mast cells have a direct and adversarial relationship. Mast cells are recruited to sites of *Candida* infection as part of the immune defense against fungal pathogens. In doing so, they degranulate, releasing mediators that drive inflammation. Chronic or recurrent *Candida* exposure in the gut—even at subclinical levels that don't produce classic thrush symptoms—can represent a persistent source of mast cell activation, another chronic low-level fire that keeps the immune system primed and the bucket full.

Symptoms suggestive of candida overgrowth include: bloating that worsens with sugar or refined carbohydrate intake, recurrent vaginal yeast infections, oral thrush, strong sugar cravings, brain fog that is particularly pronounced after eating, and a history of repeated antibiotic courses. Testing options include stool analysis with culture, organic acid testing for candida metabolites (including D-arabinitol), and antibody testing. Each has limitations, and clinical correlation matters as much as any single test.

The Broader Picture: Dysbiosis as a Chronic Trigger

IBS, SIBO, and candida overgrowth are distinct conditions, but they share a common underlying theme: a gut ecosystem that has lost its balance. Collectively, this imbalance—in which beneficial microorganisms are depleted, opportunistic or pathogenic organisms have expanded, and the gut environment has shifted toward inflammation and barrier dysfunction—is called dysbiosis.

In MCAS, dysbiosis functions as a chronic, persistent trigger that keeps the mast cell population continuously primed. It is not an episodic trigger like eating a high-histamine meal; it is a baseline condition that reduces the threshold for all other triggers and makes every exposure more likely to produce symptoms. This is why gut healing—addressed in Chapter 19—is not a peripheral part of MCAS management. For many individuals, it is the most important single intervention, because correcting the gut microbiome and restoring barrier integrity reduces the chronic baseline load on the mast cell system, raising the threshold for all other triggers simultaneously.

✦ ✦ ✦

Deeper Dive: The Gut-Immune-Mast Cell Axis

For the Science-Minded Reader

The relationship between gut health and mast cell behavior is mediated through several distinct biological pathways that are worth understanding in more detail, both because they explain the clinical observations above and because they point directly toward the most effective therapeutic targets.

The Toll-Like Receptor Pathway and Bacterial Translocation

Mast cells express a range of pattern-recognition receptors, including toll-like receptors (TLRs), that are designed to detect pathogen-associated molecular patterns—molecular signatures of bacteria, fungi, and viruses. TLR-2 and TLR-4 are particularly relevant: TLR-4, for instance, is the primary receptor for lipopolysaccharide (LPS), the outer membrane component of gram-negative bacteria. When gut bacteria or their fragments translocate across a leaky gut barrier and encounter subepithelial mast cells, TLR activation triggers mast cell degranulation through a non-IgE pathway. This is completely independent of allergy—it is an innate immune response to the perceived presence of bacteria in a location where they don't belong.

In a person with significant intestinal permeability, this TLR-mediated activation may be occurring continuously, at low grade, as a steady trickle of bacterial products crosses the barrier. Serum LPS levels, measurable in clinical testing, are often subclinically elevated in individuals with gut dysbiosis and permeability—not high enough to cause septic shock, but high enough to maintain a state of chronic immune priming. Reducing intestinal permeability and normalizing the microbiome reduces this endotoxin translocation and, with it, the chronic background activation of the mast cell network.

DAO Enzyme Activity and the Gut's Histamine Drain

Diamine oxidase (DAO) is the primary enzyme responsible for breaking down histamine in the small intestinal lumen before it is absorbed. It is produced by the enterocytes lining the small intestinal villi—the same cells that are damaged and reduced in number by intestinal inflammation, dysbiosis, and increased permeability. When the gut lining is inflamed or damaged, DAO activity falls. Less histamine is degraded before absorption, more reaches the systemic circulation, and the effective capacity of the gut's histamine clearance system is reduced.

Multiple factors impair DAO activity beyond gut inflammation: alcohol consumption, certain medications (including metformin, aspirin, some antidepressants, and several antibiotics), severe vitamin B6 or copper deficiency (both required as DAO cofactors), and the presence of DAO-inhibiting bacterial metabolites in a dysbiotic gut.[159] Conversely, supporting gut healing, reducing alcohol, ensuring adequate B6 and copper status, and addressing dysbiosis all improve DAO function.

DAO enzyme supplements—oral preparations of diamine oxidase derived from porcine kidney or plants (primarily pea sprouts)—are available and have been shown in clinical studies to reduce histamine intolerance symptoms when taken before meals.[160] They work by supplementing the gut's own degradation capacity rather than by altering the underlying cause. They are best understood as a supportive bridge measure: useful for managing symptoms while the deeper work of gut healing proceeds, but not a substitute for it. Chapter 16 covers DAO supplementation in the context of a broader supplement protocol.

The Enteric Nervous System and Mast Cell Cross-Talk

The gut has its own nervous system—the enteric nervous system (ENS), sometimes called the "second brain"—comprising an estimated two to six hundred million neurons embedded in the gut wall,[161,162] capable of operating independently of the central nervous system. The ENS and gut mast cells are in constant, intimate communication. Mast cells are positioned within micrometers of enteric nerve endings, and this proximity is functional: mast cell mediators—particularly tryptase and histamine—directly sensitize enteric neurons, lowering the threshold for pain signaling and altering gut motility. In turn, neuropeptides released by enteric nerves—including substance P and VIP (vasoactive intestinal peptide)—directly activate and modulate mast cell behavior.

This bidirectional cross-talk explains why gut symptoms in MCAS are so responsive to nervous system interventions. Practices that support vagal tone and reduce sympathetic dominance—breathwork, somatic therapies, and regular movement—have measurable effects on gut motility, mucosal inflammation, and mast cell activity in the gut wall. The gut-brain axis is not merely a metaphor. It is an active highway between two of the most mast-cell-dense environments in the body, and supporting the nervous system dimension of gut health is as important as any dietary or microbiome intervention.

Butyrate, the Gut Barrier, and Mast Cell Regulation

Butyrate, the short-chain fatty acid produced by the fermentation of dietary fiber by colonic bacteria, deserves special attention as a compound that connects microbiome health, gut barrier integrity, and mast cell regulation in a single molecule. Butyrate is the preferred fuel of colonocytes and is essential for maintaining tight junction protein expression and gut barrier function. Beyond this structural role, butyrate has direct anti-inflammatory effects: it inhibits NF-κB, a master regulator of inflammatory gene expression in immune cells, and it promotes the differentiation of regulatory T cells that suppress excessive immune responses, including mast cell over-activation.

In a dysbiotic gut where fiber fermentation is impaired and butyrate production falls, the gut barrier weakens, regulatory immune signals diminish, and the environment becomes pro-inflammatory—all of which favor mast cell activation. Restoring butyrate production through microbiome rehabilitation (increasing dietary fiber, cultivating butyrate-producing bacteria like *Faecalibacterium prausnitzii* and *Roseburia intestinalis*)[163] or through direct supplementation (sodium or calcium butyrate) supports gut barrier repair and contributes to the reduction of chronic mast cell priming from the gut.

> **The Therapeutic Implication:** *Gut healing in MCAS is not a single intervention but a layered process: reduce the microbial and dietary inputs that fill the bucket, repair the gut barrier to prevent bacterial translocation and mast cell activation, rebuild a microbiome that degrades histamine rather than producing it, and support the enteric nervous system's role in gut-immune regulation. Chapter 19 translates these principles into a practical, step-by-step gut healing protocol.*

✦ ✦ ✦

What This Means for You: Starting the Gut Healing Journey

The gut-MCAS connection can feel overwhelming at first—so many interacting variables, so many potential contributing factors. The temptation is either to do everything at once (rarely sustainable) or to become paralyzed by the complexity (equally unhelpful). What actually works is a sequential, strategic approach that addresses the most urgent issues first, then builds layer by layer.

Prioritize identifying and addressing active gut infections first. If you suspect SIBO, candida overgrowth, or other active gut infections, getting these identified and treated is the highest-priority gut intervention. Active overgrowths are producing histamine, damaging the gut barrier, and priming your mast cells continuously—no amount of probiotic support or dietary optimization will fully compensate while a significant infection is ongoing. Work with a functional medicine practitioner or integrative gastroenterologist familiar with these conditions to get appropriate testing.

Begin adjusting your probiotic choices immediately. If you are currently taking a probiotic supplement or regularly consuming fermented foods, check the strains against the histamine-producing list earlier in this chapter. Swapping a histamine-producing strain like *Lactobacillus casei* for a histamine-neutral or histamine-degrading strain like *Lactobacillus rhamnosus* or *Bifidobacterium longum* is a simple, low-risk change that can make a meaningful difference in your overall histamine load. Chapter 19 provides specific strain recommendations.

Adopt a gut-supportive dietary approach alongside your low-histamine protocol. The low-histamine diet addresses what's going in—but gut healing also requires supporting what grows there. Prioritize prebiotic fibers that feed beneficial bacteria and support butyrate production: foods like cooked and cooled potatoes, green bananas, well-tolerated cooked vegetables, and leek or onion tops (in amounts your gut can tolerate). These are often compatible with a low-histamine approach, though individual tolerance should guide the pace of introduction.

Be thoughtful about medications that affect gut integrity. If you are taking NSAIDs (ibuprofen, naproxen, aspirin) regularly, proton pump inhibitors, or antibiotics for any reason, discuss with your provider whether alternatives exist and how to mitigate gut barrier effects. This is not a suggestion to stop necessary medications—it is a prompt to be intentional about the gut consequences of long-term drug use and to prioritize gut-protective strategies if these medications are unavoidable.

Support DAO activity as a bridge measure. While the deeper work of gut healing proceeds, supporting DAO enzyme activity can help reduce histamine-related symptoms. This includes ensuring adequate dietary B6 (found in poultry, fish, potatoes, and bananas) and copper (found in shellfish, nuts, and seeds), minimizing alcohol and DAO-blocking substances, and considering supplemental DAO enzymes before meals, particularly when dietary control is more challenging.

Watch for the gut-systemic connection in your symptom tracking. As you continue your symptom journaling from Chapter 5, add notes about gut-specific events: bloating patterns, changes in bowel habits, relationships between gut symptoms and systemic reactions. Many people find that gut symptom flares reliably precede or accompany systemic mast cell flares by a day or two—a pattern that, once recognized, provides both predictive value and motivation for gut-centered interventions.

Daniel, whose story opened this chapter, eventually received a diagnosis of SIBO alongside his MCAS. Treating the bacterial overgrowth—and then rebuilding his microbiome with appropriate strains and fiber support—proved to be the single most impactful intervention in his recovery. His systemic reactivity, which had seemed to have no relationship to his gut, improved dramatically once the chronic internal histamine production was addressed. The hives became less frequent. The brain fog lifted more days than not. The gut, which had been causing trouble since childhood, finally began to heal—and as it did, it took much of the rest of his MCAS burden with it.

His gut wasn't a side issue. It was the center of the story all along.

✦ ✦ ✦

Chapter 6 at a Glance

What to Remember:

- The gut is not a peripheral player in MCAS—it is one of its most important drivers. Housing seventy percent of the body's immune tissue and the largest concentration of mast cells outside the skin, the gut's state of health directly shapes the reactivity of the entire mast cell network.
- Increased intestinal permeability (leaky gut) allows bacterial fragments and undigested proteins to reach subepithelial mast cells via toll-like receptors, triggering non-IgE mast cell activation continuously as long as permeability persists. Mast cell mediators in turn worsen permeability, creating a self-perpetuating cycle.
- Gut bacteria directly influence histamine levels. Histamine-producing bacteria—including certain *Lactobacillus* strains, *Morganella*, and *Klebsiella*—can generate a significant internal histamine burden independent of dietary intake. Histamine-degrading strains, including *Lactobacillus rhamnosus* and *Bifidobacterium longum*, provide a natural drain.
- Not all probiotics are safe for individuals with MCAS. Several widely recommended strains are histamine producers and can worsen symptoms. Strain selection is critical—not just the genus, but the specific strain.
- SIBO generates large amounts of histamine directly in the small intestine where absorption is most efficient, bypassing much of the gut's clearance capacity. It is a major hidden driver of histamine load that cannot be corrected by diet alone.
- Candida overgrowth physically penetrates the gut lining, worsens intestinal permeability, and chronically activates gut mast cells as part of the immune defense response against fungal pathogens.

- DAO enzyme activity—the gut's primary histamine-degradation mechanism—is reduced by gut inflammation, dysbiosis, alcohol, certain medications, and nutrient deficiencies. Supporting DAO activity through gut healing and targeted supplementation improves the drainage side of the histamine bucket.
- Gut healing is a sequential, layered process: identify and treat active infections, optimize microbiome composition, repair the gut barrier, support enteric nervous system function, and rebuild butyrate-producing bacterial populations. Chapter 19 provides the practical protocol.

Coming Up in Chapter 7:

Gut infections are one category of chronic immune challenge driving MCAS, but they are not the only one. For a significant number of patients, persistent infections beyond the gut—Lyme disease and its co-infections, Epstein-Barr virus and other reactivated herpesviruses, mold illness, and the complex world of biofilm-forming organisms—are keeping the mast cell system in a state of chronic activation that no dietary or microbiome intervention fully resolves. Chapter 7 explores the role of chronic infections in MCAS and what evidence-informed approaches exist for identifying and addressing them.

The Epithelial Barrier and MCAS

A Key Theory in Understanding Chronic Mast Cell Reactivity

In mast cell biology, a great deal of attention is rightly paid to triggers—the foods, chemicals, environmental exposures, and stressors that set off mast cell reactions. But an equally important and frequently overlooked question is: why are mast cells so reactive in the first place? For a significant number of individuals with MCAS, current research points to a compelling answer: a damaged epithelial barrier.

The epithelium—the cellular lining of the gut, respiratory tract, and skin—is the body's primary interface with the outside world. When functioning properly, it acts as a selective gatekeeper, allowing nutrients to pass while blocking environmental triggers, bacterial fragments, and undigested proteins from reaching the immune tissue beneath. Mast cells are strategically positioned directly below this barrier, in ideal location to respond rapidly to anything that crosses it.

When the barrier is compromised—through inflammation, dysbiosis, chronic stress, certain medications, or structural vulnerabilities such as those seen in Ehlers-Danlos Syndrome—three interconnected mechanisms drive mast cell hyper-reactivity:

- **Direct antigen penetration.** Bacterial fragments, undigested food proteins, and environmental toxins cross the breached barrier and chronically stimulate subepithelial mast cells through IgE-independent pathways—meaning standard allergy testing will not identify these activators.
- **Epithelial alarmins.** Stressed or damaged epithelial cells release signaling molecules—TSLP, IL-33, and IL-25—that directly lower the activation threshold of mast cells, making them more reactive to every trigger they subsequently encounter. This is the mechanism by which barrier damage shifts the entire mast cell system toward hyper-sensitivity, not just toward specific triggers.
- **A self-perpetuating feedback loop.** Mast cell mediators, particularly tryptase, physically degrade the tight junction proteins that hold the barrier together—worsening the permeability that activated the mast cells in the first place. Without an intervention that breaks this cycle at the level of the barrier itself, the loop continues regardless of trigger management.

This "epithelial-up" model does not replace the trigger-management strategies elsewhere in this book—it adds an upstream layer of explanation and intervention. Managing triggers reduces acute exposures. Repairing the barrier reduces the chronic background load that determines how reactive the mast cells are to every exposure. For individuals with skin, gut, and respiratory symptoms occurring simultaneously—a pattern common in MCAS—barrier dysfunction across multiple surfaces may be a primary reason the mast cell system remains in a state of chronic high alert, and barrier restoration may be among the most impactful interventions available.

CHAPTER 7

Chronic Infections

The Hidden Fires That Keep Your Mast Cells Primed

The Illness That Never Fully Ended

Nadia was twenty-two when she pulled a tick off her left thigh after a weekend camping trip in the northeast. The tick was small—one of the nymph-stage deer ticks known to carry Lyme disease—and she almost missed it. She went to urgent care, received a short course of doxycycline, and was told she'd caught it early. The blood test came back equivocal. The doctor reassured her the antibiotic course would be sufficient.

For a few months, it seemed he was right. Then the fatigue arrived—not the ordinary tiredness of a busy graduate student, but a heaviness so profound that climbing a flight of stairs required planning. Her joints began to ache in a migratory pattern that moved from her knees to her wrists to her shoulders without ever settling in one place long enough to point clearly at any diagnosis. Her memory, once sharp enough to carry her through competitive exams without much effort, began to fray at the edges. She developed episodes of flushing and heart pounding that her cardiologist attributed to anxiety. Hives appeared on her arms for the first time in her life.

Her infectious disease specialist said her Lyme had been treated. Her rheumatologist found no inflammatory arthritis. Her psychiatrist offered medication for the anxiety. None of them connected the dots: the original tick bite, the never-quite-resolved immune activation, and the slowly expanding constellation of mast-cell-mediated symptoms that were now dominating her life.

Nadia is far from alone. For a significant proportion of individuals with MCAS—estimates vary, but experienced clinicians report seeing chronic infection as a contributing or driving factor in somewhere between a third and half of their most complex cases—an unresolved or ongoing infection is the match that lit the fire. It may be Lyme disease and its co-infections, a reactivated virus from decades past, a persistent mold exposure quietly poisoning the immune system from the inside out, or a combination of all three. In each case, the mechanism is similar: chronic immune stimulation that keeps the mast cell population continuously primed, the threshold perpetually low, and the bucket permanently near-full.

Understanding the role of chronic infections in MCAS is not about adopting a particular ideological position in the deeply contested debates around Lyme disease or chronic viral illness. It is about recognizing a clinical pattern—a pattern of immune dysregulation that connects an infectious history to a mast cell phenotype—and pursuing it systematically as part of the root-cause investigation every MCAS fighter deserves.

✦ ✦ ✦

How Infections Prime Mast Cells: The Core Concept

When a pathogen enters the body—whether a bacterium, virus, or fungus—the immune system mounts a coordinated response designed to identify, contain, and eliminate the threat. Mast cells are among the first responders in this process. They express pattern-recognition receptors that detect pathogen-associated molecular patterns (the molecular signatures that distinguish microorganisms from host tissue), and when these receptors are triggered, mast cells degranulate, releasing mediators that amplify inflammation, recruit other immune cells, and begin closing off the site of invasion.

This is entirely appropriate. Mast cells are genuinely important in the defense against bacterial, viral, and fungal pathogens.[164] The problem arises when the infection is not cleared—when it persists, goes dormant, or establishes itself in tissues in ways the immune system cannot fully eradicate. In these circumstances, the mast cell response that was designed to be acute and time-limited becomes chronic.[165] The mast cells remain in a state of ongoing activation, continuously releasing subthreshold amounts of mediators that don't produce dramatic acute reactions but maintain a baseline state of immune priming and systemic inflammation. The bucket is never allowed to empty.

Three categories of chronic infection are particularly relevant to MCAS patients: tick-borne infections (primarily Lyme disease and its bacterial co-infections), viral reactivation (particularly Epstein-Barr virus and other herpesviruses), and mold illness caused by mycotoxin-producing fungi. Each operates through somewhat different mechanisms, and each requires a somewhat different approach to identification and management.

> **An Important Clarification:** *Identifying chronic infection as a potential driver of your MCAS is not the same as diagnosing yourself with Lyme disease, chronic EBV, or mold illness. These are clinical determinations that require*

> *careful evaluation by a knowledgeable practitioner. What this chapter offers is the conceptual framework for why chronic infection matters in MCAS, and the questions worth pursuing with your healthcare team.*

✦ ✦ ✦

Lyme Disease and Tick-Borne Co-Infections

Lyme disease—caused by the spiral-shaped bacterium *Borrelia burgdorferi* and transmitted primarily by the bite of infected blacklegged ticks—is the most common vector-borne infectious disease in North America and Europe. When caught early and treated adequately, most people recover completely. But for a subset of people—estimates range from ten to twenty percent of those treated—symptoms persist long after the recommended antibiotic course ends.[166] This syndrome, variably called post-treatment Lyme disease syndrome (PTLDS) or chronic Lyme disease depending on one's position in a contentious clinical debate, is one of the most contested areas in modern medicine.

That debate—whether persistent symptoms reflect ongoing infection, post-infectious immune dysregulation, or some combination—is beyond the scope of this book to resolve. What is not debated is the clinical reality that a meaningful proportion of people with a Lyme history develop a chronic multi-system illness characterized by fatigue, cognitive impairment, musculoskeletal pain, autonomic dysfunction, and a wide range of inflammatory symptoms that bear a striking resemblance to MCAS. The question of whether this results from residual bacteria, immune dysregulation left in the wake of infection, or both is important for treatment decisions but secondary to the recognition that something in the post-Lyme immune system has gone persistently wrong—and mast cells are a central part of that story.

How Borrelia Interacts with Mast Cells

Research has demonstrated that *Borrelia burgdorferi* directly activates mast cells through multiple pathways.[167] The spirochete's surface lipoproteins are recognized by TLR-1 and TLR-2 on mast cells—the same toll-like receptors discussed in Chapter 6 that respond to bacterial components crossing a leaky gut. Mast cells activated by *Borrelia* release a characteristic pattern of mediators including TNF-alpha, IL-6, and IL-33, which drive local tissue inflammation and recruit other immune cells to the site of infection. In the early phase of Lyme disease, this mast cell response is part of the appropriate immune defense. When infection persists or the immune system remains dysregulated after treatment, this mast cell activation pattern may persist indefinitely.

Particularly relevant is the neurological dimension. Borrelia has a documented tropism (a "favorite" destination in the host's body) for nervous tissue—it can infect the brain, spinal cord, and peripheral nerves, producing the cognitive impairment, mood disruption, and neuropathic pain that characterize neurological Lyme disease.[168] Mast cells in the meninges and brain parenchyma (the tissue of the brain itself), activated by both direct bacterial stimulation and the inflammatory environment of Lyme-related neuroinflammation, release mediators that worsen brain fog, amplify pain sensitization, and disrupt the autonomic nervous system. In individuals with both Lyme history and MCAS, the neurological symptoms are often the most disabling—and the most responsive to interventions that address both mast cell reactivity and underlying immune dysregulation.

Tick-Borne Co-Infections: The Hidden Companions

Borrelia does not always travel alone. The ticks that carry Lyme disease may simultaneously transmit a range of other pathogens, including *Bartonella*, *Babesia*, *Anaplasma*, and *Ehrlichia*.[169] These co-infections are critically important in the MCAS context because they are even more prone to chronicity than Borrelia itself, they are frequently missed by standard testing, and they each have distinct mechanisms of immune dysregulation that amplify mast cell reactivity.

- ***Bartonella*** – A bacterial infection increasingly recognized as a significant driver of complex chronic illness, *Bartonella* has particular affinity for endothelial cells lining blood vessels and for red blood cells.[170] It produces a pattern of immune dysregulation characterized by oscillating periods of immunosuppression and immune activation—a pattern that correlates clinically with the fluctuating, unpredictable symptom courses many complex chronic illness patients report. *Bartonella* infection has been specifically associated with mast cell activation,[171] neuropsychiatric symptoms,[172] vascular abnormalities,[173] and a stretch-mark-like skin finding called striae that appears with unusual frequency in hEDS and complex chronic illness patients.[174]
- ***Babesia*** – A protozoan parasite similar to the malaria organism, *Babesia* infects red blood cells and can persist long-term in some people.[175] Its destruction of red blood cells produces a pattern of oxidative stress and immune activation that chronically primes mast cells. Night sweats, air hunger, and cyclical symptom patterns are characteristic.
- ***Anaplasma* and *Ehrlichia*** – Bacterial infections of white blood cells that produce acute flu-like illness; chronic persistence is less well-documented but co-infection with *Borrelia* complicates immune recovery and treatment response.[176]

Testing for Lyme and co-infections is fraught with well-documented limitations. Standard two-tier testing (ELISA followed by Western blot) has limited sensitivity, particularly in chronic disease where antibody titers may have waned. Specialty laboratories offer more comprehensive Lyme panels and co-infection testing, and their clinical utility—while debated in mainstream infectious disease—is valued by many practitioners treating complex chronic illness. For individuals with MCAS who have a history consistent with tick exposure, atypical multi-system illness, and incomplete response to standard treatments, a thorough tick-borne infection workup with a knowledgeable practitioner is a reasonable and important part of the root-cause investigation.

✦ ✦ ✦

Viral Reactivation: When Old Infections Resurface

Most adults carry within them a collection of viruses they contracted years or decades ago and never fully eliminated. The herpesvirus family is the most clinically significant in this regard: Epstein-Barr virus (EBV), cytomegalovirus (CMV), human herpesvirus 6 (HHV-6), and herpes simplex viruses 1 and 2 (HSV-1 and HSV-2) all establish lifelong latency in host cells following primary infection.[177] In a healthy, well-regulated immune system, these viruses remain dormant—suppressed but not eliminated—indefinitely. In states of immune stress or dysregulation, they can reactivate, re-entering a state of active replication and renewed immune challenge.

Epstein-Barr Virus: The Most Common Viral Driver

Epstein-Barr virus deserves particular attention. EBV—the virus that causes infectious mononucleosis (glandular fever)—is carried by more than ninety-five percent of adults worldwide.[178] Primary infection typically occurs in childhood or adolescence and is followed by lifelong latency in B lymphocytes (a type of white blood cell). Under normal circumstances, the immune system maintains EBV in its dormant state without difficulty.

For a meaningful subset of people with MCAS, ME/CFS, and related conditions, EBV reactivation is a documented and clinically significant phenomenon.[179] EBV reactivation is detectable through a pattern of elevated antibody titers: specifically, elevated EBV early antigen (EA) antibodies, which indicate active viral replication, alongside elevated viral capsid antigen (VCA) IgG but absent or low VCA IgM (which would indicate recent primary infection). This pattern—sometimes called chronic active EBV—represents ongoing low-grade viral activity rather than a resolved past infection.

The mechanism connecting EBV reactivation to mast cell activation is multilayered. EBV infects B cells, and activated B cells produce immunoglobulins—including IgE—that can sensitize mast cells. EBV drives the production of pro-inflammatory cytokines including IL-6, IL-10, and TNF-alpha that directly prime mast cells. And EBV-driven immune dysregulation impairs the regulatory T cell function that normally keeps mast cell reactivity in check. In individuals with both EBV reactivation and MCAS, addressing viral reactivation often produces significant improvement in mast cell reactivity—not by treating the mast cells directly, but by removing one of the major forces keeping them primed.

HHV-6 and Cytomegalovirus

Human herpesvirus 6 (HHV-6), which causes the childhood rash illness roseola, has emerged as a significant pathogen in complex chronic illness.[180] HHV-6 has particular affinity for neurological tissue and the immune system, and its reactivation is associated with cognitive impairment, fatigue, autonomic dysfunction, and a pattern of immune dysregulation that overlaps substantially with MCAS.[181] A unique feature of HHV-6 is its capacity for chromosomal integration—in approximately about one percent (range of 0.2 percent to three percent) of the population,[182,183,184,185] HHV-6 integrates into the germline genome and is passed to offspring, producing a form of inherited HHV-6 that can reactivate under immune stress and is often missed by standard testing.

Cytomegalovirus (CMV), while less commonly reactivated than EBV or HHV-6 in otherwise healthy adults, can contribute significantly to immune exhaustion and mast cell priming in immunocompromised or chronically stressed individuals.[186,187,188] CMV has direct effects on mast cell biology through a variety of surface receptor interactions and cytokine signaling pathways.

Testing for viral reactivation requires measuring specific antibody patterns rather than simply checking for the presence of past exposure. Elevated IgG titers alone are nearly universal for herpesviruses and do not indicate reactivation. What matters is the specific antibody profile—early antigen antibodies, the ratio of IgG to IgM, and in some cases direct viral load measurement through polymerase chain reaction (PCR) testing. Specialty testing through informed practitioners is advisable; standard panels often miss the nuance needed to identify reactivation.

✦ ✦ ✦

Biofilms and Persistent Inflammation: Why Infections Are So Hard to Clear

One of the most important concepts for understanding why chronic infections are so tenacious—and why standard antibiotic courses often fail to fully resolve them—is the biofilm. A biofilm is a structured community of microorganisms enclosed within a self-produced matrix of polysaccharides, proteins, and DNA, adhered to a biological surface such as the gut lining, a joint membrane, a blood vessel wall, or virtually any tissue in the body.

Think of a biofilm as a fortress. Individual bacteria living in the open, planktonic state are relatively vulnerable to antimicrobial agents. Bacteria living within a biofilm are a different matter entirely. The extracellular matrix physically impedes antibiotic penetration, but not always antimicrobial essential oils. Bacteria within biofilms adopt altered metabolic states that make them far less susceptible to drugs designed to target actively dividing cells. Biofilm communities harbor persister cells—a dormant subpopulation capable of surviving even aggressive antibiotic treatment and repopulating the biofilm once treatment is discontinued. It is estimated that bacteria within a mature biofilm can be one hundred to one thousand times more resistant to antibiotics than their planktonic counterparts.[189,190]

Borrelia, *Bartonella*, and several other tick-borne pathogens form biofilms in host tissue. So does *Candida albicans*, *H. pylori* (the ulcer-causing gastric bacterium found at elevated rates in MCAS patients), and many of the organisms associated with SIBO. For individuals with MCAS in whom a chronic infection has been identified, biofilm disruption is often the missing piece that explains why initial treatment produced partial but incomplete improvement.

Biofilms and the Immune System: A Chronic Provocation

Biofilm-forming pathogens have a particularly problematic relationship with the immune system. The biofilm matrix partially shields the organisms inside from immune recognition, allowing them to persist in tissue while triggering enough immune activation to maintain chronic inflammation without allowing the immune system to mount a full, effective clearance response. Mast cells surrounding sites of biofilm infection are in a state of chronic, frustrated activation—responding to the ongoing infectious stimulus, releasing mediators, driving local and systemic inflammation, but unable to resolve the underlying infection.

This chronic mast cell activation at biofilm sites contributes directly to the symptom picture of persistent MCAS: tissue around the biofilm becomes chronically inflamed, mediators released by local mast cells enter the systemic circulation, and the immune system remains in a state of sustained priming. Disrupting the biofilm—physically breaking down the protective matrix to expose the organisms inside to antimicrobial agents and immune cells—is therefore an important component of treating chronic infection in MCAS patients.

Natural biofilm-disrupting compounds used in integrative medicine include N-acetylcysteine (NAC), which breaks down the disulfide bonds in biofilm matrix proteins; serrapeptase and nattokinase, proteolytic enzymes that digest the protein components of biofilm matrix; monolaurin, a fatty acid derivative with documented biofilm-disrupting properties; essential oils that penetrate the biofilm's protective layers and attack the structural integrity of the community; and certain herbal compounds including berberine, allicin (from garlic), and oregano oil. These are typically used as part of a comprehensive antimicrobial protocol rather than as standalone treatments, and their use in the context of a chronic infection should be guided by a practitioner familiar with their effects.

✦ ✦ ✦

Deeper Dive: Immune Dysregulation, Mast Cell Priming, and the Chronic Infection Cycle

For the Science-Minded Reader

Chronic infections drive MCAS through mechanisms that go beyond simple ongoing immune stimulation. Understanding the specific ways persistent pathogens dysregulate the immune system helps explain why some people with MCAS have symptom patterns and treatment responses that don't fit a straightforward mast cell stabilization approach—and why infection-directed treatment can produce dramatic improvement even in patients who have already tried extensive MCAS-specific interventions.

Th1/Th2 Immune Skewing

The immune system can be broadly divided into two functional orientations: Th1 immunity, which is oriented toward fighting intracellular pathogens like viruses and certain bacteria through cell-mediated responses; and Th2 immunity, which manages extracellular pathogens, parasites, and allergens through antibody-mediated responses and mast cell activation. In a healthy immune system, these orientations are balanced and appropriate to the threat present. Chronic infection—particularly with intracellular pathogens like *Borrelia*, EBV, and *Bartonella*—tends to suppress Th1 immunity as a survival strategy,[191] since these organisms persist within host cells and need to evade cell-mediated clearance. The consequence of Th1 suppression is compensatory Th2 upregulation.

An upregulated Th2 immune environment is precisely the environment in which mast cells thrive and over-activate.[192] Th2 cytokines—IL-4, IL-5, IL-13, and especially IL-33—promote mast cell proliferation, survival, and sensitivity. They drive IgE production, lower the threshold for mast cell degranulation, and create the inflammatory backdrop of allergic and mast-cell-mediated disease. People with chronic intracellular infections and MCAS are frequently found to have this Th2-skewed profile, which explains both their mast cell hyperreactivity and the relative ineffectiveness of Th1-type immune responses in clearing their infection.

Restoring Th1/Th2 balance—through infection treatment, immune-modulating natural compounds like medicinal mushrooms and certain herbal adaptogens, and nervous system regulation (which influences Th1/Th2 balance through autonomic-immune cross-talk)—is an important dimension of the chronic infection–MCAS treatment picture.

Molecular Mimicry and Autoimmune Activation

Certain pathogens produce proteins that closely resemble host tissue proteins—a phenomenon called molecular mimicry. When the immune system generates antibodies or T cells against these pathogen proteins, those immune responses may inadvertently target structurally similar host proteins, producing autoimmune inflammation. *Borrelia*, EBV, and several other pathogens associated with MCAS have documented molecular mimicry mechanisms that may contribute to the autoimmune features—elevated ANA titers, Sjögren's-like symptoms, thyroid autoimmunity—seen with elevated frequency in the MCAS population.

When autoimmune processes are driven by molecular mimicry, mast cells are activated through two distinct mechanisms: first, by the pathogen itself; and second, by the autoimmune inflammation the pathogen has triggered. This double activation helps explain why some people with chronic infection and MCAS have a particularly severe and treatment-resistant course—they are contending with both the infectious driver and a self-sustaining autoimmune process that continues even when the infection begins to be controlled.

Mitochondrial Dysfunction and Cellular Energy Depletion

Chronic infections—particularly EBV, HHV-6, and *Borrelia*—are documented to impair mitochondrial function:[193] the energy-producing organelles within cells are damaged or dysregulated by viral and bacterial products, reducing the cell's capacity to generate adenosine triphosphate (ATP). This mitochondrial dysfunction has direct consequences for mast cell regulation. Mast cell degranulation and mediator synthesis are energetically demanding processes, and the regulatory mechanisms that prevent excessive mast cell activation also require adequate cellular energy. When mitochondrial function is impaired, the energy budget for immune regulation shrinks—mast cells become less efficiently regulated, more prone to activation, and slower to return to a resting state after degranulation.

This mechanism helps explain the profound, disproportionate fatigue that characterizes both chronic infection and MCAS—it is not merely symptomatic but reflects a fundamental reduction in cellular energy availability. It also points toward mitochondrial support as a genuinely useful therapeutic dimension. Nutrients including coenzyme Q10, ribose, magnesium malate, and B vitamins that support mitochondrial function can improve energy status, reduce the cellular vulnerability to excessive mast cell activation, and support the recovery from chronic infection.

The Mast Cell–Pathogen Relationship: Not Always Adversarial

One nuance worth acknowledging is that the relationship between mast cells and pathogens is not simply that mast cells fight infection. Research has revealed that some pathogens have evolved to exploit mast cells for their own purposes—using mast cell products to facilitate their spread, modulate local immune responses in ways that favor pathogen survival, or redirect immune activity away from effective clearance pathways.[194] *Borrelia*, in particular, has been shown to interact with mast cell degranulation in ways that may facilitate its dissemination through host tissue.[195] This co-evolutionary complexity means that treating chronic infection in MCAS is rarely as simple as eliminating the pathogen and watching the mast cell reactivity resolve—the relationship between the infection and the mast cell phenotype may be more deeply entangled, and recovery typically requires simultaneous attention to both.

✦ ✦ ✦

What This Means for You: Pursuing the Infection Connection

If you have been working conscientiously on your MCAS—dietary adjustments, mast cell stabilizers, gut healing, nervous system support—and finding that your progress is slower or more limited than you hoped, chronic infection is one of the most important unexplored territories to consider. The signs that chronic infection may be a significant driver include:

- Onset or dramatic worsening of MCAS symptoms following a clear infectious event—a tick bite, a bout of mono, a severe viral illness, or a period of significant immune stress
- A symptom pattern that includes significant fatigue, cognitive impairment, migratory joint or muscle pain, and neurological symptoms alongside the classic mast cell picture
- Symptom fluctuations that follow cyclical patterns—monthly, or in regular intervals—suggestive of infectious cycling
- Night sweats, air hunger, or unexplained chills that accompany MCAS symptoms
- A history of significant antibiotic use without full resolution, or an antibiotic course that initially helped significantly but was followed by relapse
- Known tick exposure, particularly in Lyme-endemic areas of North America or Europe

- Previous documented EBV infection with a subsequent course that included prolonged recovery or never-quite-normal health afterward
- Living or working in a water-damaged building, or significant mold exposure history (covered more fully in Chapter 8)

Work with a knowledgeable practitioner. Chronic infection testing and treatment in the context of MCAS requires a clinician who understands both the complexity of tick-borne and viral illness and the mast cell dimension of chronic immune dysregulation. Functional medicine physicians, naturopathic doctors trained in complex chronic illness, and Lyme-literate medical doctors (LLMDs) are the practitioners most likely to have this combined knowledge base. Standard infectious disease specialists, while invaluable for acute infections, often lack training in the chronic and post-infectious presentations most relevant here.

Request a comprehensive infectious workup. Appropriate testing for the chronic infection–MCAS intersection includes: comprehensive Lyme panel with co-infections (*Bartonella, Babesia, Anaplasma, Ehrlichia*) through a specialty laboratory familiar with chronic disease presentations; EBV reactivation panel (VCA IgG and IgM, early antigen IgG, EBNA); HHV-6 IgG and ideally PCR if reactivation is suspected; CMV if immune function is otherwise compromised; and potentially *H. pylori* testing if upper gut symptoms are prominent.

Support your immune system while pursuing infection treatment. The natural immune-support interventions described later in this book—medicinal mushrooms (particularly beta-glucan-rich species like reishi, shiitake, and turkey tail), vitamin D optimization, zinc, and adaptogenic herbs—provide genuine support for Th1 immune function and help restore the immune balance that chronic intracellular infections disrupt. These are not replacements for antimicrobial treatment when infection is confirmed, but they are valuable adjuncts that improve immune competence and may reduce the immune dysregulation that perpetuates mast cell priming.

Be prepared for treatment complexity. Treating chronic infections in the context of MCAS requires particular care, because the die-off of pathogens during treatment—a phenomenon sometimes called a Herxheimer reaction or herx—can trigger significant mast cell flares as the immune system responds to the sudden release of pathogen debris and toxins. Working with a practitioner who anticipates this response, who knows how to support the mast cell system through treatment phases, and who can pace treatment appropriately for your individual tolerance is essential. Going too fast is a common and avoidable mistake.

Address biofilm disruption strategically. If chronic bacterial infection is identified, discuss biofilm disruption with your practitioner as part of the treatment protocol. Biofilm-targeting enzymes and natural compounds are typically introduced before or alongside antimicrobial treatment to improve pathogen accessibility. The timing and sequencing of this approach matters—disrupting a biofilm without adequate antimicrobial coverage can worsen symptoms temporarily as organisms are exposed. This is work best done with experienced guidance rather than independently.

Nadia's recovery began when a Lyme-literate physician ordered a comprehensive tick-borne infection panel. It confirmed active *Bartonella* alongside markers consistent with *Borrelia* exposure. A staged treatment protocol—beginning with natural immune support and biofilm disruption before introducing herbal antimicrobials, accompanied throughout by targeted mast cell stabilization—produced slow but consistent improvement over the following eighteen months. The hives faded. The flushing became infrequent. The cognitive impairment that had threatened her career retreated enough for her to return to full-time work.

She still has days that are harder than others. The bucket fills faster than it once did for a healthy twenty-two-year-old. But it empties now too—reliably, predictably—in a way it never had since that weekend camping trip changed everything. The infection had been the hidden fire. Finding it and beginning to put it out made everything else possible.

✦ ✦ ✦

Chapter 7 at a Glance

What to Remember:

- Chronic infections are a significant and underrecognized driver of MCAS in a meaningful proportion of people. They keep mast cells continuously primed through ongoing immune stimulation, immune dysregulation, and the systemic inflammatory environment that persistent pathogens create.

- Lyme disease and its tick-borne co-infections—*Bartonella, Babesia, Anaplasma*—activate mast cells through toll-like receptor pathways, drive neurological inflammation that amplifies mast cell reactivity in the brain and nervous system, and produce a post-infectious immune dysregulation that may persist long after standard antibiotic treatment.

- Viral reactivation—particularly Epstein-Barr virus, HHV-6, and CMV—represents latent infections coming back to life under immune stress. EBV reactivation drives IgE-mediated mast cell sensitization, suppresses regulatory T cell function, and produces a pro-inflammatory cytokine environment that keeps mast cell thresholds low.

- Biofilms are protective microbial fortresses that make chronic infections extremely resistant to both antibiotics and immune clearance. *Borrelia, Bartonella, Candida*, and several other organisms associated with MCAS form biofilms in host tissue, maintaining a source of chronic immune provocation and mast cell activation.
- Chronic intracellular infections skew the immune system toward a Th2 orientation—the very immune environment in which mast cells over-activate—through suppression of Th1 cell-mediated immunity. Restoring Th1/Th2 balance is an important therapeutic goal alongside direct antimicrobial treatment.
- Molecular mimicry, in which pathogen proteins resemble host tissue proteins, can trigger autoimmune responses that provide a second layer of mast cell activation independent of ongoing infection—explaining why treatment of the infection alone may not fully resolve MCAS in some patients.
- Chronic infection–associated mitochondrial dysfunction reduces the cellular energy available for immune regulation, making mast cells harder to control and contributing to the profound fatigue that characterizes this population.
- Clinical signs pointing toward chronic infection as an MCAS driver include onset after a clear infectious event, cyclical symptom patterns, significant fatigue and cognitive impairment, tick or mold exposure history, and incomplete response to standard MCAS interventions alone.

Coming Up in Chapter 8:

Chronic infection is one category of hidden load on the mast cell system—but it is not the only one. Environmental toxins, including the mycotoxins produced by indoor mold, heavy metals, and a range of chemical exposures, represent a distinct and often equally significant source of chronic mast cell priming. In Chapter 8, we explore how environmental toxins trigger and perpetuate MCAS, how to identify whether toxic burden is a factor in your case, and what evidence-informed strategies exist for reducing that burden safely and effectively.

When the Fence Collapses: Barrier Dysfunction and Chronic Reactivity

Think of a healthy epithelial barrier as a well-staffed border crossing with carefully controlled entry lanes. A dysfunctional barrier is like a section of fence that has collapsed—everything previously held back begins flooding through, and the security personnel on the other side are suddenly overwhelmed with more threats than they were ever designed to handle simultaneously.

The result is a mast cell population that is chronically, not episodically, activated—not because a specific allergen has arrived, not because an infection is present, but because the basic architecture of the barrier has failed. The mast cells beneath it are being continuously exposed to a flood of environmental signals their threshold system was never designed to process indefinitely.

This reframes how we understand mast cell hyper-reactivity. Rather than asking only *what* is triggering the mast cells, the barrier model asks: *why is the barrier allowing so many triggers through in the first place?* Reducing individual triggers helps. But if the barrier itself remains compromised, new triggers will continuously find their way through—and the mast cells beneath will remain in a state of chronic high alert regardless of how carefully triggers are managed.

The Barrier Extends Beyond the Gut

It is tempting to focus exclusively on the gut, where the research is most developed and the clinical evidence most direct. But the barrier model applies equally to the respiratory tract and the skin—and for individuals with eczema, asthma, or significant environmental sensitivities, these surfaces may be as important to address as the gut.

The respiratory epithelium normally traps inhaled particles in mucus before they reach immune tissue. When damaged—by air pollution, mold, or chronic inflammation—it becomes permeable, and the mast cells beneath begin receiving the same continuous activation signal as in a leaky gut.

The skin presents the identical pattern. Eczema is fundamentally a barrier disease, driven by deficiency of filaggrin—a protein essential to the structural integrity of the outermost skin layer. The gut-skin axis influences this, as intestinal dysbiosis primes immune cells to overreact when allergens breach a leaky skin barrier. Without structural integrity, environmental allergens and microorganisms reach the mast cells in the dermis below, triggering inflammatory cascades.

For an individual whose gut, airways, and skin barriers are all compromised simultaneously, the total mast cell burden from barrier dysfunction alone—before any individual trigger has been encountered—may be substantial enough to explain their chronic baseline reactivity.

CHAPTER 8

Environmental Toxins

Mold, Heavy Metals, and the Chemical World That Keeps Your Mast Cells Reactive

When the Building Made Her Sick

Gwen had been healthy enough for most of her forties. Demanding job, two teenagers, a full life—and the ordinary wear of all of it, but nothing she'd call illness. Then her company relocated to a newly renovated office building on the edge of the city, and something shifted.

It started with headaches she attributed to the new commute. Then a cough that her doctor treated as a respiratory infection, then as asthma, then eventually dismissed as stress-related. The fatigue that followed was in a different category from anything she'd experienced—not tiredness but a collapse of energy so complete that she would sit in her car in the parking garage for twenty minutes after work, unable to summon the will to drive home. Her thinking slowed. She began reacting to foods she had eaten without issue for decades. Hives appeared on her forearms. Her heart raced for no reason she could identify.

She saw seven doctors over two years. The diagnoses she collected included asthma, anxiety, IBS, and—eventually—MCAS. The MCAS diagnosis was accurate as far as it went. But it didn't answer the most important question: why had a healthy woman become so reactive, so suddenly, in her mid-forties?

The answer was in the building. A facilities inspection, prompted by complaints from several other employees, found extensive water damage in the walls behind the recently installed drywall—black mold colonies that had been sealed in and ventilated directly into the workspace for eighteen months. The mycotoxins produced by those mold colonies had been filling Gwen's bucket every working day. Her MCAS was not a mystery of internal biology gone wrong for no reason. It was her immune system's rational, if catastrophic, response to chronic toxic exposure.

Environmental toxins are among the most powerful and most overlooked drivers of mast cell activation. They are not the only explanation for MCAS, but for a meaningful proportion of patients—particularly those whose symptoms began or dramatically worsened following a change in environment, a home renovation, a new workplace, or a significant chemical exposure—they are the piece of the puzzle that makes everything else make sense.

✦ ✦ ✦

Toxins and Mast Cells: The Core Relationship

Before we explore specific toxin categories, it is worth understanding how environmental toxins interact with mast cells as a general principle. The relationship is not subtle—it is direct, measurable, and operates through several distinct mechanisms.

Mast cells are strategically positioned at the body's environmental interfaces: the skin, the respiratory tract, the gut lining, and the tissues surrounding blood vessels. This positioning means they are among the first cells to encounter anything that enters the body from the outside world—including toxins. Mast cells express a wide range of receptors that detect chemically damaging compounds, and when these receptors are triggered, mast cells respond as they would to any perceived threat: they activate, release mediators, and recruit the broader immune response.

In the case of a single, limited toxic exposure, this is an appropriate and self-limiting response. The problem arises with chronic or repeated exposure—living in a moldy building, having elevated heavy metals from years of accumulation, or carrying a significant body burden of industrial chemicals. In these circumstances, the mast cell response never resolves. The toxins are always present, always providing a stimulus, always keeping the bucket full. The mast cells are not overreacting to nothing; they are responding, continuously, to a genuine chemical provocation.

> **The Key Distinction:** *Environmental toxin–driven MCAS is not a malfunction of the immune system. It is an immune system responding appropriately to an inappropriate level of toxic exposure. This distinction matters enormously for treatment: reducing the toxic burden is not optional for these individuals. No amount of mast cell stabilization will provide lasting relief while the original provocation continues unabated.*

Three categories of environmental toxins are most clinically significant in MCAS: mold and mycotoxins, heavy metals, and industrial chemical exposures. Each category operates through somewhat different mechanisms and each requires somewhat different identification and remediation strategies.

✦ ✦ ✦

Mold and Mycotoxins: The Indoor Epidemic

Of all the environmental toxins implicated in MCAS, mold illness—specifically the illness caused not by mold spores themselves but by the toxic secondary metabolites that certain mold species produce, called mycotoxins—is the most prevalent and the most frequently missed.

Water-damaged buildings are far more common than most people realize. Studies have estimated that between forty and fifty percent of buildings in the United States have experienced sufficient water damage to support mold growth. When certain species of mold—particularly *Stachybotrys chartarum* (often called black mold), *Aspergillus*, *Penicillium*, *Chaetomium*, and *Fusarium*—colonize building materials, they produce mycotoxins as part of their normal biology. These mycotoxins become airborne on tiny spore and dust particles, enter the building's air system, and are continuously inhaled and ingested by the building's occupants.

The critical point for people with MCAS is this: It is the mycotoxins, not the mold spores, that drive the most significant biological damage.[196] Standard allergy testing for mold measures IgE antibody responses to mold proteins—a reaction that relatively few people develop. Mycotoxin illness is not primarily IgE-mediated. It operates through innate immune pathways, direct cellular toxicity, and—most relevantly here—direct mast cell activation. A patient can have completely negative mold allergy testing and still be seriously ill from mycotoxin exposure.

How Mycotoxins Activate Mast Cells

Mycotoxins trigger mast cell activation through multiple pathways. Trichothecene mycotoxins, produced by *Stachybotrys* and *Fusarium*, directly damage cell membranes and trigger oxidative stress, which activates mast cells through reactive oxygen species signaling.[197] Aflatoxins, produced by Aspergillus species, disrupt cellular DNA repair mechanisms and activate the innate immune response including mast cell degranulation.[198] Ochratoxin A, one of the most common mycotoxins in water-damaged buildings, impairs mitochondrial function—the same mechanism discussed in the context of chronic infections in Chapter 7—reducing the cell's capacity to regulate mast cell activity.[199]

Beyond direct mast cell activation, mycotoxins impair the systems that would normally contain mast cell reactivity. They suppress regulatory T cell function, reducing immune tolerance.[200,201,202,203,204] They damage the gut epithelium, worsening intestinal permeability and the gut-mast cell activation cycle described in Chapter 6. They impair liver detoxification pathways, reducing the body's capacity to clear not just mycotoxins themselves but the histamine and other mediators released by activated mast cells. And they drive neuroinflammation through direct toxic effects on the nervous system, worsening the central sensitization and autonomic dysregulation that characterize severe MCAS.

Recognizing Mold Illness in the MCAS Patient

The clinical pattern of mold illness overlaps substantially with MCAS—which is not coincidental, since mold illness drives MCAS in a significant proportion of affected people. Features that should heighten suspicion for mold as a driver include:

- **Pattern of symptom location** – Identify symptoms that are significantly better when away from a particular building—a workplace, a home, a school—and worse upon returning. Many patients describe feeling noticeably better on vacation or when traveling, only to relapse within days of returning home or to work.
- **Cluster of symptoms including cognitive impairment** – The cognitive effects of mycotoxin exposure—often described as a profound fogginess, word-finding difficulty, and memory disruption that feels different in character from ordinary fatigue—are among the most consistent features of mold illness.
- **History of water damage or musty odors** – Visible mold, water staining, a persistent musty smell, or a history of flooding or plumbing leaks may exist in a building where significant time is spent.
- **Unusual reactivity to chemical exposures** – Mycotoxin exposure impairs the liver's cytochrome P450 detoxification system, reducing the body's capacity to process not just mycotoxins but all chemical exposures; patients with mold illness often develop heightened reactivity to fragrances, cleaning products, and other environmental chemicals.
- **Symptoms in other building occupants** – While genetic variation in detoxification capacity means that not everyone in a water-damaged building will become equally ill, a pattern of symptoms in multiple people sharing the same space is a significant red flag.

Testing for mycotoxin exposure includes urine mycotoxin testing (available through specialty laboratories, measuring urinary metabolites of the most common indoor mycotoxins), blood tests for inflammatory markers associated with mold illness including TGF-beta-1, MMP-9, and C4a complement, and genetic testing for HLA-DR variants that affect mycotoxin detoxification capacity. Approximately twenty-five percent of the population carries HLA-DR genetic variants that influence antigen presentation and immune responsiveness, and may impair the ability to recognize and clear mycotoxins in susceptible individuals,[205,206] which explains why some people become severely ill in a water-damaged building while others in the same space remain relatively unaffected. Environmental testing of the building itself—ERMI (Environmental Relative

Moldiness Index) or HERTSMI-2 testing of dust samples—can confirm whether the physical environment is the source.

Treatment of mold illness requires, first and above all else, removal from the source. No binder, supplement, or detoxification protocol will produce meaningful lasting recovery while exposure continues. Once the individual is out of the moldy environment, a structured approach to mycotoxin clearance—using binders such as cholestyramine, activated charcoal, or bentonite clay to capture mycotoxins in the gut and prevent recirculation; supporting liver Phase 1 and Phase 2 detoxification; and addressing the downstream gut and immune damage—can produce significant improvement. This is explored further in Chapter 20 on detoxification support.

❖ ❖ ❖

Heavy Metals: Accumulating Silently, Activating Chronically

Heavy metals are a category of environmental toxin whose relevance to MCAS is often underappreciated, in part because their accumulation is typically gradual and silent—they build up in tissues over years or decades without producing acute symptoms, slowly raising the background level of chronic mast cell priming until the overall toxic burden becomes significant.

The heavy metals most relevant to MCAS patients include mercury, lead, cadmium, arsenic, and aluminum. Each has distinct sources, accumulation patterns, and mechanisms of immune disruption, but they share a common property: They are bioaccumulative, meaning the body stores them in tissues—particularly in the brain, bones, kidneys, and fatty tissue—without an efficient natural mechanism for clearance. Unlike water-soluble toxins that are readily excreted through the kidneys, fat-soluble heavy metals require specific detoxification and excretion support to remove.

Mercury: The Immune System's Nemesis

Mercury is the heavy metal with the most extensively documented effects on mast cell biology and immune function.[207] It exists in several forms, each with somewhat different toxicological profiles. Methylmercury, accumulated primarily through consumption of large predatory fish (tuna, swordfish, shark, king mackerel), is highly bioavailable and crosses the blood-brain barrier with ease. Inorganic mercury from dental amalgam fillings is released in small continuous amounts as vapor and absorbed through the respiratory tract. Ethylmercury, formerly used as a preservative in certain vaccines, has a shorter half-life but contributes to the body burden in those with significant vaccine exposure history.

Mercury activates mast cells through multiple mechanisms.[208] It directly binds to sulfhydryl groups on mast cell membrane proteins, disrupting their function and triggering degranulation. It drives the production of reactive oxygen species that further activate mast cells through oxidative stress pathways. It suppresses regulatory T cell function, removing a key brake on mast cell reactivity. And it has a documented capacity to shift immune responses toward a Th2 orientation—precisely the immune environment, as discussed in Chapter 7, in which mast cells thrive and over-activate.

Elevated mercury is detectable through hair tissue mineral analysis (HTMA), which reflects longer-term tissue accumulation, and through urine challenge testing using a chelating agent (typically DMPS or DMSA administered under medical supervision) that mobilizes mercury stores into the urine for measurement. Standard blood mercury levels reflect only recent exposure and are poor indicators of chronic body burden.

Lead, Cadmium, and Arsenic

Lead accumulates predominantly in bone, where it can remain for decades and be slowly released back into circulation during periods of physiological stress—pregnancy, menopause, illness, or extended fasting—creating a dynamic source of ongoing low-level exposure long after the original source has been removed.[209] Lead impairs DAO enzyme activity (reducing the gut's capacity to clear histamine),[210,211] disrupts the blood-brain barrier,[212] and drives neuroinflammatory pathways that amplify mast cell reactivity in the central nervous system.[213] Sources include older painted buildings, certain ceramic glazes, contaminated water from lead pipes, and occupational exposures.

Cadmium, found primarily in cigarette smoke (including secondhand smoke), certain fertilizers, and some foods grown in contaminated soil, accumulates in the kidneys and liver and impairs the very detoxification pathways needed to clear other toxins—including mycotoxins.[214] Its immune effects include disruption of T cell regulation and promotion of oxidative stress that chronically primes mast cells.

Arsenic, encountered through contaminated groundwater (a significant issue in certain geographic regions), rice and rice-based products grown in arsenic-containing soil, and some industrial exposures, is both an immune disruptor and a mast cell activator through NF-κB-mediated inflammatory signaling pathways.[215] It also impairs methylation—the biochemical process central to detoxification, neurotransmitter metabolism, and epigenetic regulation—creating a broad downstream impact on the body's capacity to manage toxic burden and regulate immune function.

✦ ✦ ✦

Chemical Exposures: The Modern Toxic Landscape

Beyond mold and heavy metals lies a broader category of chemical exposures that have become inescapable features of modern life and that, in aggregate, contribute meaningfully to the mast cell activation burden of susceptible individuals.

- **Volatile organic compounds (VOCs)** – VOCs may be emitted by building materials, paints, adhesives, synthetic carpeting, and furniture; they—including formaldehyde, benzene, and toluene—are direct respiratory mast cell activators and are particularly problematic in newly constructed or renovated spaces.[216]
- **Pesticides and herbicides** – Organophosphate pesticides impair the same acetylcholinesterase enzyme that regulates nervous system function, creating autonomic dysregulation that compounds MCAS;[217] glyphosate, the most widely used herbicide globally, disrupts the gut microbiome, impairs gut barrier function, and chelates essential mineral cofactors for detoxification enzymes.[218,219]
- **Phthalates and bisphenols** – Plasticizers found in food packaging, personal care products, and medical equipment are endocrine disruptors that alter hormonal balance—particularly estrogen signaling—in ways that directly affect mast cell sensitivity,[220] given the well-established estrogen–histamine axis discussed in Chapter 10.
- **Per- and polyfluoroalkyl substances (PFAS)** – PFAS compounds, sometimes called forever chemicals because they do not break down in the body or the environment, are found in non-stick cookware, water-repellent fabrics, food packaging, and contaminated water supplies; they impair immune function, disrupt thyroid hormone metabolism, and accumulate in liver tissue where they impair detoxification capacity.[221,222]
- **Fragrances and synthetic musks** – Perhaps the most immediately relevant chemical category for daily MCAS management, synthetic fragrance compounds in personal care products, cleaning agents, and air fresheners are among the most common acute mast cell triggers encountered in everyday life; they activate mast cells in the respiratory mucosa directly and through nervous system sensitization.[223]

The concept of total chemical body burden is important here. No single chemical exposure at typical environmental levels necessarily causes MCAS. But the combined, chronic exposure to dozens of low-level chemical stressors—in the air, food, water, and personal care products—can collectively represent a significant and persistent contribution to the mast cell trigger load. For people with MCAS who have already reduced their dietary histamine load, addressed infections, and supported their nervous system but are still not improving as expected, reducing chemical body burden is often the missing piece.

✦ ✦ ✦

Deeper Dive: How Toxins Hijack Mast Cell Regulation

For the Science-Minded Reader

Environmental toxins don't merely trigger individual mast cell activation events—they systematically impair the biological infrastructure that keeps mast cell reactivity in check. Understanding these mechanisms reveals why toxic burden reduction is not a peripheral concern but a genuine therapeutic priority.

Oxidative Stress and the NRF2 Pathway

Most of the toxins discussed in this chapter—mycotoxins, heavy metals, VOCs, pesticides—drive the production of reactive oxygen species (ROS): unstable molecules that damage cellular components including membrane proteins, mitochondrial DNA, and the tight junction proteins that maintain gut barrier integrity. This oxidative stress is a primary mechanism through which toxins prime mast cells, since ROS directly trigger mast cell degranulation through oxidative activation of the degranulation signaling cascade.

The body's primary defense against oxidative stress is the NRF2 pathway—a master regulator of antioxidant gene expression that, when activated, upregulates the production of glutathione, superoxide dismutase, catalase, and a range of other protective enzymes. Many environmental toxins specifically impair NRF2 signaling,[224] reducing the production of these protective antioxidants at exactly the moment they are most needed. Supporting NRF2 activation through dietary and supplemental approaches—including sulforaphane from cruciferous vegetables, curcumin, resveratrol, and N-acetylcysteine—is therefore a strategy that directly addresses the oxidative mechanism by which toxins prime mast cells. These interventions are discussed in the context of the supplement protocol in Chapter 16.

Impaired Detoxification and the Recirculation Problem

The liver processes toxins through a two-phase system. Phase 1 reactions, carried out primarily by cytochrome P450 enzymes, chemically modify toxins to prepare them for excretion—but these Phase 1 metabolites are often more reactive and potentially more harmful than the original compound. Phase 2 reactions conjugate (attach) these metabolites to carrier molecules—glutathione, sulfate, glucuronate, or amino acids—that make them water-soluble and ready for excretion through bile or urine.

When Phase 2 capacity is overwhelmed or impaired—by high toxic load, genetic variants in conjugation enzymes, nutrient deficiencies (glutathione synthesis requires glycine, cysteine, and glutamine; sulfation requires sulfur amino acids;

methylation requires B12, folate, and B6), or direct impairment by mycotoxins themselves—toxins and their reactive Phase 1 metabolites accumulate. They recirculate through the bloodstream, re-exposing mast cells and immune cells to provocative compounds that should have been cleared. This recirculation problem explains why some patients in moldy environments improve only partially even after removing the source: the body burden of mycotoxins already accumulated in tissue continues to cycle and provoke immune reactivity until the detoxification backlog is cleared.

The HLA-DR Genetic Factor in Mold Susceptibility

Approximately twenty-five percent of the population carries variants in the HLA-DR immune response genes that may impair the capacity to recognize and tag mycotoxins for immune clearance. In the normal immune response to mycotoxins, antigen-presenting cells display mycotoxin fragments on HLA-DR molecules, allowing the immune system to generate antibodies that facilitate toxin clearance. In individuals with susceptible HLA-DR variants, this recognition step fails—mycotoxins are not effectively tagged for clearance, they accumulate in tissues, and the immune system remains in a state of chronic low-grade activation without ever achieving resolution.

This genetic reality explains several otherwise puzzling clinical observations: why some people become profoundly ill in water-damaged buildings while others sharing identical exposure remain relatively unaffected; why some patients with mold illness have remarkably prolonged recovery timelines even after full environmental remediation; and why mold illness runs in families, with multiple members of the same household developing MCAS-like symptoms from the same exposure while other family members are spared.

Knowing whether you carry susceptible HLA-DR variants is clinically useful—it confirms that the mold connection is likely genuine and that more aggressive mycotoxin clearance support may be needed—but it is not required to act on a high clinical suspicion of mold illness. If the pattern fits, investigation and remediation are warranted regardless of genetic test results.

✦ ✦ ✦

What This Means for You: Identifying and Reducing Your Toxic Burden

The environmental toxin landscape can feel overwhelming to contemplate—mold in the walls, metals in the food, chemicals in everything. The goal is not to achieve an impossible state of zero exposure but to systematically identify your most significant sources, reduce them where you have control, and support your body's detoxification capacity so that what you can't avoid doesn't accumulate beyond your threshold.

Start with your environment, not the supplement aisle. For patients with mold illness, no detoxification protocol produces lasting improvement while exposure continues. Before investing in binders, tests, or treatments, conduct an honest assessment of the buildings where you spend the most time. Look for visible mold, water stains, musty odors, or a history of water damage. If you suspect a problematic environment, an ERMI dust test—a mail-in test that measures the DNA of mold species in settled house dust—is a relatively affordable and informative first step. If professional remediation is needed, it needs to happen before other interventions can be fully effective.

Test before treating for heavy metals. Heavy metal accumulation is not a diagnosis to assume; it is one to confirm. Hair tissue mineral analysis (HTMA) provides a useful screening picture of longer-term mineral and metal status. Provoked urine testing under medical supervision provides the most sensitive assessment of tissue metal burden. Work with a knowledgeable practitioner before initiating chelation or aggressive metal removal—mobilizing heavy metals without adequate detoxification support can temporarily worsen symptoms by recirculating metals through tissues they had previously been sequestered away from.

Reduce your daily chemical exposure systematically. The cumulative effect of daily low-level chemical exposures is real and modifiable. Practical reductions include: switching to fragrance-free personal care and cleaning products (synthetic fragrance is one of the most common daily mast cell triggers); filtering drinking water with a high-quality filter that removes heavy metals, PFAS, and agricultural chemicals; choosing organic produce for the most heavily pesticide-laden crops (the Environmental Working Group's annual Dirty Dozen list is a useful reference); replacing non-stick cookware with stainless steel or cast iron; and reducing plastic food storage in favor of glass or stainless containers, particularly for hot or fatty foods that accelerate plasticizer leaching.

Support your detoxification pathways nutritionally. The liver's detoxification capacity depends on a continuous supply of specific nutrients: glutathione precursors (N-acetylcysteine, glycine, and whey protein for those who tolerate it), B vitamins (B2, B3, B6, B12, and folate for methylation and Phase 2 reactions), sulfur-containing amino acids from cruciferous vegetables and allium family plants (garlic, onion, leek), and antioxidants that protect Phase 1 enzymes from the oxidative stress they generate. Ensuring these nutritional foundations are in place before pursuing more aggressive detoxification is both safer and more effective. Chapter 20 covers detoxification support in detail.

Use binders carefully and strategically. Binders—substances that capture toxins in the gut and prevent their reabsorption—are a useful adjunct to environmental remediation for patients with confirmed mycotoxin or chemical exposure. Cholestyramine is the most studied binder for mycotoxins and is used by practitioners specializing in mold illness; it requires a prescription and has significant nutritional implications if used long-term. Natural binders including activated charcoal, bentonite clay, and modified citrus pectin are more accessible and gentler options appropriate for general supportive use. Binders should be taken away from meals, supplements, and medications to avoid binding beneficial nutrients or therapeutic compounds.

Gwen's recovery required two things happening in parallel: getting out of the toxic building and systematically supporting her body's ability to clear the mycotoxin burden that had accumulated over eighteen months of daily exposure. The process was neither quick nor linear. For the first two months after leaving the building, her symptoms actually worsened slightly—a pattern her new physician recognized as the immune system beginning to respond now that the continuous new-exposure pressure had lifted, working through a backlog of stored toxins. By month four, the trend was unmistakably upward. By month eight, she was living a life she had feared was gone permanently.

Her MCAS hadn't been a mystery of internal biology. It had been her body doing exactly what it was built to do—protecting her from a genuine chemical threat—at a cost she couldn't sustain. Removing the threat didn't cure her instantly. But it gave her body the one thing no medication or supplement could provide: a fighting chance to find its way back.

> **A Note on Scope:** *The root cause chapters in this book describe a wide landscape of biological drivers—and if you have been reading them in sequence, you may be feeling the cumulative weight of that landscape. That response is understandable, and worth naming directly: these chapters are not a list of everything that is wrong with you. For most individuals with MCAS, one or two primary drivers account for the majority of their reactivity. The rest are background factors that matter, but not equally, and not all at once. Chapter 24 will help you identify your specific drivers. What you are building right now, through these chapters, is the map. You are not yet being asked to navigate all of it—only the portion that is yours.*

✦ ✦ ✦

Chapter 8 at a Glance

What to Remember:

- Environmental toxins are a direct and potent trigger for mast cell activation, operating through innate immune pathways that are entirely distinct from IgE-mediated allergy. Standard allergy testing does not detect most toxin-driven mast cell reactions.
- Mold illness—driven by mycotoxins produced by water-damaged building mold species including *Stachybotrys, Aspergillus, and Penicillium*—is among the most prevalent and most missed drivers of MCAS. It is the mycotoxins, not the spores, that cause the most significant biological damage.
- Approximately twenty-five percent of people carry HLA-DR genetic variants that impair mycotoxin clearance, explaining why some individuals become severely ill from mold exposure while others sharing the same environment are relatively unaffected.
- Heavy metals—particularly mercury, lead, cadmium, and arsenic—accumulate silently in tissues over years and decades, chronically activating mast cells through oxidative stress, immune dysregulation, and impairment of detoxification and DAO enzyme activity.
- Industrial chemicals including VOCs, pesticides, phthalates, PFAS, and synthetic fragrances contribute to cumulative mast cell trigger load. No single exposure is necessarily catastrophic, but the combined daily burden across multiple sources can be significant.
- Toxins impair mast cell regulation by driving oxidative stress through ROS production, disabling NRF2 antioxidant defenses, overwhelming liver detoxification capacity, and causing recirculation of reactive intermediates that maintain chronic immune priming.
- Environmental remediation comes before detoxification treatment. No binder or protocol produces lasting recovery while significant exposure continues.
- Reducing toxic burden requires a layered approach: Assess and remediate the environment, test appropriately before treating for heavy metals, reduce daily chemical exposures systematically, support detoxification pathways nutritionally, and use binders carefully and strategically as adjuncts to—not substitutes for—the foundational work.

Coming Up in Chapter 9:

Toxins from outside the body are one source of chronic mast cell priming—but some of the most powerful signals driving mast cell reactivity originate from within, in the form of a dysregulated nervous system. Chapter 9 explores the profound and bidirectional relationship between stress, trauma, the autonomic nervous system, and mast cell activation—including the emerging science of the limbic system's role in perpetuating the cycle of reactivity, and why nervous system healing is not a soft supplement to the real treatment but is a cornerstone of it.

CHAPTER 9

Nervous System Dysregulation

When Your Body's Alarm System Gets Stuck in the On Position

A Body That Forgot How to Feel Safe

Elena grew up in a household where she learned early that calm was temporary. Her father's moods were unpredictable—thunderstorm one evening, sunshine the next—and she became expert at reading the atmosphere of a room the moment she walked into it, scanning constantly for signals that told her whether it was safe to relax or time to brace. By the time she left for university, she didn't think of this skill as a trauma response. She thought of it as being perceptive. Sensitive. Good in a crisis.

She was thirty-one when the hives started. By thirty-four, she was dealing with gut pain, racing heart, brain fog, and a body that reacted to what felt like everything—perfume in an elevator, the wrong food, a difficult conversation, a night of poor sleep. She had been formally diagnosed with MCAS, and the diagnosis was accurate. What it didn't capture was the deeper pattern: a nervous system that had been running at high alert for twenty-five years, that had never learned to signal safety reliably, and that was now expressing that chronic state of vigilance as mast cell hyperreactivity throughout her body.

Her MCAS was real. Her mast cells were genuinely dysfunctional. The bucket was real, and the triggers were real. But the single most powerful thing that had been keeping her bucket perpetually full—the factor that made every other trigger hit harder and recover from more slowly—was a nervous system that had been shaped by a childhood spent never quite feeling safe.

This is not a rare story. And it is not a story about weakness, over-sensitivity, or psychological fragility. It is a story about biology—about the measurable, documented ways that chronic stress and adverse experience physically reshape the immune and autonomic systems in ways that directly lower the mast cell threshold. Understanding this connection does not diminish the reality of MCAS. It illuminates one of its most important and most treatable root dimensions.

✦ ✦ ✦

The Nervous System and Mast Cells: An Intimate Partnership

Your nervous system and your immune system are not separate departments that occasionally send memos to each other. They are deeply integrated networks that evolved together, share chemical messengers, and maintain constant bidirectional communication. Nowhere is this integration more evident than in the relationship between the autonomic nervous system and mast cells.

The autonomic nervous system—the branch of the nervous system that operates below conscious awareness—has two primary modes. The sympathetic branch is your accelerator; it activates in response to perceived threat or demand, flooding the body with adrenaline and norepinephrine, raising heart rate and blood pressure, directing blood to muscles, sharpening sensory acuity, and preparing the body for fight or flight. The parasympathetic branch is your brake; it governs rest, digestion, recovery, and repair, slowing the heart, promoting gut function, and facilitating the immune regulation and tissue healing that can only occur when the body feels safe enough to invest in maintenance rather than emergency response.

Mast cells have receptors for the chemical messengers of both branches. Norepinephrine—the primary sympathetic signaling molecule—can directly activate mast cells through adrenergic receptors.[225] Acetylcholine—the primary parasympathetic neurotransmitter, released abundantly through the vagus nerve—suppresses mast cell degranulation through muscarinic receptors.[226] This means that the autonomic state of the body determines, in a very direct biological sense, how reactive the mast cell population is at any given moment. A body in sympathetic dominance has its mast cells primed and ready. A body with healthy parasympathetic tone has its mast cells gently held in check.

> **The Fundamental Equation:** *Sympathetic dominance primes mast cells. Parasympathetic tone suppresses them. The nervous system state you live in day to day is not background noise—it is one of the primary determinants of your mast cell threshold.*

For most people, the autonomic nervous system shifts fluidly between these states as circumstances warrant—sympathetic activation during a stressful meeting, a return to parasympathetic recovery once the meeting ends. For people with MCAS, and particularly for those whose nervous systems were shaped by chronic stress, trauma, or sustained threat, this flexibility is impaired. The system gets stuck—spending far more time in sympathetic activation than the actual demands of daily life warrant, and failing to fully recover into parasympathetic rest even when the external stressor has passed. The result is a mast cell population that is chronically primed by a nervous system that never stops signaling danger.

✦ ✦ ✦

Trauma, Chronic Stress, and the Limbic System

The limbic system is a set of structures deep within the brain—including the amygdala, the hippocampus, and the hypothalamus—that processes emotional experience, encodes threat memories, and coordinates the body's stress response. The amygdala, in particular, functions as the brain's threat detection center; it evaluates incoming sensory information, compares it against a library of past experiences, and decides whether to trigger the stress response. When it detects a pattern that matches a stored threat memory, it activates the hypothalamic-pituitary-adrenal (HPA) axis and the sympathetic nervous system in milliseconds—long before the conscious brain has had a chance to evaluate whether the perceived threat is real.

In a healthy nervous system, the prefrontal cortex—the brain's rational, executive region—maintains regulatory influence over the amygdala, helping to evaluate threat signals in context and apply the brake when the amygdala fires prematurely. In a nervous system shaped by chronic stress or trauma, this regulatory influence is weakened.[227] The amygdala becomes more sensitive and more reactive, the prefrontal cortex less able to modulate it, and the HPA axis more easily triggered. Essentially, the threat-detection system becomes calibrated toward danger—not because the person is irrational or fragile, but because the nervous system has been shaped by a genuine history of threat and has updated its settings accordingly.

This recalibration has direct, measurable consequences for mast cells. Corticotropin-releasing hormone (CRH), the first signaling molecule in the HPA stress cascade, is a potent direct activator of mast cells through receptors on their surface.[228,229] Every time the amygdala fires—every time the body enters a stress response, whether the threat is real or perceived, past or present—CRH is released, and mast cells respond. In a nervous system with a chronically sensitized threat-detection system, this happens repeatedly throughout the day, providing a continuous stream of mast cell activation that has nothing to do with diet, infections, or environmental toxins and everything to do with the body's learned assessment of the world as a dangerous place.

Adverse Childhood Experiences and Biological Embedding

The research on adverse childhood experiences (ACEs)—which include abuse, neglect, household dysfunction, witnessing violence, and other significant childhood stressors—has produced one of the most important findings in modern medicine: early adversity physically alters the structure and function of the developing stress response system in ways that persist throughout life and affect physical health decades later.[230]

The ACE studies, beginning with landmark work in the 1990s and now replicated across dozens of populations, have consistently found that higher ACE scores correlate with elevated rates of autoimmune disease, inflammatory conditions, cardiovascular disease, and—increasingly evident in more recent research—mast cell–related conditions including fibromyalgia, IBS, and chronic multisystem illness.[231] The mechanism is not psychological in the dismissive sense that the word is sometimes used. It is epigenetic. Early adverse experiences alter the methylation patterns on genes regulating the HPA axis, inflammatory signaling, and immune cell behavior, creating a biological set point that is tilted toward chronic stress reactivity and immune dysregulation.[232]

This does not mean that everyone with MCAS has a trauma history—many individuals have no significant adverse experiences and develop mast cell dysfunction through entirely different pathways. And it emphatically does not mean that MCAS is caused by psychological factors in a way that makes it less real or less biological. What it means is that for a meaningful subset of people, the nervous system dimension is a primary driver that deserves the same rigorous clinical attention as diet, gut health, infections, and toxins. Treating MCAS while ignoring a chronically dysregulated nervous system is like trying to empty a bucket while one hand holds the tap open.

> **A Note on Framing:** *Understanding the nervous system's role in MCAS should feel empowering, not stigmatizing. The biological pathways are real and measurable. The therapeutic approaches—nervous system regulation, somatic therapies, limbic retraining—are evidence-informed and genuinely effective. This is medical territory, not a suggestion that the illness is imaginary or that mental effort alone will resolve it.*

✦ ✦ ✦

The Vagus Nerve: Your Body's Most Powerful Mast Cell Regulator

The vagus nerve is the longest and most complex of the cranial nerves, running from the brainstem down through the neck, chest, and abdomen, sending branches to the heart, lungs, gut, liver, spleen, and nearly every major organ. It is the primary channel of the parasympathetic nervous system—the anatomical highway through which rest-and-digest signals travel from the brain to the body and, critically, from the body back to the brain.

Approximately eighty percent of vagal fibers are afferent—they carry information upward from the organs to the brain, rather than downward.[233] This means the vagus nerve is primarily a sensory system, continuously reporting on the state of the body's internal environment. The brain uses this incoming information to assess the body's safety and allocate resources accordingly. When vagal tone is high—when the vagus is actively transmitting rich, varied signals between body and brain—the brain interprets this as a signal of safety and physiological stability, and the parasympathetic brake is applied. When vagal tone is low—as it characteristically is in people with dysautonomia, chronic stress, and MCAS—the brain receives impoverished or dysregulated body signals, cannot confidently assess safety, and defaults toward sympathetic vigilance.

The Cholinergic Anti-Inflammatory Pathway

In 2000, neuroscientist Kevin Tracey and colleagues described what is now called the cholinergic anti-inflammatory pathway: a neural circuit through which the vagus nerve directly suppresses systemic inflammation.[234] When vagal efferent fibers activate the enteric nervous system in the gut, they trigger the release of acetylcholine from enteric neurons. Acetylcholine binds to alpha-7 nicotinic receptors on macrophages and, critically, on mast cells, suppressing their capacity to produce and release pro-inflammatory cytokines and mediators.

This pathway is not metaphorical. It is a hard-wired, pharmacologically characterized circuit through which neural activity—specifically, vagal tone—directly modulates mast cell behavior at the tissue level. High vagal tone means more acetylcholine reaching mast cells, a lower probability of degranulation in response to any given stimulus, and faster recovery from activation events. Low vagal tone means less acetylcholine, more mast cell reactivity, and slower recovery. Every vagus nerve exercise, every breathing practice, every intervention that measurably improves heart rate variability (a clinical proxy for vagal tone) is directly reducing mast cell reactivity through this pathway.

This is why the nervous system practices described in Chapter 14—breathwork, vagal stimulation techniques, somatic therapies, cold water exposure, humming, and others—are not soft add-ons to the real medical treatment. They are biological interventions that address mast cell reactivity at its autonomic root. For individuals in whom nervous system dysregulation is a primary driver, these practices are often among the most powerful tools available.

Fight-or-Flight and the Amplification of Every Other Trigger

One of the most practically important consequences of chronic sympathetic dominance in MCAS is what might be called trigger amplification. The same food, scent, or environmental stimulus produces a much larger mast cell reaction when the nervous system is in a state of sympathetic activation than when it is in a parasympathetic state. This is not imagined—it reflects the direct priming effect of norepinephrine on mast cell surface receptors. A meal that would be tolerable on a calm day can trigger significant symptoms on a high-stress day not because the food has changed but because the mast cells receiving the food's histamine load are already primed by the nervous system's chemical signals.

This amplification effect explains several patterns that confuse people with MCAS enormously: why reactions seem worse during stressful periods even when diet is unchanged; why the same social situation is tolerable some days and intolerable others depending on the overall stress level; and why MCAS symptoms so reliably worsen during periods of major life stress—bereavements, relationship conflicts, workplace crises—that have no obvious dietary or environmental trigger. The nervous system is the amplifier through which every other trigger is processed. Reducing sympathetic tone doesn't eliminate triggers, but it consistently reduces the amplitude of the response to them.

✦ ✦ ✦

Deeper Dive: MRGPRX2, Neuropsychiatric Endotypes, and the Brain's Mast Cells

For the Science-Minded Reader

The nervous system–mast cell relationship extends well beyond the autonomic level into some of the most exciting and clinically relevant frontier science in MCAS research. Two areas in particular deserve attention: the MRGPRX2 receptor and its role in neuro-immune signaling, and the emerging understanding of mast cells in the central nervous system as drivers of neuropsychiatric symptoms.

MRGPRX2: The Neuropeptide Gateway

Until relatively recently, mast cell activation was understood primarily through the IgE pathway: allergen binds IgE antibodies on the mast cell surface, crosslinking occurs, degranulation follows. This model is accurate for classical allergy but fails to explain the vast majority of reactions in MCAS, which are non-IgE mediated.

A major step forward in understanding non-IgE mast cell activation came with the detailed characterization of a receptor called Mas-related G protein-coupled receptor X2, or MRGPRX2.[235] Unlike the IgE receptor, which responds to allergens, MRGPRX2 is specifically designed to respond to neuropeptides—the chemical messengers released by sensory and autonomic nerves.[236] Its natural ligands—a specific molecule produced by the body (or found in nature) that fits into a matching receptor on a cell, much like a key fits into a lock—include substance P, the neuropeptide released by sensory nerve fibers during pain and stress; compound 48/80, a synthetic polymer compound; and a range of basic compounds including certain antibiotics, neuromuscular blocking agents, and fluoroquinolones, which explains why some individuals with MCAS have dramatic reactions to these medications through a pathway entirely independent of allergy.

The clinical significance of MRGPRX2 is substantial. It provides a mechanistic explanation for why physical sensations—pain, pressure, heat, cold, and vibration—trigger mast cell reactions in people with MCAS; substance P is released from sensory nerves in response to all of these stimuli, and substance P activates mast cells via MRGPRX2.[237,238] It explains why emotional distress, which triggers neuropeptide release through the nervous system, is a reliable mast cell activator even in the absence of any external chemical trigger. And it provides a target for understanding why certain medications—particularly some antibiotics and contrast dyes used in imaging—trigger mast cell reactions in people with MCAS at rates far exceeding their IgE-mediated allergy potential.

Importantly, MRGPRX2 activation does not produce the same mediator profile as IgE-mediated degranulation. MRGPRX2-triggered reactions tend to release more neuropeptides and certain cytokines with a different inflammatory profile than classic IgE reactions,[239] which may help explain why some people with MCAS present with neurological and pain-predominant symptoms rather than the classic allergic picture of hives and anaphylaxis. The neuropeptide-MRGPRX2 axis bridges the nervous system and the mast cell system in a way that makes their inseparability at the molecular level unmistakably clear.

Central Nervous System Mast Cells and Neuropsychiatric Endotypes

Mast cells are not confined to peripheral tissues. They are present in the brain—specifically in the meninges (the membranes surrounding the brain), the hypothalamus, the thalamus, the hippocampus, and the choroid plexus.[240] These central nervous system mast cells are relatively few in number compared to peripheral mast cell populations, but their location—adjacent to the blood-brain barrier, in direct communication with neurons and microglia—gives them disproportionate influence over brain function.

Researchers including Dr. Leonard Weinstock have theorized and documented what might be called neuropsychiatric endotypes of MCAS: presentations in which mast cell mediators released within the central nervous system—or peripherally produced mediators that cross the blood-brain barrier—drive a constellation of neurological and psychiatric symptoms that can dominate the clinical picture.[241] In these individuals, brain fog, anxiety, depression, cognitive impairment, and autonomic dysregulation are not merely secondary consequences of a body in distress; they are primary expressions of mast cell activity in or near the brain itself.

The mechanisms are several. Histamine, released by CNS mast cells or crossing the blood-brain barrier from peripheral sources, acts on H1 and H3 receptors in the brain to disrupt neurotransmitter balance, impair cognitive processing, and alter circadian rhythm and sleep architecture. Tryptase released by meningeal mast cells activates protease-activated receptors (PARs) on neurons and microglia, promoting neuroinflammation and sensitizing pain pathways. Cytokines including IL-6, IL-1 beta, and TNF-alpha, produced by activated CNS mast cells, drive microglial activation and the neuroinflammatory state that underlies depression, anxiety, and brain fog in ways that are increasingly well-characterized in the neuroinflammation literature.

The autonomic nervous system dimension is also central here. The hypothalamus—where mast cells are concentrated in the brain—is the master coordinator of autonomic function. Mast cell activation in the hypothalamus can directly disrupt the autonomic set point, altering baseline heart rate, blood pressure regulation, temperature control, and the HPA axis stress response.[242] This hypothalamic mast cell involvement may be one of the primary mechanisms through which MCAS produces the dysautonomia and autonomic symptoms that bring so many patients to cardiology and neurology before ever reaching a diagnosis.

The practical implication of this emerging science is significant. For individuals with MCAS whose most disabling symptoms are neurological or psychiatric in character—severe anxiety, depression, cognitive impairment, or autonomic instability that doesn't respond adequately to peripheral mast cell stabilization—the central nervous system dimension may need to be directly addressed. Interventions that support the blood-brain barrier's integrity (omega-3 fatty acids, phosphatidylserine, and anti-inflammatory compounds with CNS penetration including curcumin and luteolin), reduce neuroinflammation, and support central mast cell stability are an important dimension of treatment for this subset of individuals.

✦ ✦ ✦

What This Means for You: Healing the Nervous System as Medical Treatment

If the nervous system–mast cell connection resonates with your experience—if you recognize the pattern of symptoms worsening with stress and emotional arousal, of never feeling truly rested or safe, of reactions that seem to have no dietary or environmental explanation—then nervous system regulation belongs at the center of your treatment plan, not at the periphery.

This is medical work. It is not simply relaxation or positive thinking. The practices that genuinely improve vagal tone, reduce HPA axis hyperreactivity, and shift the autonomic set point toward safety produce measurable, biological changes in mast cell reactivity. Chapter 14 is devoted to these practices in practical detail. Here, it is worth establishing the principles that guide them.

Treat the nervous system like any other organ requiring rehabilitation. Just as a damaged gut lining requires consistent, sustained effort to repair, a nervous system calibrated toward chronic threat requires consistent, sustained practice to recalibrate. Sporadic efforts produce sporadic results. The most effective nervous system interventions work through neuroplasticity: the brain's capacity to form new neural pathways in response to repeated experience. This takes time, measured in weeks to months, and requires regularity more than intensity.

Heart rate variability is your nervous system report card. Heart rate variability (HRV)—the natural variation in the interval between heartbeats—is the most accessible and well-validated clinical measure of autonomic balance and vagal tone. Higher HRV indicates greater autonomic flexibility and stronger parasympathetic tone; lower HRV indicates sympathetic dominance and reduced vagal influence. Monitoring HRV through a wearable device provides real-time feedback on your autonomic state, helps you identify which practices most effectively shift your nervous system toward recovery, and gives you objective evidence of progress over time.

Recognize the feedback loop between symptoms and nervous system state. MCAS symptoms themselves activate the sympathetic nervous system—a racing heart, hives, gut pain, and the terror of an unpredictable body are inherently threatening experiences that the nervous system responds to by raising the alarm. This creates a vicious cycle: mast cell activation triggers sympathetic arousal, which further primes mast cells, which produce more symptoms. Breaking this cycle requires learning to meet symptoms with a nervous system response of relative calm rather than fear—not by denying the symptoms or dismissing them, but by developing the physiological capacity to activate the parasympathetic brake even while experiencing discomfort. This is the core skill taught in somatic therapies and limbic retraining approaches.

Address trauma with appropriate support. For patients whose nervous system dysregulation has roots in adverse experience, trauma-informed therapy can be genuinely transformative for MCAS. Somatic Experiencing, EMDR (Eye Movement Desensitization and Reprocessing), sensorimotor psychotherapy, and Internal Family Systems therapy are among the evidence-informed approaches that work at the level of the nervous system rather than purely at the cognitive level—addressing the embodied, physiological patterns of threat response that drive mast cell reactivity in ways that talking therapies alone often cannot reach.[243]

This is not a requirement for every MCAS patient, but for those with significant adverse histories, it may be the single most powerful intervention available.

Sleep is nervous system medicine. The glymphatic clearance of inflammatory debris, the restoration of HPA axis sensitivity, the consolidation of learning and memory, and the repair of autonomic tone all occur primarily during deep and REM sleep.[244] For individuals with MCAS whose nervous systems are stuck in sympathetic dominance, sleep is both compromised by that dysregulation and essential for resolving it. Prioritizing sleep hygiene, addressing histamine-driven sleep disruption through appropriate supplementation (discussed in Chapter 16), and using nervous system practices in the evening to support the parasympathetic transition into sleep create a virtuous cycle in which better sleep supports better nervous system regulation, which supports better sleep.

Elena's healing did not begin with a dietary change or a new supplement. It began when a therapist who understood both MCAS and somatic work helped her recognize that her body had been running a survival program for two and a half decades, and that the hives, the gut pain, and the racing heart were not random attacks—they were the body's learned prediction that the world was dangerous, expressed through the mast cell network that sits at the body's environmental interfaces.

Learning to feel safe in her body—literally, physiologically—was the hardest and the most transformative work she did. It didn't happen overnight. But as her nervous system gradually found a new set point, everything else responded. The bucket capacity grew. The threshold for reactions rose. The same foods she'd been avoiding for three years became manageable. Her world, which had been contracting steadily for half a decade, began to expand again.

The nervous system is not a soft variable in the MCAS equation. For many people, it is the equation itself.

✦ ✦ ✦

Chapter 9 at a Glance

What to Remember:

- The autonomic nervous system and mast cells are in constant, direct biological communication. Sympathetic activation (via norepinephrine) primes mast cells toward degranulation; parasympathetic tone (via acetylcholine through the vagus nerve) suppresses it. The nervous system state you live in shapes your mast cell reactivity as directly as your diet.
- Chronic stress and adverse experience physically reshape the limbic system, sensitizing the amygdala's threat-detection function and

weakening prefrontal regulation. This recalibration keeps the HPA axis chronically activated, flooding the body with CRH that directly activates mast cells throughout the day regardless of external triggers.

- Adverse childhood experiences are epigenetically embedded in immune and autonomic function, producing measurable increases in inflammatory reactivity and mast cell priming that persist into adulthood. This is a biological finding, not a psychological explanation, and it points toward specific, evidence-informed treatment approaches.
- The vagus nerve mediates the cholinergic anti-inflammatory pathway—a hard-wired circuit through which vagal tone directly suppresses mast cell mediator production at the tissue level. Improving vagal tone through breathwork, somatic practices, and other nervous system interventions is a direct biological intervention for mast cell reactivity.
- Sympathetic dominance amplifies the response to every other trigger category—food, environment, infection, and toxin. The same stimulus produces a larger mast cell reaction in a sympathetically dominant nervous system than in a parasympathetically balanced one, explaining why MCAS reactions are reliably worse during high-stress periods.
- The MRGPRX2 receptor on mast cells responds directly to neuropeptides including substance P, released by sensory nerves in response to pain, pressure, heat, cold, and emotional stress. This receptor provides the molecular mechanism through which physical sensation and emotional experience activate mast cells independently of allergy or prior sensitization.
- Mast cells in the central nervous system—particularly in the meninges, hypothalamus, and hippocampus—drive neuropsychiatric endotypes of MCAS including anxiety, depression, cognitive impairment, and autonomic dysregulation through histamine, tryptase, and cytokine release within or near the brain. Peripheral mast cell stabilization alone may be insufficient for this patient subset.
- Nervous system healing is medical treatment: consistent practice of vagal tone–building techniques, trauma-informed therapy where indicated, HRV monitoring for biofeedback, and sleep prioritization all produce measurable, biological improvements in mast cell reactivity. Chapter 14 provides the practical protocols.

Coming Up in Chapter 10:

The nervous system is one internal driver of mast cell reactivity—but it is not the only one. Hormones, particularly estrogen, have direct and powerful effects on mast cell sensitivity that help explain one of the most consistent clinical observations in MCAS: why the condition disproportionately affects women, why symptoms track the menstrual cycle with such reliability, and why hormonal transitions—puberty, pregnancy, perimenopause—are so frequently the trigger points for onset or dramatic worsening. Chapter 10 explores the estrogen–histamine axis, thyroid dysfunction, and adrenal imbalance as hormonal drivers of MCAS that are often correctable once identified.

CHAPTER 10

Hormones and MCAS

The Estrogen–Histamine Axis, Thyroid Dysfunction, and the Adrenal Connection

The Calendar She Kept

Fiona was thirty-eight when she noticed the pattern. She had been tracking her MCAS symptoms for four months—her allergist had suggested it as a way to identify food triggers—and the journal was filling up with data she hadn't expected. Not food reactions, primarily. A calendar.

Every month, between days twenty-one and twenty-eight of her cycle, everything got worse. The hives that were manageable the rest of the month became daily. The gut pain that she'd mostly learned to live with became genuinely debilitating. The brain fog descended like a weather system. Her heart raced at rest. She reacted to foods that had been fine the week before. And then, reliable as a tide, the first day of her period arrived—and within twenty-four hours the whole picture cleared, dramatically, as if someone had turned down the volume on her immune system.

She took the journal to her gynecologist, who was sympathetic but puzzled. The gynecologist informed her that MCAS can definitely fluctuate, but didn't know why it tracked Fiona's cycle so precisely. She referred Fiona to her immunologist, who offered a similar expression of thoughtful uncertainty. Nobody connected the biological dots between estrogen, progesterone, and mast cell reactivity—because it is a connection that is genuinely underappreciated in conventional medical training, despite being documented in the research literature for decades.[245,246]

The estrogen–histamine axis is one of the most clinically important and most consistently overlooked dimensions of MCAS—particularly for women, who represent the overwhelming majority of MCAS diagnoses. But hormonal influences on mast cell biology extend well beyond estrogen. Thyroid hormones regulate mast cell function at the cellular level,[247] and thyroid dysfunction—

whether overt or subclinical—can dramatically worsen mast cell reactivity. Adrenal function shapes the cortisol response that is supposed to counterbalance the inflammatory effects of mast cell activation but frequently fails to do so adequately in chronically stressed individuals with MCAS.

Understanding the hormonal dimension of MCAS does not require a deep background in endocrinology. It requires knowing which questions to ask—and being willing to look at the body as an integrated system in which immune function and hormonal balance are not separate conversations.

✦ ✦ ✦

The Estrogen–Histamine Axis: A Two-Way Street

Of all the hormonal relationships in MCAS, none is more directly impactful or more frequently relevant than the relationship between estrogen and histamine.[248] This relationship is bidirectional—estrogen influences histamine, and histamine influences estrogen—creating a feedback loop that can amplify both hormonal imbalance and mast cell reactivity simultaneously.

How Estrogen Primes Mast Cells

Mast cells express estrogen receptors—both the classical nuclear estrogen receptors (ERα and ERβ) and membrane-bound receptors that mediate rapid, non-genomic responses to estrogen signaling.[249] When estrogen binds to these receptors, it increases mast cell sensitivity in several ways: it upregulates the expression of IgE receptors on the mast cell surface, making the cell more responsive to IgE-mediated triggers; it lowers the threshold for degranulation in response to substance P and other neuropeptides via MRGPRX2; it promotes the survival and proliferation of mast cells in estrogen-rich tissue environments; and it directly enhances the release of histamine from mast cell granules.

The clinical consequence of this estrogen–mast cell relationship is a body that becomes significantly more mast-cell-reactive as estrogen levels rise. This explains with elegant precision why MCAS symptoms reliably worsen in the late luteal phase of the menstrual cycle—the days before menstruation, when estrogen has been dominant and progesterone is beginning its premenstrual fall. This demonstrates why pregnancy, which produces some of the highest estrogen levels in a woman's life, is a common trigger for MCAS onset or dramatic worsening—and why some women experience profound postpartum improvement as estrogen levels drop, while others who breastfeed maintain elevated estrogen and find their symptoms persist. It explains why perimenopause—a period of irregular, often high and fluctuating estrogen levels before the final estrogen decline of menopause—is one of the most common trigger points for new or dramatically worsened MCAS.

> **A Pattern Worth Recognizing:** *If your MCAS symptoms reliably worsen in the week before your period, improve within a day or two of menstruation beginning, and correlate with other hormonal transitions in your history, estrogen dominance or estrogen–progesterone imbalance is very likely contributing to your mast cell reactivity. This is not a coincidence to dismiss—it is a clinically actionable signal.*

How Histamine Drives Estrogen Dominance

The relationship runs in the other direction too, which is what makes the estrogen–histamine axis a genuine self-amplifying loop rather than a simple one-way influence. Histamine directly stimulates the ovaries to produce more estrogen—it acts on H1 and H2 receptors in ovarian tissue, increasing estradiol synthesis.[250] And excess histamine reduces progesterone production, tipping the hormonal balance further toward estrogen dominance.[251]

In a person with MCAS and significant mast cell mediator release, this histamine-to-estrogen pathway means that the very mediators being overproduced by reactive mast cells are actively promoting the hormonal environment—estrogen dominance—that makes mast cells more reactive. Left unaddressed, this cycle is self-perpetuating: mast cell activation produces histamine, histamine promotes estrogen production, elevated estrogen further primes mast cells, which produce more histamine.

This cycle is also relevant to understanding why some women with MCAS find that hormonal contraceptives—particularly those with high estrogen content or progestins that convert to estrogen-like compounds in the body—worsen their symptoms significantly. And it illuminates why natural progesterone, which has mast-cell-stabilizing properties and counterbalances estrogen's mast-cell-sensitizing effects, is sometimes a useful therapeutic consideration for women with MCAS and clear hormonal cycling of symptoms.

Progesterone's Protective Role

If estrogen is the mast cell sensitizer, progesterone is to some degree its counterbalance. Progesterone has documented anti-inflammatory and mast-cell-stabilizing effects; it reduces mast cell sensitivity to IgE-mediated triggers, downregulates the expression of mast cell surface receptors including the IgE receptor, and promotes the production of anti-inflammatory prostaglandins that dampen mast cell reactivity.[252] In the mid-luteal phase of a healthy menstrual cycle—when both estrogen and progesterone are present—the estrogen-driven mast cell priming is partially offset by progesterone's stabilizing influence.

When progesterone falls prematurely in the late luteal phase, or when progesterone production is chronically insufficient (a pattern sometimes called luteal phase defect or relative progesterone deficiency, common in women with chronic stress, hypothyroidism, or significant gut dysfunction), the estrogen–progesterone balance tips toward estrogen dominance and the mast-cell-sensitizing effects of estrogen are unchecked. This is the hormonal picture underlying the late-luteal MCAS flare pattern—and it is a picture that is potentially addressable through progesterone support, stress reduction, and the gut and liver health interventions that improve estrogen metabolism and clearance.

Estrogen Metabolism and the Liver–Gut Axis

Estrogen does not simply rise and fall in a vacuum—it is metabolized, conjugated, and cleared through the liver and gut in a process that, when functioning well, keeps estrogen levels appropriately regulated and clears used estrogen efficiently from the body. When liver Phase 2 conjugation is impaired—by nutrient deficiencies, high toxic burden, genetic variants in conjugation enzymes, or the same mycotoxin exposures discussed in Chapter 8—used estrogen may be inadequately cleared and recirculated, contributing to estrogen dominance. When the gut microbiome contains a high burden of bacteria expressing the enzyme beta-glucuronidase (which cleaves the conjugate from processed estrogen in the gut, freeing it for reabsorption rather than excretion), circulating estrogen is further elevated.

This is sometimes called the estrobolome effect—the influence of the gut microbiome on estrogen metabolism and circulating estrogen levels. Addressing the gut microbiome, supporting liver detoxification with supplements like DIM (diindolylmethane, from cruciferous vegetables), calcium D-glucarate, and B vitamins, and reducing the beta-glucuronidase burden in the gut through probiotic support and dietary fiber are all strategies that address the hormonal root of estrogen-driven MCAS by improving estrogen clearance rather than simply suppressing estrogen itself.

✦ ✦ ✦

Thyroid Dysfunction: The Metabolic Gatekeeper of Mast Cell Reactivity

The thyroid gland produces hormones—primarily thyroxine (T4) and triiodothyronine (T3)—that regulate metabolic rate in virtually every cell of the body. When thyroid function is optimal, cellular energy production, immune regulation, gut motility, and neurotransmitter balance all run at the correct tempo. When thyroid function is impaired, these processes slow down—or, in certain forms of thyroid dysfunction, become erratic—in ways that have direct consequences for mast cell behavior and overall MCAS symptom severity.

Thyroid dysfunction and MCAS co-occur at rates significantly above chance. There are several reasons for this. First, the same autoimmune and inflammatory processes that drive MCAS—chronic immune dysregulation, elevated pro-inflammatory cytokines, molecular mimicry—also increase the risk of Hashimoto's thyroiditis, the autoimmune condition that is the most common cause of hypothyroidism in the developed world. Second, thyroid hormones directly influence mast cell function at the cellular level. And third, the downstream consequences of hypothyroidism—slowed gut motility, impaired liver detoxification, reduced mitochondrial efficiency, and increased susceptibility to infections—each worsen MCAS through the mechanisms discussed throughout this book.

How Hypothyroidism Amplifies MCAS

When thyroid hormone levels are low—whether from Hashimoto's autoimmune destruction of the thyroid, iodine or selenium deficiency, chronic stress suppression of the pituitary's thyroid-stimulating hormone production, or other causes—several MCAS-relevant consequences follow.

Gut motility slows, worsening constipation and the conditions that favor SIBO and dysbiosis—the very gut imbalances discussed in Chapter 6 that drive histamine production and impair gut barrier integrity. Liver detoxification slows, reducing the clearance of estrogen, mycotoxins, and other toxins that prime mast cells. Mitochondrial function falls with the overall metabolic slowdown, reducing cellular energy for immune regulation. And the immune system's regulatory capacity diminishes, allowing mast cells to operate with less constraint.

Perhaps most directly relevant: Thyroid hormone T3 has specific effects on mast cell granule content and degranulation threshold.[253] Mast cells in hypothyroid environments have been shown in research models to be more easily triggered and to release more histamine per activation event than mast cells in euthyroid (normal thyroid) conditions.[254] Correcting hypothyroidism—even subclinical hypothyroidism, where TSH is only mildly elevated and T4 is technically within range but low-normal—can produce surprisingly significant improvements in MCAS symptom severity for people in whom thyroid function is a contributing factor.

Thyroid Autoimmunity: The Hashimoto's–MCAS Overlap

Hashimoto's thyroiditis deserves specific attention because it represents the intersection of thyroid dysfunction and autoimmune inflammation in a combination that is particularly relevant to MCAS. In Hashimoto's, the immune system generates antibodies against thyroid peroxidase (TPO) and thyroglobulin, driving chronic inflammatory destruction of thyroid tissue. This chronic autoimmune inflammation produces the same kind of cytokine environment—elevated IL-6, TNF-alpha, and

Th2-skewed immune activity—that primes mast cells. Individuals with Hashimoto's and MCAS are therefore dealing with both the metabolic consequences of reduced thyroid function and the immune consequences of ongoing autoimmune inflammation, each of which amplifies the other.

Importantly, standard thyroid assessment often misses the full picture in these individuals. A TSH test within the normal reference range does not rule out Hashimoto's—TPO and thyroglobulin antibodies should be measured directly. And the functional medicine approach of optimizing free T3 (the active form of thyroid hormone) rather than simply normalizing TSH may be relevant for people whose symptoms persist despite technically normal TSH values. The conversion of T4 to active T3 depends on selenium, zinc, and adequate gut function—all factors commonly impaired in MCAS—which means that standard T4 replacement may not be sufficient if conversion is impaired.

> **Testing Recommendation:** *A comprehensive thyroid assessment for individuals with MCAS should include TSH, free T4, free T3, reverse T3, TPO antibodies, and thyroglobulin antibodies. Relying on TSH alone misses both conversion problems and the autoimmune component that may be driving mast cell priming independently of the metabolic effects of thyroid hormone deficiency.*

✦ ✦ ✦

Adrenal Imbalance: Cortisol, Mast Cells, and the Chronic Stress Paradox

The adrenal glands produce cortisol—the body's primary stress hormone and one of its most important anti-inflammatory regulators. In an acute crisis, cortisol rises rapidly, suppressing the immune response sufficiently to prevent the inflammatory cascade from becoming self-destructive while the body deals with the immediate threat. Once the threat has passed, cortisol falls and the immune system returns to normal operation. This regulation is elegant and essential.

In chronic stress—the kind that most people with MCAS know intimately—this elegant system develops a paradoxical dysfunction. The HPA axis, chronically activated by persistent stressors (physical, immune, emotional, environmental), runs at high output for extended periods. The adrenal glands, designed for acute surges rather than sustained high-output production, become less efficient over time. The result can take two forms: cortisol excess in the earlier stages of chronic stress, and cortisol insufficiency—sometimes called adrenal fatigue in functional medicine, though the more precise term is HPA axis dysregulation or hypocortisolism—in later stages or in patients with prolonged illness.

The Cortisol–Mast Cell Relationship

Cortisol (a glucocorticoid) suppresses mast cell activation and mediator release, giving it functional mast cell–stabilizing effects.[255,256,257] Through glucocorticoid receptors on mast cells, cortisol reduces the expression of IgE surface receptors, lowers sensitivity to degranulation triggers, reduces the synthesis of inflammatory mediators including histamine and leukotrienes, and accelerates the return to a resting state after an activation event. This is precisely why corticosteroids—pharmacological versions of cortisol—are among the most rapidly effective treatments for anaphylaxis and severe mast cell reactions: they essentially override the mast cell activation signal through the same pathway that endogenous cortisol uses under normal circumstances.

When cortisol production is insufficient—as it is in HPA axis dysregulation—the natural mast cell stabilizing influence of cortisol is diminished. Mast cells that would ordinarily be held in relative check by adequate cortisol become more reactive. Reactions are more severe and more prolonged. Recovery from activation events takes longer. The same triggers that would produce a modest, self-limiting reaction in a person with healthy cortisol output produce exaggerated, difficult-to-resolve reactions in someone with cortisol deficiency.

This explains a clinical pattern that puzzles many individuals with MCAS: why symptoms are often worst in the morning, when cortisol should be at its daily peak but, in HPA axis dysregulation, may be low or poorly timed; why illness, emotional stress, or significant physical exertion reliably triggers prolonged flares rather than the self-limiting reactions a healthy cortisol response would produce; and why some patients find that short courses of low-dose corticosteroids produce dramatic temporary improvement far beyond what would be expected from their anti-inflammatory effects alone—because they are supplying what the body's own cortisol system is failing to provide.

The Cortisol–Histamine Bidirectional Loop

As with estrogen and histamine, the cortisol–mast cell relationship is bidirectional in ways that create self-reinforcing cycles. Histamine released by activated mast cells directly stimulates the adrenal glands to produce more cortisol—an attempt by the body to self-regulate the mast cell reaction. In a healthy system with adequate adrenal reserve, this works: histamine rises, cortisol follows, mast cell activation is dampened. In a person with depleted adrenal function, the cortisol response to histamine is blunted or delayed—the mast cell activation proceeds further than it should before the brake is applied, and recovery is prolonged.

At the same time, the chronic activation of the HPA axis by MCAS-driven systemic inflammation contributes to the adrenal depletion that impairs the cortisol response. This is another of MCAS's self-perpetuating loops. Mast cell activation triggers histamine, histamine demands cortisol, chronic cortisol demand depletes adrenal reserve, impaired cortisol response allows mast cell activation to proceed further—which demands more cortisol, and so the cycle continues.

DHEA and the Adrenal Balance

Cortisol is not the only adrenal hormone relevant to MCAS. DHEA (dehydroepiandrosterone) and its sulfate form DHEA-S are adrenal androgens that serve as precursors to sex hormones and have independent anti-inflammatory and immune-modulating effects. DHEA levels typically fall with the same HPA axis depletion that impairs cortisol, and low DHEA is associated with increased inflammatory reactivity and reduced immune regulation.[258] The cortisol-to-DHEA ratio is a useful functional measure of adrenal balance—a high ratio (high cortisol relative to DHEA) suggests early chronic stress; a low ratio with both hormones reduced suggests later-stage HPA axis dysregulation. Healthy FPA axis resilience is indicated by a cortsiol:DHEA ratio of 5:1 to 6:1; elevated/acute stress 10:1 to 19.9:1; and maladaptive/chronic stress greater than 20:1. Finally, advanced dysregulation is more nuanced being variable and often both numbers being low.

Supporting adrenal function through adaptogenic herbs—including ashwagandha, rhodiola, eleuthero, and holy basil—is discussed in Chapter 17. The foundational interventions are the same ones that support the nervous system: adequate sleep, reduced chronic stressors, blood sugar stability, and the gradual reduction of the total inflammatory burden that places ongoing demand on the HPA axis.

✦ ✦ ✦

Deeper Dive: The Full Hormonal Picture in MCAS

For the Science-Minded Reader

The hormonal influences on mast cell biology extend into several additional areas that are worth understanding for the complete clinical picture. Three deserve mention for the science-minded reader.

Insulin Resistance and Mast Cell Priming

Insulin resistance—a state in which cells respond less efficiently to insulin, requiring the pancreas to produce more of it to maintain blood glucose control—has documented connections to mast cell biology.[259] Elevated insulin levels promote mast cell survival and alter how they behave. It can shift them away from releasing histamine suddenly and instead toward producing other types of inflammatory signals.[260] The chronic low-grade inflammation that accompanies insulin resistance—characterized by elevated TNF-alpha, IL-6, and C-reactive protein—provides an additional pro-inflammatory backdrop that primes mast cells. And blood sugar instability itself, through the adrenaline surges that accompany hypoglycemic episodes, activates mast cells via the same adrenergic pathway discussed in Chapter 9.

For people with MCAS who also have insulin resistance or metabolic syndrome—a combination that is more common than chance would predict, given the shared inflammatory drivers—blood sugar stabilization through dietary carbohydrate management, regular balanced meals, physical activity, and targeted supplementation (including berberine, chromium, and alpha-lipoic acid) reduces mast cell priming from the metabolic dimension alongside the hormonal and immune dimensions.

Testosterone's Complex Role

Testosterone's relationship to mast cells is more nuanced than estrogen's and less consistently documented in the clinical literature, but it is worth acknowledging. In general, androgens including testosterone have mast-cell-stabilizing effects similar to progesterone—they reduce mast cell sensitivity and promote anti-inflammatory immune orientations.[261,262,263] This is consistent with the clinical observation that MCAS is significantly less common and typically less severe in men than in women, and that women with higher androgen levels (as in polycystic ovary syndrome, or PCOS) sometimes have somewhat attenuated estrogen-driven mast cell cycling despite the other health challenges PCOS presents.

In men with MCAS, low testosterone—hypogonadism, which may be primary or secondary to chronic illness and HPA axis dysregulation—can worsen mast cell reactivity and is worth assessing, particularly in men whose MCAS onset or worsening coincides with documented testosterone decline.

The Hormone–Gut–Mast Cell Triangle

A unifying theme in the hormonal dimension of MCAS is the central role of gut health in hormonal balance. Estrogen metabolism and clearance depend critically on gut microbiome composition and liver function.[264,265] Thyroid hormone conversion from T4 to active T3 depends partly on gut bacteria and on the reduction of intestinal inflammation.[266] Cortisol production and regulation are influenced by gut microbiome signaling through the gut–brain axis. And the gut itself is the largest mast-cell-dense environment in the body, responding directly to the hormonal changes that mast cells are driving.

This triangle—hormones shaping gut function, gut health shaping hormone metabolism, and both interacting with mast cell populations throughout—underscores a theme that runs through all of this section of the book. These root causes are not independent variables. They are a web. Addressing them in isolation, one at a time, is less effective than understanding how they amplify each other and targeting the intersections where intervention has the highest leverage. For many people, improving gut health improves both estrogen clearance and thyroid hormone conversion simultaneously—two hormonal improvements from one foundational intervention.

✦ ✦ ✦

What This Means for You: A Hormonal Assessment Framework

If you are a woman with MCAS, the hormonal dimension is almost certainly relevant to your experience. If you are a man with MCAS, hormonal assessment—particularly thyroid and cortisol—is still an important part of the root-cause picture. Here is how to approach this territory systematically.

Track the hormonal pattern in your symptom journal. For women, note where you are in your menstrual cycle on every journal entry for at least two to three months. Clear cyclical patterns—particularly late-luteal worsening and early-menstrual improvement—point directly to the estrogen–histamine axis as a significant driver. The same tracking applies to pregnancy history, postpartum course, and perimenopausal transitions. Patterns across years are as informative as patterns across weeks.

Request a comprehensive hormonal panel. A full assessment relevant to MCAS should include: estradiol and progesterone measured at appropriate cycle phases (typically days two to four (day three is ideal) for baseline estrogen and FSH, and day twenty-one for luteal progesterone; and in the morning between 7:00 and 9:00 ideally); full thyroid panel including TSH, free T4, free T3, reverse T3, and both thyroid antibodies; morning cortisol and ideally a four-point salivary cortisol curve to assess the diurnal pattern; DHEA-S; and fasting insulin and glucose to assess metabolic status. This is a broader panel than most physicians routinely order, and making the case for its relevance in the context of MCAS is part of the patient advocacy skills discussed in Chapter 24.

Support estrogen clearance through gut and liver health. Before reaching for hormonal interventions, ensure that the foundations of estrogen clearance are in place: a healthy gut microbiome with adequate fiber intake to reduce beta-glucuronidase activity, cruciferous vegetables or DIM supplementation to support Phase 2 liver conjugation of estrogen, and adequate B vitamins and magnesium for methylation of estrogen metabolites. These dietary and gut-health strategies address the accumulation of estrogen that drives mast cell sensitization at its source, rather than downstream.

Consider the thyroid–gut–conversion triangle. If thyroid testing reveals low or low-normal free T3 despite adequate T4 and normal TSH, consider T4-to-T3 conversion as a potential issue—particularly if gut inflammation, selenium deficiency, or elevated reverse T3 are present. Selenium (two to three Brazil nuts daily, or a supplemental 200 mcg dose) is the most important nutrient for healthy T4-to-T3 conversion, and correcting deficiency often produces significant improvement in conversion efficiency. Zinc, adequate protein intake, and gut healing support the same conversion process.

Address adrenal function through foundation before supplementation. The most sustainable path to healthy adrenal function begins with reducing the demands on the HPA axis: consistent sleep, blood sugar stability through regular balanced meals, reduction of chronic stressors, and treatment of the underlying infections, toxins, and gut dysfunction that are placing ongoing demands on the adrenal stress response. Adaptogenic herbs can support the recovery of adrenal function once the load is being reduced, but they are adjuncts to the foundational work, not substitutes for it.

Be thoughtful about hormonal contraceptives. For women with MCAS and clear menstrual-cycle-driven symptom patterns, hormonal contraceptives deserve careful consideration. High-estrogen preparations may worsen the estrogen–histamine axis significantly.[267] Progestin-only preparations vary considerably in their mast-cell effects depending on which progestin is used and how it metabolizes. If hormonal contraception is medically necessary or strongly preferred, working with an informed gynecologist to choose a preparation least likely to worsen estrogen dominance is important. Natural bioidentical progesterone cream or low-dose oral progesterone is sometimes explored as a therapeutic option for women with MCAS and documented luteal phase progesterone insufficiency, though this should always be guided by appropriate testing and clinical supervision.

Fiona's journal had given her something invaluable: objective evidence of a hormonal pattern that her physicians had not recognized. Once her functional medicine practitioner reviewed the data and ordered a comprehensive hormonal panel, the picture became clear: low luteal progesterone, elevated TPO antibodies consistent with early Hashimoto's, and a morning cortisol that was half what it should have been for the time of day. Three hormonal abnormalities, each amplifying the others, each feeding directly into her mast cell reactivity.

Addressing all three—progesterone support in the luteal phase, selenium and dietary changes for Hashimoto's, and foundational adrenal support through stress reduction and adaptogens—didn't produce overnight transformation. But by her fourth month of treatment, the late-luteal flares that had dominated her life for three years had become noticeably milder. By her eighth month, she barely needed to check the calendar. Her body had found a more stable hormonal ground, and her mast cells had settled with it.

The hormones were not the whole story. They rarely are in MCAS. But they were the piece of the story that, once addressed, made everything else work better.

✦ ✦ ✦

Chapter 10 at a Glance

What to Remember:

- Estrogen directly primes mast cells by upregulating IgE surface receptors, lowering the degranulation threshold, and enhancing histamine release. This explains why MCAS symptoms reliably worsen in the premenstrual phase, and why hormonal transitions—pregnancy, postpartum, perimenopause—are common trigger points for MCAS onset or dramatic worsening.
- The estrogen–histamine relationship is bidirectional: histamine stimulates ovarian estrogen production while simultaneously reducing progesterone, creating a self-amplifying cycle of estrogen dominance and mast cell reactivity that requires intervention at multiple points to break.
- Progesterone has mast-cell-stabilizing effects that partially counterbalance estrogen's sensitizing influence. Relative progesterone deficiency—common in chronic stress and gut dysfunction—removes this protective counterbalance and worsens the late-luteal MCAS flare pattern.
- Estrogen clearance depends on gut microbiome composition (estrobolome) and liver detoxification capacity. Supporting both through gut healing and liver-supportive nutrients (DIM, calcium D-glucarate, B vitamins) reduces the estrogen accumulation driving mast cell sensitization at its source.
- Thyroid hormone T3 has direct mast-cell-stabilizing effects; hypothyroidism—including subclinical and Hashimoto's-driven hypothyroidism—amplifies MCAS through impaired gut motility, slowed liver detoxification, reduced mitochondrial efficiency, and diminished immune regulation. Comprehensive thyroid assessment including antibodies and free T3 is essential.
- Cortisol is a natural mast cell stabilizer through glucocorticoid receptors on mast cells. HPA axis dysregulation reduces the cortisol response available to counterbalance mast cell activation, explaining more severe and prolonged reactions, and creates a bidirectional loop in which mast cell activation further depletes adrenal reserve.

- Insulin resistance adds a metabolic dimension to mast cell priming through insulin receptor signaling and the pro-inflammatory background of metabolic syndrome. Blood sugar stabilization reduces mast cell reactivity from this dimension.
- The gut is the central hub of the hormonal–mast cell triangle: it governs estrogen clearance through the estrobolome, influences thyroid hormone conversion through gut integrity and microbiome signaling, and regulates cortisol regulation through gut–brain axis communication. Gut healing simultaneously addresses multiple hormonal drivers.

Coming Up in Chapter 11:

The root causes explored in Chapters 5 through 10 are largely environmental and functional—things that happen to the body or in the body that can be identified and addressed. But beneath all of them lies another layer: the genetic and epigenetic architecture that determines how vulnerable a given individual is to these influences in the first place. Chapter 11 explores DAO enzyme genetics, MTHFR and methylation, the somatic mutation hypothesis, and why understanding your genetic predispositions is not a counsel of fatalism but an invitation to more precisely targeted healing.

CHAPTER 11

Genetic and Epigenetic Factors

Why Your DNA Sets the Stage . . . and Why It Doesn't Write the Whole Story

The Family That Reacted to Everything

When Miriam brought her daughter Zoe to an MCAS specialist for the first time, she sat in the waiting room filling out the intake questionnaire and realized, with a slow, widening sense of recognition, that she was describing herself. The foods that triggered Zoe's hives were the same foods Miriam had quietly avoided for thirty years without knowing why. The fatigue that had derailed Zoe's sophomore year of high school was the same fatigue that had shadowed Miriam's twenties and that she had long ago made her peace with, chalking it up to "just the way I am." Zoe's gut pain, her racing heart, her sensitivity to fragrances, her brain fog after a difficult week—all of it mapped, symptom for symptom, onto a version of Miriam's own history.

Miriam's mother had been the same way. "Sensitive," the family had always said of her. Sensitive stomach, sensitive skin, sensitive to stress. She'd had hives for most of her adult life, a heart that raced inexplicably, and a list of foods she'd learned by experience not to eat. Nobody had ever given her a diagnosis. The word MCAS had not existed in medicine when she was raising her children.

Three generations. Three women. One unrecognized biological thread running through all of them.

Genetics in MCAS is not a simple story. It does not follow the tidy patterns of single-gene disorders where one mutation reliably produces one disease. The genetic landscape of MCAS is more like a mosaic: multiple small predispositions—variants in enzymes that clear histamine, in receptors that regulate mast cell activation thresholds, in the cellular machinery that maintains DNA integrity in mast cells themselves—that individually have modest effects but in combination, and in the presence of the right environmental triggers, create a body that is significantly more vulnerable to mast cell dysregulation than average.

Understanding this genetic landscape does not produce fatalism. It produces precision. Knowing which biological predispositions are at play allows interventions to be targeted more accurately, expectations to be set more realistically, and the particular levers most likely to move your individual system to be identified and pulled. Genes set the stage. They do not determine the performance.

✦ ✦ ✦

DAO Enzyme Genetics: When the Drain Is Built Narrow

In Chapter 6 we met diamine oxidase (DAO) as the gut's primary histamine-clearing enzyme—the drain through which dietary histamine is degraded before it can be absorbed into the bloodstream. We discussed how gut inflammation, dysbiosis, and certain medications reduce DAO activity and impair this clearance. But for some people, the drain was built narrower than average from the beginning. This is the story of DAO enzyme genetics.

The gene encoding DAO—called AOC1 (amine oxidase copper-containing 1)—exists in multiple variants across the human population. Certain single nucleotide polymorphisms, or SNPs (pronounced "snips"), in the AOC1 gene produce a DAO enzyme that is less catalytically efficient—it processes histamine more slowly, or is produced in lower quantities, or is more sensitive to inhibition by common dietary and pharmacological DAO blockers.[268] These variants are not rare; population studies have found that meaningful proportions of individuals carry at least one SNP associated with reduced DAO activity, and in some Northern European populations the frequency of at-risk variants is surprisingly high.[269]

Importantly, reduced DAO genetic capacity does not automatically produce histamine intolerance or MCAS. It creates a narrower margin. A person with genetically reduced DAO who eats a low-histamine diet, maintains a healthy gut, and keeps their overall mast cell load low may never experience significant symptoms. The same person who eats a diet rich in aged cheeses and fermented foods, drinks alcohol regularly, has SIBO from impaired gut motility, and is managing significant chronic stress may find their bucket overflowing constantly—because the drain that was already narrower than average is now further impaired by every additional factor working against it.

> **The Practical Implication:** *If you carry reduced-DAO genetic variants, you will likely need to be more diligent than average about the histamine content of your diet, more attentive to gut health as a foundational priority, and more careful about DAO-blocking medications and substances. This is not a life sentence of extreme restriction—it is a calibration of how tightly you need to manage your drain to keep the bucket from overflowing.*

Supporting DAO Activity Regardless of Genetics

Whether reduced DAO activity stems from genetic variants, gut inflammation, nutritional deficiency, or all three, the support strategies are the same. DAO requires copper and vitamin B6 as cofactors for its catalytic function—deficiency of either reduces enzyme activity independent of genetic capacity. Vitamin C, iron, and riboflavin (B2) also support DAO function in secondary pathways. Certain probiotic strains, particularly *Lactobacillus rhamnosus*, have been shown to upregulate DAO gene expression in the gut epithelium.[270] And healing the gut lining—restoring the enterocyte populations where DAO is produced—is the foundational DAO support strategy that no supplement fully substitutes.

DAO enzyme supplements themselves are available over the counter and can meaningfully supplement the gut's clearance capacity when taken before histamine-containing meals. They do not correct the underlying genetics or the gut damage that reduces DAO expression, but they can provide practical relief while deeper healing work proceeds. Testing for DAO genetic variants is available through specialty genetics laboratories and increasingly through consumer genomics platforms that allow raw data analysis through third-party interpretation tools.

✦ ✦ ✦

Somatic Mutations: The Mast Cell's Own Genetic Drift

One of the most intellectually fascinating and clinically important advances in MCAS research over the past decade is the emerging understanding, pioneered most prominently by Dr. Lawrence Afrin, that the mast cell population itself may carry acquired genetic mutations that fundamentally alter its behavior. This hypothesis—that MCAS often stems from somatic mutations in a subset of mast cells—represents a paradigm shift in how we understand the condition, and its implications reach into every aspect of MCAS management.

To understand why this matters, it helps to distinguish between two types of genetic change. Germline mutations are inherited—they are present in every cell of the body from conception, passed down from parents, and are the kinds of genetic variants that appear in conditions like cystic fibrosis or Huntington's disease. Somatic mutations, by contrast, are acquired—they arise in individual cells during a person's lifetime as a result of errors in DNA replication, exposure to mutagens, impaired DNA repair, or simply the accumulation of damage over time. Somatic mutations affect only the descendants of the cell in which they arose, not the entire body.

Cancer is the most familiar consequence of somatic mutation: a cell acquires mutations that disable its growth controls and it proliferates uncontrollably. Systemic mastocytosis—the clonal mast cell disease most familiar to hematologists—is driven by a specific somatic mutation (D816V in the c-Kit gene) that causes mast cells to proliferate excessively and accumulate in organs.[271] Dr. Afrin's insight is that MCAS represents a subtler version of this same process: somatic mutations in a subset of mast cells that do not cause proliferation (so the cell counts remain normal, and standard mastocytosis markers may be normal) but do cause the affected mast cells to behave aberrantly—activating inappropriately, releasing mediators in wrong combinations, responding to stimuli that should not trigger them, and failing to return to a resting state efficiently after activation.

What Somatic Mutations Mean in Plain Language

Imagine your mast cell population as a large workforce of security guards. The vast majority are well-trained and professional—they respond to real threats, use proportionate force, and stand down when the situation is resolved. But scattered through the workforce are a small number of guards who acquired faulty programming at some point during their career: they raise alarms without real cause, use excessive force when they do respond, and never fully disengage. The other guards around them—hearing repeated alarms—begin to respond as though there must be a genuine threat, amplifying the disruption.

This is the somatic mutation model of MCAS. A subset of mast cells, carrying acquired mutations that alter their behavioral programming, drive chronic inappropriate activation that then primes the broader mast cell population. These mutant cells are not cancerous—they are not proliferating out of control. They are simply dysfunctional in their signaling behavior, in ways that are difficult to detect with standard testing because they don't elevate cell counts or produce the dramatic tryptase elevations associated with mastocytosis.

The mutations themselves—when researchers have been able to identify them—tend to occur in genes encoding the signaling pathways that regulate mast cell activation and degranulation: kit receptor variants other than the classical D816V, mutations in Ras pathway components, alterations in genes that regulate the expression of mast cell surface receptors.[272,273] The pattern mirrors what is seen in other low-burden clonal blood disorders, and the analogy to cancer biology is intentional; mutations accumulate, often starting early in life, in individuals whose DNA repair machinery is subtly impaired, and the accumulation of these mutations in the mast cell lineage eventually crosses a threshold of behavioral disruption that produces clinical MCAS.

Implications for Comorbidities: The Somatic Mutation Hypothesis Extended

Dr. Afrin has extended this somatic mutation model to help explain one of the most puzzling features of MCAS: why it so consistently co-occurs with hEDS, fibromyalgia, chronic fatigue, IBS, and POTS.[274] His hypothesis is that the same impairment in DNA repair machinery that allows somatic mutations to accumulate in mast cells may also produce somatic mutations in other cell types throughout the body—connective tissue cells, autonomic neurons, gut epithelial cells—producing a mosaic of subtly dysfunctional cellular populations across multiple tissues simultaneously.

This would explain why decades of germline genetic research have failed to find the causative gene for hEDS; the connective tissue changes may not be germline at all, but rather the product of somatic mutations in fibroblasts and connective tissue cells that are specific to certain individuals and cannot be detected in standard blood-based genetic testing. It would illustrate why people with MCAS are individually unique in their symptom patterns and trigger profiles—because their particular mosaic of somatic mutations differs from every other person's. And it would shed light on the family clustering observed in conditions like Miriam's family—not because a single causative gene is passed down, but because the tendency toward impaired DNA repair and somatic mutation accumulation is inherited, predisposing multiple family members to related but individually unique expressions of cellular dysfunction.

> **Established vs. Emerging Science:** *The somatic mutation hypothesis for MCAS is a compelling and clinically influential framework, but it remains an area of active and developing research. It is presented here as the most coherent theoretical model for MCAS pathogenesis currently available—one that explains the most clinical observations and has the most implications for personalized treatment—while acknowledging that formal proof through large-scale genomic studies is still accumulating.*

✦ ✦ ✦

Hereditary Alpha-Tryptasemia: A Genetic Amplifier

Among the genetic factors in MCAS, hereditary alpha-tryptasemia (HαT) is the most recently characterized and in some ways the most directly actionable.[275,276,277] First described in detail in 2016 by Dr. Jonathan Lyons and colleagues at the National Institutes of Health, HαT is a genetic trait caused by the duplication of one or more copies of the TPSAB1 gene, which encodes the alpha form of tryptase—one of the primary proteins stored in mast cell granules.

Normally, humans carry two copies of TPSAB1. In HαT, individuals carry three or more copies, producing elevated amounts of alpha-tryptase. Because tryptase exists as a tetramer—four protein subunits assembled together—the extra alpha-tryptase subunits produce unusual alpha/beta-tryptase mixed tetramers with different functional properties than normal tryptase. These abnormal tetramers activate protease-activated receptor 2 (PAR2) more efficiently than normal tryptase, increasing vascular permeability and enhancing sensitivity to pressure and vibration. The result is a biological state of amplified mast cell signaling that affects the entire mast cell population, not just a subset.

Prevalence and Clinical Significance

HαT is not rare. Studies estimate that it is present in approximately four to six percent of people of Northern European descent—meaning that in a room of one hundred people, four to seven of them carry this trait without knowing it.[278,279] In MCAS patient populations, the frequency is significantly higher than in the general population, confirming that HαT is a meaningful genetic risk factor for developing clinically significant mast cell dysfunction.

The clinical consequences of HαT are wide-ranging. Elevated baseline tryptase—typically above 8 ng/mL and sometimes significantly higher—is the most measurable feature, and it is important to recognize that elevated tryptase in HαT does not indicate systemic mastocytosis. This distinction matters enormously for diagnosis: people with HαT and MCAS who present with elevated tryptase may receive unnecessary bone marrow biopsies or prolonged hematology workups looking for mastocytosis, when the elevated tryptase is simply a reflection of their genetic tryptase burden.

Beyond the diagnostic implications, HαT produces a pattern of symptoms that overlaps substantially with MCAS: severe anaphylaxis with triggers that seem disproportionately minor, connective tissue abnormalities that resemble hEDS, autonomic symptoms including POTS-like orthostatic intolerance, neuropsychiatric features including anxiety and cognitive impairment, and gastrointestinal inflammation. Many of these symptoms appear to result directly from the enhanced PAR2 activation and increased vascular permeability that the abnormal alpha/beta tryptase tetramers produce.

HαT and Non-IgE Pathway Amplification

One of the most clinically important features of HαT is its interaction with non-IgE mast cell activation pathways—particularly the MRGPRX2 receptor discussed in Chapters 1 and 9. The abnormal tryptase tetramers produced in HαT appear to enhance MRGPRX2 sensitivity, which means that individuals with HαT react more dramatically to neuropeptide signals, physical stimuli, and medications that activate mast cells through this pathway. This helps explain why HαT-positive individuals tend to have more severe anaphylactic reactions, more pronounced reactivity to medications, and a higher rate of idiopathic (trigger-unknown) mast cell events than the general MCAS population.

Testing for HαT is now available through clinical genetics laboratories and some academic medical centers. The test involves sequencing of the TPSAB1 gene to identify extra copies. For MCAS patients with elevated baseline tryptase, severe or disproportionate anaphylactic reactions, a family history of similar presentations, or connective tissue abnormalities alongside their mast cell symptoms, HαT testing is a meaningful addition to the diagnostic workup. There is currently no specific treatment that targets HαT itself, but knowing it is present refines risk stratification, helps avoid misdiagnosis as mastocytosis, and guides the intensity of mast cell stabilization and emergency preparedness that is appropriate for the individual.

✦ ✦ ✦

MTHFR and Methylation: The Body's Master Control Switch

Methylation is one of the body's most fundamental biochemical processes—a chemical reaction in which a methyl group (one carbon atom bonded to three hydrogen atoms) is added to a molecule, altering its function. Methylation controls gene expression, detoxifies harmful compounds, produces neurotransmitters, metabolizes histamine through the HNMT enzyme pathway, builds and repairs cell membranes, and regulates the immune system's inflammatory tone. It is, quite literally, one of the master control processes of human biology.

The methylation cycle depends on a series of enzyme-driven reactions, and one enzyme in particular—methylenetetrahydrofolate reductase, mercifully abbreviated as MTHFR—sits at a critical junction in the pathway. MTHFR converts folate into its active form (5-methyltetrahydrofolate, or 5-MTHF), which is required to convert homocysteine to methionine—a transformation that generates the universal methyl donor S-adenosylmethionine (SAM). Without adequate MTHFR function, the entire methylation cascade is impaired upstream.

MTHFR Variants: How Common and How Significant

Variants in the MTHFR gene are among the most common genetic polymorphisms in the human population.[280] The two most clinically relevant variants are C677T and A1298C. The C677T variant, when present in two copies (homozygous), reduces MTHFR enzyme activity by approximately sixty to seventy percent compared to normal.[281] When present in one copy (heterozygous), activity is reduced by approximately forty percent. The A1298C variant has somewhat milder effects on MTHFR function but compounds C677T's impact when both are present as compound heterozygosity.

The frequency of the MTHFR C677T variant varies by ethnicity but is common worldwide. Approximately ten to fifteen percent of many populations (especially European and some Asian groups) are homozygous (TT), and forty to sixty percent carry at least one copy of the variant.[282,283] These are not rare disease-causing mutations—they are common population variants that create a spectrum of methylation capacity. Most people with MTHFR variants live without dramatic health consequences. But in the context of MCAS—where impaired histamine clearance, immune dysregulation, and accumulated toxic burden are already stressing the system—reduced methylation capacity adds another layer of vulnerability that, once addressed, can meaningfully improve the clinical picture.

MTHFR, Histamine, and the HNMT Connection

The most direct connection between MTHFR and MCAS is through histamine metabolism. While DAO handles histamine clearance in the gut lumen, a separate enzyme—histamine N-methyltransferase (HNMT)—is responsible for breaking down histamine inside cells and in the systemic circulation. HNMT methylates histamine, rendering it inactive for excretion. This methylation reaction depends on SAM as the methyl donor—the very compound whose production is impaired when MTHFR function is reduced.

Impaired MTHFR function therefore reduces not only the gut's DAO-adjacent clearance systems but also the systemic, intracellular histamine clearance that HNMT provides. An individual with both reduced DAO genetic capacity and MTHFR impairment is working with two partially blocked histamine drains simultaneously—a combination that significantly lowers the threshold at which histamine accumulates to symptom-producing levels.

Beyond histamine metabolism, impaired methylation reduces the capacity to detoxify heavy metals (mercury methylation is a key step in its excretion), produces lower levels of SAM (which has documented mood-regulating and anti-inflammatory properties), impairs the production of glutathione (the body's master antioxidant and a critical molecule for detoxification), and dysregulates inflammatory gene expression by altering the epigenetic methylation patterns on DNA that control immune function.[284] In the complex MCAS patient, MTHFR variants are rarely the sole cause of anything—but they are a frequently present amplifier of nearly every other vulnerability.

Supporting Methylation Without Overwhelming a Sensitized System

The natural response to learning about MTHFR impairment is to supplement with methylfolate and methylcobalamin—the active forms of folate and B12 that bypass the MTHFR enzyme's conversion step. This is a valid and often helpful approach, but it requires care in the MCAS population. Some individuals with significant histamine sensitivity and methylation impairment react to methylfolate supplements with increased anxiety, palpitations, or paradoxical worsening of symptoms—a phenomenon sometimes attributed to overmethylation or to the mobilization of toxins that were previously sequestered. Starting at very low doses (fractions of standard doses) and increasing slowly is the appropriate approach for sensitized individuals.

Folinic acid (a different active folate form that doesn't require MTHFR but also doesn't directly push methylation as hard as methylfolate)is sometimes a better-tolerated starting point. Often labeled as calcium folinate, folinic acid is synthesized in a lab, but bioidentical and readily recognized by the body. While 5-MTHF (methylfolate) is the "end result" of folate metabolism, folinic acid sits one step back in the cycle, which changes how your body reacts to it. Folinic acid acts as a "speed limiter" that allows your body to convert folate at its own natural pace, helping you avoid the jitters and anxiety often triggered by the more aggressive methylfolate. It is also more versatile, providing the essential building blocks for DNA repair and cellular healing without over-taxing your metabolic system. For people with methylation deficiencies and co-occurring sensitivities (like certain COMT gene variations), methylfolate can feel like "too much, too fast," whereas folinic acid keeps the nervous system calm.

Riboflavin (B2) is a cofactor for MTHFR itself and can improve enzyme function even in the presence of genetic variants, sometimes producing significant improvement at modest doses of 100 to 400 milligrams daily. Magnesium, zinc, and adequate protein intake support the broader methylation cycle alongside folate and B12 supplementation.

◆ ◆ ◆

Deeper Dive: Epigenetics and Why Genes Are Not Destiny

For the Science-Minded Reader

The word epigenetics literally means "above genetics"—it refers to changes in how genes are expressed without changes to the underlying DNA sequence itself. Epigenetic regulation is the mechanism by which the same DNA blueprint produces dramatically different outcomes depending on how its instructions are read, silenced, or amplified in response to experience and environment.

The epigenome—the full complement of chemical modifications that regulate gene expression across the genome—is not fixed at birth. It is dynamically shaped throughout life by diet, stress, toxin exposure, infections, sleep, exercise, social relationships, and virtually every aspect of lived experience.[285] This is why identical twins, who share the same DNA, become progressively more different in their health profiles as they age: their epigenomes diverge in response to different life experiences, and these epigenetic differences alter gene expression in ways that produce different biological phenotypes.

Epigenetic Mechanisms Relevant to MCAS

Three primary epigenetic mechanisms are most relevant to understanding MCAS vulnerability and recovery.

DNA methylation—the addition of methyl groups to cytosine bases in the DNA sequence, typically at CpG sites—is the most studied epigenetic mark. When a gene's promoter region is heavily methylated, the gene is generally silenced; when it is demethylated, the gene can be expressed. The methylation patterns that regulate inflammatory genes, immune cell differentiation, and mast cell surface receptor expression are all subject to epigenetic modification by the factors discussed throughout Chapters 5 through 10: chronic stress alters the methylation of HPA axis genes; adverse childhood experiences alter the methylation of immune regulatory genes; toxic exposures alter the methylation of detoxification genes. This is the biological mechanism through which experience becomes physiology.

Histone modification is a second epigenetic layer. The proteins around which DNA is wrapped (histones) can be chemically modified in ways that loosen or tighten the DNA packaging, making genes more or less accessible to the transcription machinery. Butyrate—the short-chain fatty acid produced by a healthy gut microbiome—is a potent histone deacetylase inhibitor, meaning it keeps histones in a configuration that favors anti-inflammatory gene expression. This is one mechanism through which gut health directly shapes immune cell behavior at the epigenetic level.

MicroRNA regulation—in which small non-coding RNA molecules modulate the translation of messenger RNA into protein—is a third layer that is increasingly recognized as central to immune regulation. Specific microRNAs regulate the expression of mast cell surface receptors, the production of inflammatory mediators, and the sensitivity of the HPA axis. Dietary factors including omega-3 fatty acids, curcumin, resveratrol, and green tea catechins modulate microRNA expression in ways that have documented anti-inflammatory and mast-cell-modifying effects.

Why Epigenetics Makes Recovery Possible

The most important clinical implication of epigenetics for individuals with MCAS is this: Because epigenetic marks are dynamic and responsive to experience, the biological programming that predisposes to mast cell hyperreactivity is not permanently fixed. It can be shifted. Consistently.

Studies of dietary intervention, exercise, stress reduction, and targeted supplementation show measurable epigenetic changes in immune cell populations within weeks to months of sustained practice.[286,287,288] The nervous system interventions described in Chapter 9—breathwork, somatic therapies, vagal tone training—produce documented epigenetic changes in inflammatory gene expression. Gut healing changes the epigenetic milieu of mucosal immune cells through butyrate and microbiome-derived signals. Methylation support through B vitamins directly adds methyl groups to the epigenome, shifting gene expression patterns in ways that reduce inflammatory tone.

This is why the phrase "genes are not destiny" is not wishful thinking in MCAS. It is a mechanistic statement about epigenetic plasticity. The genetic variants that create narrower DAO drains, lower mast cell thresholds, or impair DNA repair machinery set the parameters of individual vulnerability—but the epigenome translates those parameters into actual biological outcomes, and the epigenome responds to everything you do, eat, think, and experience. Recovery in MCAS is not about overcoming genetics. It is about systematically shifting the epigenetic expression of a genetic vulnerability toward health.

✦ ✦ ✦

What This Means for You: Using Genetic Knowledge Without Being Defined By It

Genetic testing in MCAS is a tool for precision, not a verdict. Used appropriately, it helps elucidate why certain interventions matter more for you than for the average person, why certain symptoms have been lifelong rather than acquired, and why family members show similar patterns. Here is how to engage with this information constructively.

Consider genetic testing strategically, not comprehensively. Consumer genomics platforms like 23andMe provide raw genetic data that, when analyzed through third-party interpretation tools designed for health applications, can reveal DAO variants, MTHFR polymorphisms, and a range of other relevant SNPs. This is a reasonable and relatively affordable starting point. More targeted clinical testing—HαT through a genetics laboratory, comprehensive MCAS-relevant SNP panels through functional medicine laboratories—provides higher accuracy for the variants that matter most. The goal is not to find every possible genetic variant but to identify the specific vulnerabilities most relevant to your clinical picture.

Use genetic information to calibrate your foundational interventions. If DAO variants are present, gut healing and DAO enzyme support become higher priorities than they might be for someone without these variants. If MTHFR impairment is confirmed, methylation support through active B vitamins becomes a specific, targeted intervention rather than a general supplement. If HαT is present, the intensity of mast cell stabilization warranted is higher and emergency preparedness (including access to epinephrine) should be discussed with your physician. Genetics tells you where to focus your effort, not whether the effort is worthwhile.

Understand that the same genetic variants respond to the same foundational interventions. The beauty of the epigenetic model is that regardless of which specific genetic variants you carry, the foundational interventions that improve epigenetic expression of immune regulation are consistent: gut healing (butyrate and microbiome support), methylation nutrition (B vitamins, magnesium, adequate protein), anti-inflammatory diet (omega-3 fatty acids, polyphenols, cruciferous vegetables), nervous system regulation (vagal tone, stress reduction), adequate sleep, and toxin burden reduction. You may need to calibrate the intensity or sequencing based on your genetic picture, but the direction of intervention is universal.

Share what you learn with your family. MCAS has significant genetic and epigenetic components that cluster in families—as Miriam and Zoe discovered. If you have children, siblings, or parents with similar symptom patterns, the understanding you develop about your own biology may be the most valuable gift you can offer them: the possibility of earlier recognition, more targeted intervention, and a shorter road to a diagnosis that took you years to find.

Reframe genetic findings as levers, not limits. Every genetic variant that reduces DAO capacity, impairs methylation, amplifies tryptase signaling, or lowers the mast cell threshold is also a specific point where targeted support can make a measurable difference. The narrower your DAO drain, the more powerfully gut healing and DAO supplementation improve your histamine clearance. The more impaired your methylation, the more significantly active B vitamins shift your biochemical picture. Genetic variants are not solely vulnerabilities—they are also the map to the interventions most likely to help you specifically.

Miriam left that initial appointment with her daughter carrying something she had not expected: not anxiety about the genetic thread running through her family, but relief—relief that there was a biological explanation that was coherent, that honored the reality of what three generations of women in her family had experienced, and that pointed toward real interventions rather than more years of "sensitive" as the only available label.

She made an appointment for herself the following week. At fifty-three, she was not too late. Her own genetics had not changed. But her epigenome—her body's dynamic, responsive translation of those genetics into daily biology—was still writing new chapters. She intended to influence how they read.

◆ ◆ ◆

Chapter 11 at a Glance

What to Remember:

- MCAS has a significant genetic architecture that is not the simple single-gene inheritance of classic genetic diseases, but a mosaic of multiple predisposing variants—in enzymes, receptors, and cellular repair machinery—that together lower the threshold for mast cell dysfunction in response to environmental triggers.
- DAO enzyme variants (in the AOC1 gene) reduce histamine clearance capacity in the gut, narrowing the margin before histamine accumulates to symptom-producing levels. These variants create a narrower drain rather than no drain—making dietary management, gut healing, and DAO cofactor support more important, not impossible.
- Somatic mutations in the mast cell population itself—acquired during a person's lifetime in a subset of mast cells—may represent the most fundamental driver of MCAS for many patients. These mutations alter mast cell behavioral programming without increasing cell numbers, explaining why standard mastocytosis markers are typically normal and why MCAS presentations are so individually variable.
- Dr. Afrin's somatic mutation hypothesis extends to comorbidities; the same impaired DNA repair machinery that allows mast cell mutations to accumulate may produce somatic mutations in connective tissue cells, autonomic neurons, and gut epithelium—offering a unifying biological explanation for the MCAS–hEDS–dysautonomia triad.
- Hereditary alpha-tryptasemia (HαT), caused by extra copies of the TPSAB1 gene, is present in four to six percent of Northern European populations and significantly higher proportions of MCAS patients. It produces elevated baseline tryptase, amplified PAR2 and MRGPRX2 signaling, and a more severe, reactive mast cell phenotype. HαT testing is appropriate for people with elevated baseline tryptase, severe anaphylaxis, or connective tissue features alongside MCAS.
- MTHFR variants—present in up to forty percent of the population—impair the methylation cycle, reducing systemic histamine clearance through HNMT, impairing detoxification of heavy metals and toxins, lowering glutathione production, and dysregulating inflammatory gene expression. Active B vitamin supplementation (methylfolate, methylcobalamin) bypasses the impaired conversion step, though sensitized individuals should start at very low doses.

- Epigenetics—the dynamic regulation of gene expression by methylation, histone modification, and microRNA—is the mechanism through which genetics translates into biology and through which interventions produce recovery. The epigenome responds to diet, gut health, nervous system state, toxin burden, sleep, and life experience, making biological change genuinely possible despite genetic predispositions.
- Genes set the stage but do not determine the performance. Every genetic variant relevant to MCAS is also a specific point where targeted intervention can make a measurable difference—making genetic knowledge a precision tool for more effective treatment rather than a verdict of permanent limitation.

Coming Up in the Next Section of the Book:

With a thorough understanding of what MCAS is, how it presents, and the full landscape of root causes and triggers that drive it, we are ready to move from understanding to action. The next section of the book opens with one of the most important principles in MCAS management: why stabilizing the mast cell system must come before fixing its root causes, and how to build the healing baseline from which deeper recovery becomes possible. Chapter 12 lays out the strategy of stabilizing before repairing—the foundation on which everything else in this book is built. If the preceding chapters have felt like a long inventory of complexity, Chapter 12 marks the turn. From this point forward, the book belongs entirely to what is actionable, what is achievable, and what people with MCAS are already doing to build lives that are larger than this condition. The biology you have just spent eleven chapters understanding is now yours to use.

CHAPTER 12

Stabilizing Before Fixing

Why Calming the System Must Come Before Repairing Its Root Causes

The Renovation That Made Everything Worse

James had done his research. By the time he arrived at his first functional medicine appointment, he had spent three months reading about MCAS, identifying his root causes, and designing what he thought was a comprehensive recovery plan. He had purchased a bottle of quercetin, a probiotic, a DAO enzyme supplement, an herbal antimicrobial protocol for suspected SIBO, a methylfolate supplement for his MTHFR variants, a heavy-duty liver support formula, and a binder for suspected mycotoxin exposure. He was ready, as he put it, to address everything at once.

The next six weeks were among the worst of his illness. The herbal antimicrobials for SIBO triggered a severe Herxheimer-like reaction that kept him house-bound for days. The methylfolate produced anxiety and palpitations so intense he stopped sleeping. The liver support formula—containing several botanicals his mast cells hadn't encountered before—triggered hives daily. His gut, already inflamed and sensitized, reacted to the new probiotic strains with cramping and bloating. The quercetin, which should have been his most reliable ally, seemed to be contributing to the noise.

He called his practitioner in despair. "I thought I was doing everything right," he said. "I've addressed every root cause I could find."

The practitioner's response was gentle but direct. "You tried to fix the house while it was on fire," she said. "The first step in any renovation is making sure the structure is stable enough to work on. Right now, your mast cells are so reactive that every new thing you introduce becomes another trigger. We need to calm the system down first—create a healing baseline—before we start adding things in."

James's experience is one of the most common and most avoidable mistakes in MCAS management. The impulse to address root causes comprehensively and immediately is completely understandable—after years of unexplained suffering and a hard-won diagnosis, the desire to do everything, right now, is powerful. But in a highly reactive mast cell system, this impulse consistently backfires. The very interventions meant to heal become additional triggers, the bucket overflows from the weight of too many new inputs, and the person is left sicker and more discouraged than before.

The principle of stabilizing before fixing is not a counsel of passivity. It is a strategy of sequencing—doing things in the right order so that each step makes the next one possible. It is, for most individuals with MCAS, the difference between a recovery trajectory that gradually improves and one that circles in expensive, exhausting frustration.

◆ ◆ ◆

Why the Order of Operations Matters

Imagine trying to repaint a room while the windows are broken and rain is blowing in. You could use the finest paint available, apply it with perfect technique, and choose exactly the right color—and it would peel off within days, because the underlying conditions make it impossible for the paint to adhere. The quality of the intervention is irrelevant when the environment cannot support it.

MCAS operates by a similar logic. When the mast cell system is in a state of high reactivity—when the bucket is chronically full, the threshold is low, and every new input is processed as a potential threat—the environment is not yet capable of supporting the deeper repair work that addresses root causes. Herbal antimicrobials, even gentle ones, involve compounds the reactive mast cell system may identify as foreign provocations. Aggressive detoxification mobilizes toxins that, moving through an inflamed gut and overwhelmed liver, trigger mast cell activation along their excretion route. New probiotic strains, new supplement compounds, even therapeutic foods can all add to the reactive load of a system that is already at its limit.

The stabilization Phase 1s about changing the environment first. It is about lowering the water level in the bucket far enough that the mast cells have room to breathe—enough margin between their current activation state and their threshold that introducing new interventions doesn't immediately push them over the edge. Once that margin exists, root cause treatment becomes possible because the system is resilient enough to tolerate it. Without that margin, even the most precisely targeted interventions fail because the system has no capacity to receive them.

> **The Core Principle:** *You cannot effectively repair a system that is actively in emergency mode. Stabilization creates the physiological space in which repair becomes possible. It is not a delay in treatment—it is the first, most essential phase of treatment.*

This principle has a parallel in conventional medicine that most people intuitively understand. A surgeon does not repair a broken leg in a patient who is actively hemorrhaging. First, they stabilize the patient—control the bleeding, maintain blood pressure, ensure the airway—and only once stability is achieved do they proceed to the repair. The repair is not less important than the stabilization. But without stabilization first, the repair cannot succeed.

In MCAS, stabilization means doing enough to calm mast cell reactivity that the system stops running in constant emergency mode—not achieving perfect health, not resolving every symptom, but creating a functional baseline from which deeper work can begin. What does this look like in practice?

✦ ✦ ✦

The Stabilization Phase: What It Involves and What It Doesn't

Stabilization is defined by what it emphasizes and by what it deliberately does not attempt. Understanding both is essential to avoiding the most common pitfalls.

What Stabilization Emphasizes

The stabilization phase focuses on three categories of intervention that have the highest probability of reducing reactivity without introducing new triggers: dietary simplification, low-risk mast cell support, and trigger-load reduction.

Dietary simplification in the stabilization phase means adopting a clean, low-histamine approach focused on fresh, simply prepared whole foods while eliminating the most common trigger categories. This is not about perfection—it is about removing the largest dietary contributors to the mast cell load while the system settles. The low-histamine dietary approach is covered in detail in Chapter 13, but the stabilization version is intentionally conservative: fresh proteins (pasture-raised chicken or turkey, never-aged, grass-fed beef, local wild-caught or commercially frozen fish, and cage-free organic eggs when tolerated), well-tolerated vegetables (onions, zucchini, carrots, green beans, cucumber, and leafy greens like romaine or butter lettuce) and grains (white rice, quinoa, freshly cooked potatoes, or sometimes gluten-free grains), limited food variety to reduce the number of novel inputs the immune system must evaluate. New foods are introduced slowly and one at a time once the baseline is established.

Low-risk mast cell support means starting with the most well-tolerated, thoroughly researched, and genuinely mast-cell-stabilizing compounds before attempting anything more complex. Quercetin (125 mg/day), buffered vitamin C (100 mg/day), and magnesium glycinate (100 mg/day) are the foundational starting points for most people—compounds with decades of safety data, well-characterized mechanisms, and the lowest likelihood of producing paradoxical reactions in sensitized individuals. These are introduced one at a time, at low doses, with careful observation before adding anything further.

Trigger load reduction means systematically identifying and removing the most significant non-dietary contributors to the mast cell bucket: addressing obvious environmental exposures (fragrances, chemical products, mold if identified), supporting sleep quality, reducing avoidable stressors, and applying the nervous system practices from Chapter 14 consistently. These changes cost nothing biochemically—they don't introduce new compounds the reactive system must process—but they can meaningfully lower the baseline activation level within days to weeks.

What Stabilization Deliberately Does Not Attempt

Equally important is what the stabilization phase holds back. This is often the harder part for motivated, knowledgeable individuals who have identified real root causes and are eager to address them.

- **Aggressive antimicrobial protocols** – Whether pharmaceutical or herbal, die-off reactions in a highly reactive system can be severe and difficult to control. SIBO treatment, Lyme disease protocols, candida eradication programs—all of these are appropriate interventions for the right patient at the right time, but the right time is not when the mast cell system is operating at maximum reactivity. These are Stage 3 and 4 interventions in the stabilize–support–repair–rebuild framework, not Stage 1.
- **Heavy-duty detoxification protocols** – Binders, chelation, and aggressive liver-support programs that mobilize significant toxin loads are best undertaken once the gut barrier has been partially healed and the mast cell system has sufficient stability to handle the transient increase in circulating toxins that detoxification inevitably involves.
- **Multiple new supplements introduced simultaneously** – Even beneficial compounds become confounding variables when introduced together. If a reaction occurs—and in a reactive system, reactions are common—it is impossible to identify which new addition caused it, making it impossible to make rational decisions about what to continue and what to discontinue.

- **Aggressive dietary restriction beyond what is necessary** – The counterintuitive risk of extreme dietary restriction in MCAS is nutritional depletion and the development of anticipatory anxiety around food that can worsen the nervous system dimension of reactivity. The goal is a clean, simplified diet—not the most restricted diet imaginable.
- **Major lifestyle changes implemented simultaneously** – The total stress load of rapid, comprehensive lifestyle change is itself a mast cell trigger. Pacing change is not weakness—it is the recognition that the nervous system and immune system need time to adapt to new inputs, and that adaptation requires stability, not overwhelm.

> **A Realistic Timeframe:** *The stabilization phase typically takes four to twelve weeks, depending on the severity of reactivity at baseline. For highly reactive individuals—those experiencing daily significant reactions, anaphylaxis-level events, or profound systemic symptoms—twelve weeks of deliberate stabilization before beginning root cause treatment is not conservative. It is wise. For those with more moderate reactivity who have already been managing some aspects of their condition, stabilization may be achieved in four to six weeks.*

✦ ✦ ✦

Creating a Healing Baseline: The Four Markers of Readiness

How do you know when stabilization has been sufficient—when the healing baseline has been established well enough to begin addressing root causes? There are no laboratory tests that answer this question definitively, but there are four practical markers that experienced practitioners and patients both recognize as indicators of readiness.

Marker One: Reaction Frequency and Severity Have Reduced

The first and most important marker is a meaningful reduction in how often reactions occur and how severe they are when they do. This doesn't mean reactions have stopped entirely; in moderate-to-severe MCAS, that goal is too far away to serve as a readiness threshold. It means the pattern has shifted noticeably: fewer reactions per week, reactions that are less intense and shorter in duration, a baseline state that feels meaningfully calmer than it did at the start of the stabilization phase. If reactions are still occurring daily with significant severity after twelve weeks of sincere stabilization efforts, this signals either that the stabilization approach needs adjustment or that a significant trigger is still active and unaddressed.

Marker Two: You Can Identify a Reliable Safe Zone

A healing baseline includes the identification of a personal safe zone: a set of foods, environments, and daily practices within which you consistently feel better rather than worse. This safe zone may be narrow at first—perhaps only a small list of well-tolerated foods and a carefully managed home environment—but its existence is significant. It demonstrates that the mast cell system, when given consistent, low-trigger conditions, can achieve a degree of calm. The safe zone is the platform from which expansion becomes possible. Without it, every new intervention is attempted on unstable ground.

Marker Three: Sleep Has Improved

Sleep is one of the most sensitive indicators of overall mast cell load; histamine is a wakefulness-promoting neurotransmitter and excess mast cell mediator activity reliably disrupts sleep architecture. When the stabilization Phase 1s working, sleep is typically one of the first things to improve—not necessarily to perfect, but meaningfully better. Longer stretches of uninterrupted sleep, more restorative deep sleep, and waking feeling at least somewhat refreshed rather than already exhausted are all signs that the mast cell burden has genuinely reduced. Conversely, persistent severe sleep disruption despite consistent stabilization efforts is a sign that the baseline has not yet been established.

Marker Four: Cognitive Function and Emotional Resilience Have Partially Returned

Brain fog, anxiety, and emotional dysregulation are among the first symptoms to worsen when the mast cell system is under heavy load and among the first to improve when the load reliably lifts. When individuals in the stabilization phase begin to notice that they can think more clearly on good days, that the pervasive anxiety has quieted to a manageable background rather than a constant foreground, and that they are able to engage with the work of their own healing with some degree of equanimity rather than constant dread—this is a meaningful marker of improved neurological and immune stability. It is a signal that the central nervous system mast cell burden has reduced sufficiently that the brain can begin to function more normally.

✦ ✦ ✦

The Four-Stage Framework: Stabilize, Support, Repair, Rebuild

The stabilization Phase 1s the first stage in a four-stage framework that provides the organizing structure for MCAS recovery. Understanding all four stages from the beginning helps set realistic expectations and prevents the discouragement that comes from measuring early-stage progress against end-stage goals.

Stage 1: **Stabilize** – Calm the reactive system. Reduce trigger load across all categories. Introduce only low-risk, well-tolerated mast cell supports. Establish the healing baseline—the safe zone from which all further work proceeds. Duration: four to twelve weeks, depending on baseline reactivity.

Stage 2: **Support** – With the baseline established, begin targeted support for the systems most compromised by MCAS: gut barrier repair, nervous system regulation, nutritional repletion, hormonal balance, and specific mast cell stabilization through the supplement and dietary protocol described later in the book. Introduce interventions one at a time, observe responses carefully, and pace additions to the capacity of the system. Duration: three to six months, overlapping with Stage 3 as readiness allows.

Stage 3: **Repair** – Address identified root causes systematically and in order of clinical priority. SIBO treatment, viral reactivation management, Lyme and co-infection protocols, mycotoxin clearance, heavy metal removal—these deeper interventions are now possible because the system has enough stability to tolerate them without catastrophic reactivity. Each root cause intervention is paced to the individual's tolerance, with mast cell stabilization maintained throughout as the safety net. Duration: highly variable, from months to years depending on the complexity and number of root causes identified.

Stage 4: **Rebuild** – Expand dietary tolerance, increase environmental exposure range, reintroduce activities and social engagements that the illness had restricted, and establish a sustainable long-term lifestyle that maintains the progress achieved. The goal of rebuilding is not a return to a pre-illness baseline that may not have been optimal even then—it is the construction of a more informed, more intentional relationship with the body's needs and capacities. Duration: ongoing.

These stages are not rigidly sequential. Most individuals begin some Stage 2 support work—particularly nervous system regulation and sleep optimization—during the stabilization phase, because these interventions are low-risk and their calming effects actively support stabilization. And Stage 4 rebuilding begins long before Stage 3 repair is complete: expanding dietary tolerance and gradually widening the safe zone happens incrementally throughout the recovery process, not all at once at the end.

What the framework provides is a mental model for sequencing decisions. When uncertain about whether to introduce a new intervention, the question to ask is: which stage does this belong to, and have I completed enough of the preceding stage to support it? This question prevents the most common sequencing error—jumping to Stage 3 root cause treatment before Stage 1 stabilization is genuinely achieved.

> **A Note on Individual Variation:** *The four-stage framework is a guide, not a rigid protocol. Some patients move through Stage 1 in weeks and are ready for Stage 2 and 3 work much sooner than others. Some spend six months in Stage 2 support before the system is stable enough for aggressive root cause treatment. The pace is determined by biology, not by willpower or ambition, and honoring that reality is part of the work.*

✦ ✦ ✦

Deeper Dive: The Biology of Why Sequencing Matters

For the Science-Minded Reader

The clinical wisdom of stabilizing before fixing is grounded in specific biological mechanisms that explain why a reactive mast cell system responds poorly to interventions that would be well-tolerated in a less reactive one—and why creating a stable baseline genuinely changes how the body responds to subsequent treatment.

Mast Cell Priming States and Treatment Tolerance

As discussed in Chapter 5, mast cells exist on a spectrum from resting to primed to activated. A primed mast cell responds to stimuli that a resting cell would ignore, releases more mediators per activation event, and recovers to a resting state more slowly. The priming state is not merely a matter of immediate trigger exposure—it reflects the cumulative activation history of the cell, the inflammatory cytokine environment it inhabits, and the epigenetic programming that determines its baseline sensitivity.

When treatment is introduced into a highly primed mast cell system, the new compounds—however beneficial their intended effects—are evaluated by immune cells whose threat threshold is already critically low. Novel compounds, even natural ones, can activate mast cells through pattern recognition receptors, through direct receptor interactions, or through the inflammatory signaling cascades that their metabolism generates. A mast cell system running at sixty percent of its reaction threshold will process new inputs very differently from one running at twenty percent. Stabilization is the process of lowering the operating level from sixty percent toward twenty—creating the headroom that allows treatment to be received as support rather than attack.

The Gut Barrier and Treatment Absorption

A second biological reason for the sequencing principle involves the gut barrier. When intestinal permeability is high—as it typically is in active MCAS, given the mast-cell-mediated damage to tight junctions discussed in Chapter 6—supplements and herbal compounds are absorbed differently than they would be through an intact barrier. Partially digested supplement proteins, lipopolysaccharides mobilized by compounds that alter gut bacteria, and biofilm-disrupting agents that release bacterial fragments into a leaky gut all become additional activators of the subepithelial mast cell population. Partial gut barrier healing—achieved through dietary simplification, glutamine, zinc carnosine, and other gut-healing compounds that are introduced early in Stage 2 support—meaningfully improves the gut's capacity to process treatment compounds without immune reactivity.

This explains the clinical observation that many supplements tolerated poorly by highly reactive patients become well-tolerated after three to six months of foundational work. The supplement hasn't changed. The gut's capacity to process it has.

The Nervous System's Role in Treatment Response

The autonomic nervous system dimension of treatment tolerance is perhaps the most underappreciated. As established in Chapter 9, sympathetic dominance primes mast cells and reduces their threshold for activation. In a nervous system running in chronic sympathetic overdrive, new treatments—particularly those that require metabolic processing, that produce temporary detoxification symptoms, or that directly affect the nervous system through gut-brain axis signaling—are processed in a context of heightened reactivity. The same intervention that produces a mild, transient adaptation response in a parasympathetically balanced nervous system can produce a significant, alarming reaction in a chronically sympathetically dominant one.

Building vagal tone and parasympathetic capacity during the stabilization phase—through consistent breathwork, gentle movement, and sleep prioritization—does not merely improve subjective wellbeing. It measurably shifts the autonomic context in which all subsequent treatment occurs, reducing the probability of adverse reactions and improving the body's capacity to benefit from interventions rather than simply reacting to them.

✦ ✦ ✦

What This Means for You: Building Your Stabilization Plan

Translating the principle of stabilization into daily practice requires a concrete plan. The following provides the framework for the first four to twelve weeks—a starting point to be individualized based on your personal trigger pattern, severity of reactivity, and the guidance of any practitioners working with you.

Week one: Assess and simplify. Before adding anything, spend the first week removing. Clear fragranced products from your immediate environment. Switch to the simplified low-histamine dietary approach described in Chapter 13. Stop any supplements or herbal protocols you are currently taking that were introduced without systematic observation—these can be reintroduced later, one at a time, with proper assessment. This subtraction-first week is not about deprivation; it is about creating a clean slate from which you can observe what your body does when the trigger load is reduced.

Week two: introduce your first mast cell support. With a clean baseline established, introduce a single low-risk mast cell stabilizing compound. For most people, quercetin is the appropriate starting point: begin at a quarter of the standard dose (typically 125 mg rather than 500 mg), taken with a meal. Observe for five to seven days before assessing your response and considering a dose increase or the addition of a second compound. If you react, reduce the dose further or switch to vitamin C as an alternative first support. One compound at a time, observed carefully, is the non-negotiable rule of the stabilization phase.

Begin nervous system practices from the start. Nervous system regulation is the one category of intervention appropriate to begin in full during the stabilization phase, because it introduces no new biochemical inputs. Diaphragmatic breathing for five to ten minutes morning and evening, a simple vagal toning practice (humming, cold water to the face, or slow exhale emphasis), and consistent sleep and wake times all begin shifting the autonomic environment within days to weeks. These are not substitutes for biochemical stabilization—they are its necessary complement.

Track everything, but simply. Use the symptom tracker from Chapter 5 during the stabilization phase, noting daily: overall reactivity on a scale of 1 to 10, specific symptoms and their severity, any dietary changes or new exposures, sleep quality, and stress level. Review weekly rather than daily—the trend over time is more meaningful than day-to-day fluctuation. Look for the gradual lowering of average reactivity that signals the bucket is draining. Individual bad days are expected and do not indicate failure.

Communicate with your healthcare team. The stabilization Phase is not something to undertake in isolation, particularly if you are managing significant comorbidities, taking prescription medications that interact with mast cell biology, or have a history of severe anaphylactic reactions. A practitioner familiar with MCAS can help assess whether your stabilization strategy is appropriately calibrated, identify any persistent triggers that are preventing progress, and guide the transition from Stage 1 to Stage 2 support at the right moment.

Reframe slow progress as appropriate progress. The stabilization phase requires a specific kind of patience—not passive waiting, but active, attentive, consistent effort in a narrow range of interventions while resisting the pull toward doing more. The bucket doesn't empty overnight. The mast cell priming state built over months or years of high trigger load doesn't resolve in a week. Every day that the system is given low-trigger conditions and gentle support is a day the priming state is walking back toward baseline. The progress is real even when it isn't dramatically visible. Trust the biology, and keep showing up for the work.

James returned to his practitioner eight weeks after their first conversation, having spent those weeks doing exactly the opposite of what he'd initially tried: less, not more. A simplified low-histamine diet. One mast cell stabilizer introduced at a time. Daily breathwork. No aggressive protocols of any kind. The difference was striking enough that even he was surprised. The daily hives had become occasional. His sleep had improved by something he could only describe as a category change. His gut, which had been in near-constant distress, had quieted.

"I feel like I finally have a foundation," he said. "Like the house is stable enough to work on."

It was. The renovation—the real work of addressing his root causes—could now begin. Not because his MCAS was resolved, but because his body had enough stability to receive the work that needed doing next. That stability had been built not by doing everything at once, but by doing the right things, in the right order, one careful step at a time.

✦ ✦ ✦

Chapter 12 at a Glance

What to Remember:

- Stabilization must precede root cause treatment in MCAS. A highly reactive mast cell system cannot effectively receive or tolerate the interventions needed to address its underlying drivers—it is in emergency mode, and every new input is processed as a potential threat rather than support.
- The renovation analogy is apt: trying to repair a house while it is on fire doesn't work. First stabilize the structure—calm the mast cell system—then proceed to the deeper repair work. The order of operations is not optional.
- Stabilization focuses on three things: dietary simplification to a clean low-histamine approach, introduction of low-risk well-tolerated mast cell supports one at a time, and systematic reduction of the most significant trigger loads across food, environment, stress, and sleep.
- Stabilization deliberately withholds aggressive antimicrobial protocols, heavy-duty detoxification, multiple simultaneous new supplements,

extreme dietary restriction beyond what is necessary, and sweeping lifestyle changes introduced all at once.

- The four markers of a healing baseline are meaningful reduction in reaction frequency and severity, identification of a reliable personal safe zone, improvement in sleep quality, and partial return of cognitive clarity and emotional resilience.
- The four-stage framework—Stabilize, Support, Repair, Rebuild—provides the organizing structure for MCAS recovery. Each stage creates the conditions that make the next one possible. Jumping stages consistently produces the frustrated, circling pattern that many people with MCAS know too well.
- The biology of sequencing: Highly primed mast cells respond to new compounds as threats; a compromised gut barrier absorbs treatments with greater immune reactivity; and a sympathetically dominant nervous system amplifies adverse reactions. Stabilization addresses all three, changing how the body receives subsequent treatment.
- Nervous system regulation—breathwork, vagal toning, sleep consistency—is the one intervention category appropriate to pursue fully during the stabilization phase because it introduces no new biochemical inputs while actively supporting the autonomic environment in which all treatment occurs.

Coming Up in Chapter 13:

With the stabilization framework established, we turn to one of its most practical and immediate components: the low-histamine lifestyle. Chapter 13 goes beyond a simple list of foods to avoid and explores the full landscape of dietary and non-dietary triggers, the principles of food storage and preparation that dramatically affect histamine content, and how to approach the low-histamine diet as a flexible, sustainable foundation for long-term MCAS management—not a permanent state of extreme restriction.

CHAPTER 13

The Low-Histamine Lifestyle

Food, Freshness, and the Full Environment of Calm

The List That Changed Everything—and Nothing

The first thing most people do when they receive an MCAS diagnosis, or when they discover that histamine intolerance may be driving their symptoms, is search the internet for a list of foods to avoid. Within minutes they have found one. Often several. And they are immediately confronted with a problem: the lists don't agree.

One list includes tomatoes as a high-histamine food. Another lists them only as a histamine liberator, which is a different category. A third omits them entirely. Avocados appear on most lists, but then so do spinach and leftovers and fermented anything and alcohol and vinegar—and suddenly what looks like a manageable set of restrictions has expanded to cover most of what was in the refrigerator. One source says strawberries are fine; another brands them trigger foods for life. The information is real. The confusion is also real.

Clare had this experience. She spent her first week of low-histamine eating in a state of near-paralysis—terrified of making the wrong choice, eating mostly plain rice and steamed chicken because those felt safe, and gradually becoming both undernourished and more anxious about food than she'd ever been in her life. By the end of the week her symptoms hadn't improved. Her stress had quadrupled. And she'd developed what she could only describe as a dread of mealtimes.

The problem wasn't the low-histamine approach itself. The problem was treating it as a list to be followed with perfect compliance rather than a set of principles to be understood and applied with intelligence and flexibility. The low-histamine lifestyle—done well—is not a rigid, fear-driven elimination protocol. It is a way of thinking about food and environment that reduces the histamine bucket without making life smaller than it needs to be.

This chapter is about doing it well.

✦ ✦ ✦

Understanding the Low-Histamine Approach: Principles Over Lists

Before engaging with any specific food guidance, it helps to understand the underlying principles that determine why certain foods are problematic and others are not. With these principles in hand, navigating unfamiliar foods, eating in new environments, and making real-life dietary decisions becomes possible without a laminated reference card in every pocket.

Principle One: Histamine Accumulates With Time

The most important principle in low-histamine eating is freshness. Histamine does not exist in meaningful quantities in freshly caught fish or freshly cooked meat. It accumulates as proteins break down under bacterial action over time. This process begins the moment an animal product is harvested and continues throughout storage, transport, aging, curing, smoking, fermenting, and cooking—and it accelerates dramatically at room temperature compared to refrigeration.

This is why the same food can be perfectly tolerable one day and problematic the next. A piece of tuna eaten at a restaurant where the fish was delivered that morning is a completely different food, histamine-wise, from the same species eaten at a restaurant where it has been sitting in a display case for two days. Freshly cooked chicken breast eaten immediately is very different from leftover chicken breast reheated the next evening. The food hasn't changed. The time has.

The practical consequence of this principle is transformative. Rather than simply banning a category of food, it changes when and how that food is prepared and eaten. Fresh unaged red meat, prepared immediately and eaten the same day, is well-tolerated by many people with MCAS. The same meat, aged, marinated overnight, or left as leftovers, is a significant trigger. The problem is not the meat—it is the time.

> **The Freshness Rule:** *When in doubt, fresh wins. Fresh proteins cooked immediately and eaten without storage are among the most reliably tolerated foods in the low-histamine approach, regardless of the protein source. Cook what you need for one meal, eat it, and avoid storing cooked proteins whenever possible during the stabilization phase.*

Principle Two: Not All Triggers Work the Same Way

As introduced in Chapter 5, foods affect the histamine bucket through several distinct mechanisms, and understanding the difference helps explain why reactions are so inconsistent and why identical lists are not useful for everyone.

High-histamine foods contain histamine that was already formed before you ate them—primarily through bacterial action on the amino acid histidine. Aged cheeses, fermented foods, cured meats, most fish that isn't extremely fresh, alcohol, vinegar, and most fermented condiments fall into this category. These foods add histamine directly to your system regardless of what else is happening in your body.

Histamine-liberating foods do not contain significant histamine themselves but trigger the release of histamine from body stores through mechanisms that are not fully characterized but appear to involve direct mast cell interaction or complement activation.[289] Strawberries, citrus fruits, pineapple, papaya, tomatoes, egg white, chocolate, shellfish, and certain food additives fall into this category. Their effect is highly individual and dose-dependent—a small amount may be tolerable while a larger amount triggers symptoms, and the same amount may be fine on a low-bucket day and problematic on a high-bucket day.

DAO-blocking foods and substances reduce the gut's capacity to clear dietary histamine by inhibiting the DAO enzyme, effectively narrowing the drain. Alcohol is the most potent DAO blocker encountered in everyday life, followed by certain teas, energy drinks, and some medications. These don't add histamine but prevent its removal, which raises the effective load equivalently.

Knowing which category a food falls into helps calibrate your response. A high-histamine food like aged parmesan adds directly to the bucket every time, regardless of circumstances. A histamine liberator like strawberries may be manageable in small amounts on a good day when the bucket is low. A DAO blocker like alcohol is particularly problematic in combination with other triggers, even in small amounts. These are different problems requiring different solutions.

Principle Three: The Diet Is a Tool, Not a Permanent Identity

The low-histamine diet, particularly in its strictest form, is appropriate for the stabilization phase and the early weeks of Stage 2 support. It is not meant to be a permanent, maximally restrictive state of being. As the gut heals, mast cell reactivity reduces, DAO activity improves, and the overall trigger load drops, dietary tolerance reliably expands. Foods that were genuinely intolerable during peak reactivity often become manageable—and occasionally even well-tolerated—after six to twelve months of foundational work.

Treating the low-histamine diet as a permanent identity produces two problems. First, it tends toward progressive restriction. Every new reaction gets attributed to something that was previously tolerated, and the list of forbidden foods expands until the diet is nutritionally inadequate. Second, it creates a relationship with food characterized by fear rather than information—and the fear itself, through the nervous system mechanisms described in Chapter 9, contributes to mast cell reactivity around mealtimes in ways that make reactions more likely regardless of what is actually being eaten.

The goal is to use the low-histamine approach intelligently during the period when it is most needed, track which specific foods affect you personally, and reintroduce foods one at a time as your overall system stabilizes. Your personal low-histamine diet should get smaller over time, not larger.

✦ ✦ ✦

Food Storage, Freshness, and Preparation: The Practical Details

The freshness principle is the most powerful dietary tool in low-histamine management—and it is entirely about how food is handled rather than which foods are eliminated. These practices apply during the stabilization phase and, to a lesser degree, throughout the recovery process.

Proteins: The Highest-Stakes Category

Animal proteins are where freshness matters most, because they are the primary substrate for the bacterial histamine production that makes high-histamine foods problematic. In practical terms, this means:

- **Buy local and fresh, cook the same day** – Ideally purchase fresh meat, poultry, and fish on the day you intend to cook them. If this isn't possible, freeze immediately after purchase and defrost only what you need.
- **Avoid leftovers during stabilization** – Cooked proteins left in the refrigerator accumulate histamine rapidly—a chicken breast that was fine at dinner becomes a meaningful trigger source by lunch the next day. Cook in single-meal quantities and eat immediately during the stabilization phase; leftovers can be reintroduced cautiously later.
- **Choose frozen over "fresh" fish from display cases** – Unless you have direct knowledge that the fish was caught and delivered that day, commercially "fresh" fish in display cases often has a histamine load well above what freshly caught fish would have. Commercially frozen fish—caught and frozen at sea—typically has lower histamine than the display case alternative.
- **Avoid canned, smoked, cured, aged, or fermented animal products entirely during stabilization** – This covers canned tuna, smoked salmon, deli meats, pepperoni, salami, aged cheeses, and fermented fish sauces. These are the highest-histamine foods in the typical diet and reliable triggers regardless of bucket level.

- **Handle raw proteins with speed** – Minimize the time animal proteins spend at room temperature during preparation. Take them from refrigerator to pan, not from refrigerator to counter to preparation to pan an hour later.

Fruits and Vegetables: Context-Dependent

Most fresh vegetables are low-histamine and well-tolerated by the majority of individuals with MCAS. The exceptions are the histamine-liberating and high-histamine vegetables that appear consistently on trigger lists:

- **Highest concern** – tomatoes, spinach, eggplant, avocado (also a liberator for many), fermented vegetables (sauerkraut, kimchi), and pickled vegetables of all kinds
- **Histamine liberators to monitor individually** – strawberries, citrus fruits (orange, lemon, lime, grapefruit), pineapple, papaya, raspberries, and banana (the riper, the more problematic for some)
- **Generally well-tolerated** – most other fresh vegetables and fruits, particularly apples, pears, mango (unripe), blueberries, melon, grapes, carrots, broccoli, cauliflower, zucchini, sweet potato, green beans, peas, cucumber, and leafy greens other than spinach

Ripeness matters more than most people expect. Overripe fruits have higher histamine content than the same fruit eaten at peak ripeness, because bacterial activity increases as fruit softens and begins to break down. During stabilization, aim for produce at peak freshness and avoid anything bruised, overripe, or beginning to turn.

Grains, Legumes, and Starches

Grains and starchy foods are among the most reliably tolerated foods in the low-histamine approach for most individuals. White rice, quinoa, organic oats (for those without oat sensitivity), millet, and most simple starches including potatoes and sweet potatoes are well-tolerated and nutritionally useful anchors during the stabilization phase. Sourdough bread—while beloved as a gut-health food—is fermented and therefore a source of biogenic amines including histamine, making it inappropriate during stabilization. Fresh baked goods made with baking powder or yeast (rather than sourdough cultures) are generally better tolerated.

Legumes are individually variable. Many people with MCAS tolerate well-cooked fresh or frozen legumes without difficulty; others react, particularly to those with higher oxalate content (soybeans, navy beans, black beans, peanuts) or those that are canned (canned beans accumulate histamine during storage). Fresh-cooked dried beans or lentils, prepared the same day, are a better option than canned during stabilization.

Condiments, Sauces, and Flavoring

This is where many people inadvertently undermine an otherwise careful low-histamine approach. The condiment category is dominated by fermented, aged, or vinegar-based products that are among the most concentrated histamine sources in the kitchen:

- **Avoid entirely during stabilization** – Vinegar and all vinegar-based condiments (ketchup, mustard, mayonnaise, most salad dressings, pickles, relish, hot sauce, soy sauce, Worcestershire sauce, fish sauce, teriyaki sauce), fermented sauces, and anything labeled "aged."
- **Use with care** – Lemon juice is technically high in citric acid and acts as a histamine liberator for some; fresh herbs are generally safe but dried herbs and spices accumulate histamine over time—use fresh herbs generously and replace dried spice jars that have been open more than six months.
- **Generally safe** – High-quality cold-pressed olive oil, fresh garlic and onion (well-tolerated by most), fresh herbs, sea salt, coconut aminos as a soy sauce alternative, and mild fresh salsa if made entirely from well-tolerated ingredients and eaten immediately.

✦ ✦ ✦

Beyond the Plate: Non-Food Triggers in the Low-Histamine Lifestyle

The low-histamine lifestyle is not only about food. The bucket, as Chapter 5 established, is filled by everything—and the non-food triggers are often as significant as dietary ones, particularly for people who have already made substantial dietary adjustments and are puzzled by persistent reactions.

Temperature and Physical Environment

Both heat and cold can directly trigger mast cell degranulation through temperature-sensitive receptors on the mast cell membrane. Hot showers or baths, saunas, hot tubs, and rapid movement between very warm and cool environments are common and underappreciated triggers. Many people with MCAS find that they can tolerate warm showers much better than hot ones, and that keeping the bathroom from steaming significantly reduces post-shower reactions. Conversely, sudden cold—plunging into cold water, stepping into strong air conditioning from summer heat—can equally trigger degranulation.

Managing temperature stability in daily life is a practical and immediately actionable intervention. Lukewarm showers rather than hot, layering clothing to avoid sudden temperature swings, pre-cooling the car before getting in during summer, and sitting near climate control systems in restaurants rather than directly under them are all small adjustments that collectively reduce the temperature-trigger contribution to the daily bucket.

Fragrances, Chemicals, and Air Quality

The respiratory mucosa is densely populated with mast cells, and airborne chemical exposure is one of the most direct non-dietary routes of mast cell activation. During the stabilization phase, creating a fragrance-reduced home environment is one of the highest-return low-risk changes available:

- **Replace scented personal care products** – Shampoo, conditioner, body wash, lotion, deodorant, and laundry detergent are all available in fragrance-free versions that work as well as their synthetically scented counterparts; these changes immediately and permanently reduce daily chemical exposure.
- **Remove air fresheners, scented candles, and plug-in diffusers** – These are among the most concentrated airborne chemical triggers in many homes; even "natural" scented candles produce volatile organic compounds when burned that can activate respiratory mast cells.
- **Switch to fragrance-free cleaning products** – Most major cleaning tasks can be accomplished with fragrance-free commercial products, diluted white vinegar (used externally only—not consumed), or simple soap and water.
- **Ventilate when cooking** – Certain cooking processes—high-heat searing, browning, or cooking histamine-producing foods—release volatile compounds that can be inhaled; opening windows and using extractor fans during cooking reduces this exposure.
- **Be strategic about public environments** – Perfume and fragrance exposure in enclosed public spaces—elevators, waiting rooms, offices—is a significant and largely uncontrollable trigger source for many individuals with MCAS. Seating near ventilation or choosing timing that reduces exposure (early morning in a gym rather than peak hours, for instance) are practical accommodations.

Stress, Exertion, and Lifestyle Triggers

Stress and exercise as mast cell triggers were covered in depth in Chapters 5 and 9, but their inclusion in the low-histamine lifestyle deserves explicit acknowledgment because they are so frequently the silent variable that undermines otherwise careful dietary management. A person who eats a perfectly low-histamine diet but consistently skips meals (blood sugar instability is a stress trigger), overdrives workouts, or works through chronic sleep deprivation is operating with a bucket that is never getting an opportunity to truly empty.

The low-histamine lifestyle, fully lived, includes attention to the following:

- **Meal timing and blood sugar stability** – Eating at consistent intervals, not skipping meals, and including adequate protein and fat at each meal to blunt blood sugar swings that trigger sympathetic activation and mast cell priming.
- **Exercise pacing** – Movement is therapeutic and important—but during stabilization it should be gentle, consistent, and below the threshold that triggers post-exertional reactions. Walking, gentle swimming, restorative yoga, and light cycling are often well-tolerated; high-intensity interval training, heavy lifting, and prolonged cardio are Stage 3 and 4 territory for most reactive patients.
- **Sleep consistency** – The same sleep and wake time seven days a week, including weekends, stabilizes the circadian cortisol rhythm that has direct effects on mast cell reactivity. Social jetlag—sleeping in significantly on weekends—disrupts this rhythm and can produce measurable increases in Monday and Tuesday reactivity.
- **Social and emotional environment** – Not every stressor is controllable, but identifying and reducing unnecessary ones—conflicts, obligations, relationships, or media consumption that reliably produce sympathetic arousal without proportionate benefit—reduces the emotional contribution to the bucket in ways that are both underrated and genuinely effective.

✦ ✦ ✦

Deeper Dive: The Science of Histamine in Food

For the Science-Minded Reader

Histamine in food is not a single, fixed quantity. It is a dynamic variable shaped by microbiology, chemistry, temperature, time, and the composition of the food itself. Understanding these dynamics explains why food histamine data from research literature is often inconsistent—measurements taken at different times post-harvest, at different storage temperatures, and in different food processing conditions will produce dramatically different histamine concentrations for the same food category.

The Microbiology of Histamine Formation

Histamine formation in food is primarily a microbial process. Bacteria possessing the enzyme histidine decarboxylase convert the amino acid histidine—abundant in animal muscle proteins—to histamine as a metabolic byproduct. The bacteria most prolific in this conversion include species of *Morganella*, *Hafnia*, *Klebsiella*, *Enterobacter*, and certain *Lactobacillus* strains.[290,291] Their activity is temperature-dependent: Histamine formation is negligible below 4°C (refrigerator temperature) but accelerates rapidly above 10°C and reaches dramatic rates at room temperature and above.[292,293] This is why the time-temperature history of a food—not just whether it has been refrigerated—determines its histamine content.

Fish are the highest-risk category because they naturally carry high loads of free histidine and because the spoilage bacteria that colonize fish surfaces are particularly efficient histamine producers. The phenomenon of "scombroid fish poisoning"—a form of food poisoning characterized by flushing, hives, and gastrointestinal symptoms that mimics allergy—is simply histamine toxicity from poorly handled fish.[294] For individuals with MCAS, what causes poisoning at high doses causes reactions at much lower doses, making fish handling and freshness especially critical.

The Role of Biogenic Amines Beyond Histamine

Histamine is the best-known biogenic amine in food, but it is not the only one relevant to MCAS. Tyramine, putrescine, cadaverine, and phenylethylamine are biogenic amines found in many of the same high-histamine foods—aged cheeses, fermented products, cured meats, wine—and they interact with mast cell biology through overlapping mechanisms.[295,296,297] Tyramine, in particular, is a potent vasoactive amine that competes for DAO clearance.[298] When multiple biogenic amines are present simultaneously, they compete for the same degradation pathways, effectively raising the concentrations of all of them above what would be predicted from any single amine alone.

This interaction explains why the combination of high-histamine foods produces reactions disproportionate to what any individual food would be expected to cause. A small glass of red wine (high in both histamine and tyramine) paired with aged cheese (again, high in both) and processed meat (adding further biogenic amines) creates a combined biogenic amine load that saturates DAO and HNMT clearance rapidly—even in people who might tolerate any one of these foods in isolation.

Oxalates and Salicylates: The Often-Overlooked Triggers

Oxalates and salicylates are naturally occurring plant compounds that act as triggers for a subset of people with MCAS through mechanisms distinct from histamine. Oxalates—found in high concentrations in spinach, almonds, peanuts, beets, and dark chocolate—can promote mast cell activation through crystal-induced inflammation and possibly through their effects on gut barrier integrity.[299] Salicylates—found in many fruits, vegetables, herbs, and spices—directly influence inflammatory prostaglandin pathways in ways that can trigger mast cell mediator release.[300] This may be due to a heightened sensitivity to triggers like salicylates.

Not every person with MCAS is sensitive to oxalates or salicylates, and identifying whether these are contributing factors requires systematic observation rather than automatic elimination. If a patient has carefully reduced dietary histamine without adequate improvement, and if their diet is high in oxalate-rich or salicylate-rich foods, these are worth investigating as secondary contributors. Functional medicine practitioners experienced in MCAS can help assess whether a trial of oxalate or salicylate reduction is warranted.

✦ ✦ ✦

What This Means for You: Building Your Low-Histamine Practice

The low-histamine lifestyle, understood as a set of principles and practices rather than a list of prohibitions, becomes manageable—even liberating—once the framework is clear. Here is how to put it into practice without the paralysis that felled Clare's first week.

Start with the freshness rule, not the food list. Before memorizing any list of forbidden foods, implement the freshness rule: cook fresh proteins the day of purchase, eat them at the meal they are prepared for, and avoid leftovers. This single change removes the largest histamine contributors from most people's diets and produces noticeable improvement within days for the majority of MCAS patients. It is the highest-return dietary intervention available and it applies to what you already eat, not to an entirely foreign set of foods.

Use the three-category framework to interpret your reactions. When a food reaction occurs, ask yourself: Is this a high-histamine food (it contains histamine regardless of circumstances), a histamine liberator (it releases histamine from stores and may be dose- or context-dependent), or a DAO blocker (it reduces your clearance capacity)? Different answers suggest different solutions—completely avoiding a high-histamine food, managing dose and timing for a liberator, or eliminating DAO blockers from the meal rather than the food that accompanied them.

Create a simple, rotating safe meal template. Rather than approaching every meal as a new decision with potential for error, build a small rotation of safe, simple meals that you know your system tolerates. Two or three protein options (fresh chicken, fresh fish, fresh beef), three or four vegetable options, two starch options, and a handful of safe seasonings. Use these as your foundation during stabilization, then add variety gradually as your system stabilizes. Structure reduces decision fatigue and the anxiety that makes every meal feel high-stakes.

Address your immediate environment alongside your diet. In the first week, swap your most commonly used scented products for fragrance-free alternatives. Replace scented laundry detergent—because everything you wear and sleep on carries that scent—first, then personal care products. This environmental simplification works synergistically with dietary changes to lower the overall bucket level rather than addressing diet while leaving a significant non-dietary contributor unchanged.

Track food reactions with a three-day window. Mast cell reactions to food are not always immediate. Some reactions—particularly gut symptoms and brain fog—can appear six to twenty-four hours after the triggering food was eaten, making attribution difficult without systematic tracking. Note everything eaten and note symptoms over a three-day window, looking for patterns across the following day, not just within the hour. This longer tracking window often reveals connections that immediate-reaction tracking misses.

Plan for social eating before it happens. Eating in social situations—restaurants, dinner parties, travel—is the most common source of accidental high-histamine exposure during the stabilization phase, and the stress of navigating it can itself fill the bucket. Research restaurant menus in advance and identify two or three safe options before arriving. Carry low-histamine snacks when traveling. Communicate dietary needs clearly but without lengthy explanation; most restaurants can prepare a simple fresh protein with steamed vegetables and olive oil without difficulty. Planning ahead transforms social eating from anxiety-provoking to manageable.

Clare's second attempt at the low-histamine approach looked completely different from her first. Armed with principles rather than a prohibitive list, she spent her first week implementing the freshness rule, swapping her scented cleaning products, and building a rotation of five simple safe meals. She wasn't perfect—she made mistakes, had a reaction to something she thought was safe, and had to track back to figure out what had caused it. But she was eating varied, nutritious food, she was not afraid of mealtimes, and by week three her baseline reactivity had dropped enough that she could feel, for the first time, the bottom of her bucket.

That feeling—of a bucket that is not perpetually at the rim—is what the low-histamine lifestyle is designed to create. Not perfection. Not permanent extreme restriction. Just enough space to breathe, and to begin the deeper work that makes lasting recovery possible.

✦ ✦ ✦

Chapter 13 at a Glance

What to Remember:

- The low-histamine approach is a set of principles, not a list to follow with perfect compliance. Understanding why certain foods are problematic—through which mechanism they fill the bucket—produces far better outcomes than memorizing prohibitions.
- Freshness is the single most important dietary principle in low-histamine management. Histamine accumulates over time in animal proteins under bacterial action, meaning the same food can be a significant trigger or a safe choice depending entirely on how long it has been stored, how it has been handled, and how it was prepared.
- Three mechanisms distinguish food triggers: High-histamine foods add histamine directly; histamine liberators trigger histamine release from body stores and are dose- and context-dependent; DAO-blocking foods reduce histamine clearance capacity. Understanding which category a food falls into shapes the management strategy.
- Avoiding leftovers—particularly cooked proteins—during the stabilization Phase is one of the highest-return, easiest-to-implement dietary changes available to most people tackling MCAS.
- The non-food dimension of the low-histamine lifestyle includes temperature management, fragrance and chemical exposure reduction, exercise pacing, meal timing for blood sugar stability, sleep consistency, and emotional environment. These non-dietary factors frequently account for reactions that seem to have no dietary explanation.
- The low-histamine diet is a tool for the stabilization and early support phases—not a permanent identity. Dietary tolerance expands as the gut heals, mast cell reactivity reduces, and overall trigger load drops. The goal is a diet that gets progressively less restrictive over time, not more.
- Biogenic amines beyond histamine—tyramine, putrescine, cadaverine—compete for the same clearance pathways and interact to produce combined loads greater than any single amine alone. This explains disproportionate reactions to combinations of high-histamine foods.
- Building a simple, rotating safe meal template during stabilization reduces decision fatigue and food anxiety, both of which contribute to mast cell reactivity through the nervous system mechanisms described in Chapter 9.

Coming Up in Chapter 14:

Diet is one dimension of the healing baseline—but it works most powerfully in combination with nervous system regulation, the subject of Chapter 14. Breathwork, vagal exercises, somatic practices, and sleep optimization are not soft add-ons to the real treatment; they are biological interventions that directly reduce mast cell reactivity through the autonomic and cholinergic pathways described in Chapter 9, and they belong at the center of any comprehensive MCAS management plan. Chapter 14 makes these practices concrete, accessible, and immediately usable.

CHAPTER 14

Nervous System Regulation

Breathwork, Vagal Exercises, Somatic Practices, and Sleep: A Practical Guide

The Five Minutes That Changed Her Mornings

For the first three years of her MCAS, Theresa woke up already reactive. Before she had eaten a single bite of food, before she had encountered a single environmental trigger, her body was already running at what she described as a low-level hum of alarm. Her heart beat just slightly too fast. Her gut was already tense. The quality of her attention was already that particular kind of hypervigilance—scanning for threat, braced for the next reaction—that had become so familiar she could no longer remember what it felt like not to feel it.

Her practitioner suggested she try a simple morning breathing exercise before getting out of bed. Five minutes of slow, extended-exhale breathing—in for four counts, out for eight—before her feet hit the floor. Nothing else. No supplements, no dietary changes, just five minutes of deliberate breathing.

Theresa was skeptical. She had read enough about MCAS by this point to know that her problem was biological, not a matter of insufficient relaxation. Suggesting she breathe more slowly felt, frankly, a little dismissive.

She tried it anyway.

By the end of the first week, she noticed something she could not easily explain: her mornings were different. Not transformed, not symptom-free, but measurably calmer in those first hours. The hum of alarm had dropped by a register. She reacted less to her morning coffee—a food she'd been considering eliminating. She moved through the shower and the preparation for the day with less bracing and more ease.

By the end of the month, she understood what had happened. The breathing hadn't been a distraction or a placebo. It had been activating her vagus nerve, directly increasing parasympathetic tone, and through the cholinergic anti-inflammatory pathway described in Chapter 9, it had been physically reducing the activation state of her mast cells before her day had even begun. She had been changing her biology with her breath, five minutes at a time, before she did anything else.

This chapter is the practical counterpart to the science of Chapter 9. Everything covered here has a biological mechanism. None of it is incidental. And the practices are simple enough to begin today.

✦ ✦ ✦

Why Nervous System Regulation Is Medical Treatment

Before moving into the practices themselves, it is worth restating the framework from Chapter 9 in practical terms—because if you understand why these practices work, you will practice them with commitment rather than tentative compliance.

Sympathetic nervous system activity—the fight-or-flight response—directly primes mast cells through norepinephrine acting on adrenergic receptors on the mast cell surface. A body in sympathetic dominance has a lower mast cell activation threshold, produces more mediators per activation event, and recovers from reactions more slowly. Every hour spent in chronic sympathetic dominance is, biologically, an hour spent with the mast cell bucket filling from the inside.

Parasympathetic activity—mediated primarily through the vagus nerve—directly suppresses mast cell reactivity through the cholinergic anti-inflammatory pathway: acetylcholine released by vagal efferent fibers binds to alpha-7 nicotinic receptors on mast cells and macrophages, reducing mediator release and dampening inflammatory signaling. Every intervention that measurably increases vagal tone—and several are described in this chapter—is directly lowering mast cell reactivity through this pathway.

Heart rate variability (HRV), the most accessible clinical measure of vagal tone and autonomic flexibility, is strongly and reproducibly improved by consistent practice of the interventions in this chapter. Higher HRV correlates with lower inflammatory marker levels, better immune regulation, lower cortisol reactivity, and improved quality of life across chronic illness populations. It is not a soft outcome measure. It is a direct biological indicator of how well the body can regulate its own mast cell activity.

> **The Core Commitment:** *Twenty minutes of daily nervous system practice—spread across morning and evening if needed—is the minimum effective amount for meaningful autonomic change. Less than this produces inconsistent results. Consistency matters far more than perfection: five minutes every day outperforms forty minutes once a week.*

✦ ✦ ✦

Breathwork: The Most Direct Vagal Intervention Available

Breathing is the only autonomic function under both conscious and unconscious control—the bridge between the voluntary and involuntary nervous systems. This gives deliberate breathing a unique and powerful capacity to influence the autonomic state: by consciously slowing and deepening the breath, you can directly shift the autonomic balance toward parasympathetic dominance within minutes.

The mechanism is precise. Slow breathing—particularly with exhalation longer than inhalation—stimulates the vagus nerve directly through baroreceptors in the chest wall and through respiratory sinus arrhythmia, the natural coupling of heart rate to the breathing cycle. Inhalation slightly increases heart rate as the sympathetic branch accelerates the heart; exhalation slows it as the parasympathetic branch applies the brake.[301] When exhalation is deliberately extended, more time is spent in the parasympathetic phase of each breath cycle, and the cumulative effect across five to ten minutes of practice is a measurable shift in autonomic balance and a measurable increase in HRV.

Practice One: Extended-Exhale Breathing

This is the simplest, most portable, and most immediately effective vagal breathing technique—the one that changed Theresa's mornings. It requires no equipment, no special posture, and can be practiced anywhere.

Extended-Exhale Breathing: Step by Step

Position: Sit comfortably or lie down. Rest one hand on your belly and one on your chest.

Inhale slowly through the nose for a count of 4, allowing the belly to rise first, then the chest.

Exhale slowly through the nose or pursed lips for a count of 6 to 8. The exhale should be longer than the inhale.

At the end of the exhale, pause briefly before the next inhale—do not force this, just allow a natural moment of stillness.

Continue for 5 to 10 minutes. If counting feels effortful, aim simply for an exhale that is noticeably longer than the inhale.

Use: Every morning before rising. Also during any pre-reaction warning signs, before meals, and as an evening wind-down practice.

If you notice light-headedness during this practice, you are breathing too deeply. The goal is slow, not deep. Keep the breath natural in volume—just slow the rhythm and extend the exhale.

Practice Two: Resonance Frequency Breathing

Resonance frequency breathing, also called coherent breathing or heart rate variability biofeedback breathing, involves breathing at a specific rate—approximately five to six breaths per minute (a cycle of about ten to twelve seconds)—that produces maximum HRV and the strongest parasympathetic response. For most adults, this translates to an inhale of five seconds and an exhale of five seconds, though individual resonance frequency varies slightly.

Resonance Frequency Breathing: Step by Step

Set a gentle timer or use a breathing app that guides a 5-second inhale and 5-second exhale rhythm.

Breathe in through the nose for 5 seconds, allowing the belly to expand.

Breathe out through the nose for 5 seconds, allowing the belly to fall.

Continue for 10 to 20 minutes for the full HRV benefit. Even 5 minutes produces measurable autonomic shifts.

Use: Ideal for the primary daily practice session; particularly valuable when using a wearable HRV monitor to observe the biofeedback effect in real time.

Practice Three: Physiological Sigh

The physiological sigh is a naturally occurring breathing pattern—a double inhale through the nose followed by a long, slow exhale—that the body produces spontaneously to deflate alveoli that have collapsed during shallow breathing. Research by Andrew Huberman and colleagues at Stanford has demonstrated that a single intentional physiological sigh produces the fastest and most reliable acute reduction in physiological arousal of any single breathing maneuver studied, measurable within one to two breath cycles.[302]

Physiological Sigh: Step by Step

Take a full inhale through the nose.

At the top of the inhale, take a second, shorter sniff through the nose to fully expand the lungs.

Release in a long, slow, complete exhale through the mouth or nose—allow all the air to leave unhurriedly.

Repeat once or twice. Two to three physiological sighs are typically sufficient to produce a noticeable shift in arousal level.

Use: Ideal for acute moments—the first sign of a reaction, a stressful event, a moment of anxiety or hyperarousal. Think of it as your emergency calm-down tool.

✦ ✦ ✦

Vagus Nerve Exercises: Stimulating the Brake Directly

Beyond breathing, several direct physical practices stimulate vagal afferent fibers in ways that produce measurable increases in parasympathetic tone. These exercises work through the anatomical pathways of the vagus nerve itself—the ear, the throat, the chest, and the gut—and are easy to integrate into daily routines without requiring significant time or equipment.

Humming and Gargling

The vagus nerve innervates the muscles of the larynx and pharynx. Activating these muscles through humming, gargling, singing, or chanting creates vibrations that directly stimulate vagal afferent fibers, increasing parasympathetic signaling. This is one of the fastest and most accessible vagal exercises available.

Humming Practice

Choose any comfortable note or hum along to music you enjoy.

Hum for 1 to 2 minutes, allowing the vibration to resonate in the chest and throat.

For gargling: take a mouthful of water and gargle vigorously for 30 to 60 seconds, twice daily.

Use: Morning routine, shower, car commute. Even 60 seconds of humming contributes measurable vagal activation.

Cold Water Exposure

Cold water applied to the face—particularly splashing cold water on the forehead, eyes, and cheeks—activates the diving reflex, a powerful parasympathetic response mediated through the vagus nerve that produces an immediate slowing of heart rate and reduction in sympathetic tone. This is the same reflex marine mammals use to conserve oxygen during diving; in humans, it produces a rapid and measurable shift toward parasympathetic dominance.

Cold Water Facial Immersion

Fill a bowl with cold water (not ice water—cold tap water is sufficient). Alternatively, use the cold setting on a running tap.

Splash cold water onto your face several times, focusing on the forehead and cheeks, or briefly submerge the lower face in the bowl.

Hold breath naturally during immersion—this enhances the diving reflex.

Duration: 10 to 30 seconds is sufficient. This does not need to be prolonged to be effective.

Use: Particularly valuable during acute mast cell reactions or high-stress moments when rapid autonomic downshift is needed. Also useful as a morning practice to shift the nervous system from sleep to waking without sympathetic surge.

A note for people with MCAS: cold water exposure activates the vagus nerve powerfully in most people, but in highly reactive patients, strong cold stimulation can occasionally trigger mast cell reactions through MRGPRX2 receptor activation by temperature change. Begin gently—cool rather than very cold—and observe your individual response before increasing intensity.

Valsalva Maneuver and Bearing-Down Breath

The Valsalva maneuver—used medically to quickly slow a racing heart—involves bearing down as if having a bowel movement while keeping the breath held briefly. The bearing-down phase stimulates vagal afferents through increased intrathoracic pressure, producing a parasympathetic response that slows heart rate within seconds. A gentler version involves simply exhaling against slightly closed lips (bearing out rather than bearing down) for five to ten seconds.

Modified Valsalva Breath

Take a comfortable breath in.

Exhale against slightly pursed lips or a lightly closed airway, as if gently bearing down or resisting the airflow.

Maintain this gentle pressure for 5 to 10 seconds, then release and breathe normally.

Repeat 2 to 3 times.

Use: Especially valuable during episodes of palpitations or tachycardia. Can be used discreetly in any setting.

Auricular (Ear) Vagal Stimulation

A specific branch of the vagus nerve—the auricular branch, sometimes called the Arnold nerve—innervates a small region of the outer ear, primarily the cavum concha (the bowl-shaped area just outside the ear canal) and the cymba concha (the area above the ear canal). Gentle stimulation of this area produces direct vagal activation that is measurable on HRV monitoring.

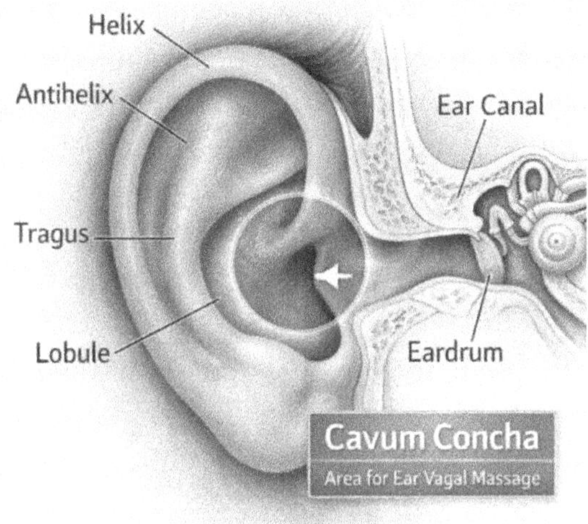

Ear Vagal Massage

Using one or both index fingers, gently press and massage the bowl-shaped hollow of the outer ear (the cavum concha) using small circular motions.

Continue for 1 to 2 minutes on each side. Gentle pressure is sufficient—this should feel pleasant, not uncomfortable.

Some people find that exhaling during the massage enhances the calming effect.

Use: Morning or evening routine; during or after stressful situations; as a quiet, unobtrusive practice that can be used in almost any context.

✦ ✦ ✦

Somatic Practices and Limbic Retraining

Breathwork and vagal exercises work primarily from the bottom up—they shift the physiological state directly, and the nervous system's sense of safety follows the body. Somatic practices and limbic retraining approaches work complementarily from multiple directions simultaneously, addressing the body's stored patterns of threat response that perpetuate sympathetic dominance even in the absence of current external stressors.

Somatic Awareness: Learning to Feel the Body Differently

Somatic practices begin with a deceptively simple skill: the capacity to notice sensations in the body without immediately interpreting them as threat. For many people with MCAS, bodily sensations have been associated with danger for so long that even neutral or mildly uncomfortable sensations—a small change in heart rate, a minor shift in gut feeling, a brief skin sensation—automatically trigger the sympathetic alarm response. This learned association between sensation and danger is self-reinforcing: the sympathetic response to the sensation creates more uncomfortable sensations, which trigger more alarm, in the cycle described in Chapter 9.

Learning to observe bodily sensations with curiosity rather than fear—to approach the body as a source of information rather than a site of threat—is a core somatic skill that gradually interrupts this cycle. It is practiced by pausing periodically throughout the day to notice what sensations are present in the body, naming them neutrally ("there is tightness in my chest," "my hands feel warm"), and then choosing, deliberately, to stay with the sensation for a moment rather than immediately reacting to it. Over time, this practice trains the nervous system to expand its tolerance for bodily experience without escalating into alarm.

The Body Scan

The body scan is one of the most accessible somatic practices and one of the most well-researched interventions for reducing chronic pain, anxiety, and inflammatory reactivity. It involves systematically directing attention through different regions of the body, noticing sensations without judgment, and releasing held tension as it is discovered.

Simple Body Scan Practice

Lie down comfortably or sit in a supported position. Close your eyes if comfortable.

Begin at the top of the head. Spend 10 to 20 seconds simply noticing any sensations present—warmth, tingling, tension, or neutrality. Do not try to change anything; just notice.

Move slowly downward: forehead, eyes and jaw, neck and shoulders, chest, belly, lower back, hips, thighs, knees, calves, feet. Spend 10 to 20 seconds with each area.

When you encounter tension or discomfort, try exhaling slowly while imagining the breath moving through that area, then allow the exhale to carry some of the tension away. Do not force relaxation—invite it.

Duration: 10 to 20 minutes. A shorter version of 5 minutes scanning just the major body regions is useful as a quick reset during the day.

Use: Evening practice before sleep; also helpful during the recovery period after a mast cell reaction, when the nervous system remains activated after the acute event.

Orienting Responses: Signaling Safety to the Nervous System

The orienting response is a fundamental nervous system behavior. When a genuine threat resolves, mammals—including humans—naturally look around their environment, taking in sensory information that signals that the current situation is safe. This deliberate environmental scanning activates the social engagement system (the ventral vagal complex in Polyvagal Theory terms) and signals the brainstem's threat-detection centers that the emergency is over.

For individuals with MCAS whose nervous systems have lost the capacity to signal safety reliably, deliberately practicing the orienting response teaches the nervous system to access this signal on demand.

Orienting Practice

Sit comfortably and allow your gaze to soften—unfocus slightly rather than staring at any particular point.

Slowly allow your eyes to move around the room, taking in whatever is there without any agenda. You are simply looking around, letting the environment come to you.

As you do this, notice: is there anything in this immediate environment that is an actual threat right now? Usually the answer is no. Allow that recognition to register in the body, not just the mind.

Let the jaw soften, the shoulders drop, the breath slow. These are the body's natural responses when the nervous system receives a safety signal.

Duration: 2 to 5 minutes. This is particularly useful at the beginning of a meal (to reduce anticipatory sympathetic activation around food) and before sleep.

Limbic System Retraining

For people whose nervous system dysregulation has deep roots—whether in adverse childhood experiences, chronic illness, or prolonged high-symptom periods that have conditioned the limbic system to associate ordinary activities with danger—structured limbic retraining programs may offer the most powerful available intervention.

Programs such as the Dynamic Neural Retraining System (DNRS) developed by Annie Hopper and the Gupta Program developed by Ashok Gupta are structured neuroplasticity-based programs designed specifically for people with chronic multi-system conditions including MCAS, ME/CFS, and multiple chemical sensitivities. These programs work through the principle of directed neuroplasticity: repeatedly and consistently activating positive, safety-associated, neural pathways while interrupting and redirecting the habitual threat-response pathways that maintain the illness cycle. They require significant daily practice—typically one to two hours per day for several months—but have produced documented recovery in patients who had not responded adequately to purely physiological approaches.

These programs are not appropriate for everyone with MCAS, and they are not a replacement for addressing physical root causes. But for individuals whose condition is significantly maintained by nervous system sensitization—particularly those who find that reactions occur disproportionately to apparent physical triggers, who have a strong history of anxiety and hypervigilance alongside their physical symptoms, or who have been unable to make progress despite careful physical management—they represent a potentially transformative therapeutic option. Information about these programs is available through their respective websites, and both offer free introductory materials.

✦ ✦ ✦

Sleep Optimization: The Nervous System's Nightly Reset

Sleep is not passive. It is the most biochemically active phase of the daily cycle—the period during which the glymphatic system clears inflammatory debris from the brain, the HPA axis restores its cortisol sensitivity, the immune system consolidates its regulatory function, and the autonomic nervous system undergoes its deepest recovery. For people with MCAS, restorative sleep is not a luxury; it is a clinical necessity.

The challenge is that MCAS creates conditions that undermine exactly the sleep it requires. Histamine is a powerful wakefulness-promoting neurotransmitter that disrupts sleep architecture—particularly the transitions into and maintenance of deep slow-wave sleep and REM sleep. Sympathetic dominance maintains a state of physiological arousal that makes falling asleep difficult and sustaining sleep harder. And the anxiety and hypervigilance of a nervous system calibrated to threat produce the classic MCAS sleep pattern: difficulty falling asleep, frequent waking, light unrefreshing sleep, and waking already activated.

Sleep Hygiene Fundamentals for MCAS

The foundational sleep practices for people dealing with MCAS overlap with general sleep hygiene recommendations but have several modifications specific to this group:

- **Consistent sleep and wake times, including weekends** – It is the most powerful single sleep intervention available; consistent timing stabilizes the cortisol circadian rhythm that has direct effects on morning mast cell reactivity. Even one night of significantly altered sleep timing disrupts this rhythm for two to three days afterward.

- **Light exposure management** – Morning bright light (ideally outdoor natural light), within thirty minutes of waking, anchors the circadian clock and boosts daytime serotonin production—the precursor to melatonin. Evening light dimming and blue-light reduction from screens in the two hours before bed protects melatonin onset. Blue-light blocking glasses used after sundown are a practical tool for those who cannot eliminate screen use in the evening.
- **Temperature** – Core body temperature naturally drops to initiate sleep onset; keeping the bedroom cool—ideally between 65 and 68 degrees Fahrenheit (18 to 20 degrees Celsius) for most people—supports this cooling and improves both sleep onset and deep sleep quality. Conversely, overheating during sleep—particularly under heavy blankets or in a warm room—is a mast cell trigger and a common cause of fragmented MCAS-associated sleep.
- **Histamine and meal timing** – The gut is most histamine-active in the later evening as food continues to be processed. Eating the final meal of the day at least three hours before sleep reduces the histamine load during sleep-onset and reduces the likelihood of histamine-driven sleep disruption. High-histamine foods in the evening meal are particularly problematic for sleep quality.
- **Alcohol avoidance** – Even small amounts of alcohol are among the most potent disruptors of deep and REM sleep architecture, in addition to being powerful DAO blockers and direct mast cell activators. For MCAS patients with sleep problems, alcohol is the single dietary change most likely to produce immediate, dramatic improvement in sleep quality.

Supplements and Natural Supports for MCAS Sleep

Several natural compounds specifically support sleep in the context of histamine intolerance and MCAS, addressing the histamine-driven sleep disruption rather than simply producing sedation:

- **Magnesium glycinate** – Magnesium is an NMDA receptor antagonist—it reduces neurological excitability—and glycinate (or bisglycinate) is the most absorbable and most calming of the magnesium forms.[303] Taking 200 to 400 mg thirty to sixty minutes before bed supports both nervous system calming and sleep quality without the morning grogginess associated with heavier sedative approaches and is well-tolerated by the majority of people with MCAS.
- **Low-dose melatonin** – Melatonin is a natural hormone but it is not sedative in the conventional sense; it signals the brain that nighttime has

arrived. Low doses (0.5 to 1 mg, much lower than the 5 to 10 mg commonly sold) taken thirty to sixty minutes before desired sleep onset are more physiologically appropriate than high doses, which can cause morning grogginess and paradoxical effects in sensitive individuals. Regular use of higher-dose melatonin supplements (often greater than 1 mg) may lead to reduced responsiveness over time in some individuals (melatonin tolerance), potentially altering the body's sensitivity to both supplemental and endogenous melatonin.

- **L-theanine** – This is an amino acid found in green tea that promotes relaxation without sedation through GABA-A receptor modulation; taking 100 to 200 mg at bedtime supports the nervous system transition into sleep and reduces sleep-onset anxiety and is generally very well tolerated in MCAS.
- **Quercetin** – The same compound used as a daytime mast cell stabilizer has documented benefits for sleep quality through its effects on histamine signaling in the brain; some practitioners time a portion of the quercetin dose to the evening to reduce overnight histamine activity.
- **Vitamin B6** – B6 supports both DAO enzyme function and the production of serotonin and melatonin in the pineal gland; deficiency specifically impairs sleep quality and is common in individuals with MCAS with gut dysfunction. Taking 25 to 50 mg of the active form (pyridoxal-5-phosphate or P5P) in the evening is a safe and often useful addition.
- **Tart cherry extract** – Tart cherries (especially Montmorency) naturally contain small amounts of melatonin. They also contain proanthocyanidins/polyphenols that may reduce inflammation and increase tryptophan availability, which leads to higher serotonin and melatonin levels. Juice (240 mL; 8 ounces) is most commonly used in clinical trials, but you can also take concentrate (30–60 mL), or capsules (480–1,000 mg/day). It's generally considered well tolerated in many individuals with MCAS, but its minor salicylate content may trigger symptoms in people whose buckets are nearly full.

Evening Nervous System Wind-Down Routine

The most effective sleep intervention is not a single supplement or practice—it is a consistent evening routine that signals to the nervous system, over the course of sixty to ninety minutes before bed, that the day's demands are ending and safety is present. This routine uses the practices already described in this chapter in a sequenced evening application:

Sample Evening Wind-Down Routine (sixty to ninety minutes before sleep)

Sixty minutes before bed, dim lights, reduce screens or use blue-light blocking glasses. Do light, non-stimulating activity (gentle reading, conversation, gentle stretching).

Forty minutes before bed, take magnesium glycinate and any other bedtime supplements.

Thirty minutes before bed, do ten minutes of extended-exhale breathing or resonance frequency breathing, practiced lying down or in a comfortable seated position.

Twenty minutes before bed, do a body scan practice (ten to fifteen minutes), moving attention through the body and releasing held tension.

Ten minutes before bed, do an orienting practice—a brief visual scanning of the safe, familiar bedroom environment. Take low-dose melatonin if using.

At lights out: Allow the breath to slow and the eyes to close. If thoughts are active, return attention gently to the sensation of breathing, not to the content of the thoughts.

✦ ✦ ✦

Deeper Dive: HRV Monitoring and Biofeedback

For the Science-Minded Reader

Heart rate variability biofeedback—using real-time HRV measurement to observe and train the autonomic nervous system—is the most scientifically validated nervous system intervention currently available for chronic inflammatory and stress-related conditions. Multiple randomized controlled trials have demonstrated that consistent HRV biofeedback training reduces inflammatory markers, improves emotional regulation, reduces anxiety and depression, improves cognitive function, and measurably reduces symptom burden in populations including IBS, fibromyalgia, and chronic fatigue—all conditions with overlapping biology to MCAS.[304,305,306,307]

HRV monitoring devices range from clinical-grade chest straps to consumer-grade wrist wearables, with varying accuracy. The most widely used consumer platforms for HRV biofeedback include HeartMath (a chest-strap or ear-clip sensor paired with a guided biofeedback app that provides real-time coherence feedback during resonance frequency breathing) and Polar H10 or similar chest straps paired with apps such as Elite HRV or HRV4Training. Wrist-based wearables including

Garmin, Oura Ring, Galaxy Watch, and Apple Watch now provide morning resting HRV measurements that, while less precise than chest-strap measurements, provide useful trending data over weeks and months.

For individuals with MCAS, the most valuable use of HRV monitoring is not achieving a specific score but observing the direction of trend over time in response to their nervous system practices. A rising trend in resting morning HRV across weeks of consistent practice is objective biological evidence that vagal tone is improving and the autonomic environment for mast cell regulation is shifting in the right direction. This kind of objective feedback can be powerfully motivating for people whose progress feels slow or invisible from symptom observation alone—the HRV trend often shows improvement weeks before dramatic symptom reduction becomes apparent.

HRV also serves as a practical tool for pacing: measuring HRV before exercise, social engagement, or other higher-demand activities provides real-time information about whether the autonomic system has sufficient reserve for the planned activity. A significantly lower-than-baseline HRV reading suggests the nervous system is already stressed and the planned activity may push toward reactivity; a normal or above-baseline reading suggests adequate reserve to proceed. For individuals who struggle with post-exertional reactions, HRV-guided pacing is a more physiologically accurate tool than calendar-based pacing alone.

✦ ✦ ✦

What This Means for You: Building Your Daily Practice

The nervous system practices in this chapter become effective through consistency, not intensity. The goal is not to achieve peak performance at any single practice session—it is to show up daily, consistently, and gradually shift the autonomic set point over weeks and months. Here is how to build a sustainable daily practice.

Start with two anchor practices. Choose one morning practice and one evening practice and commit to them for four weeks before adding anything else. The morning practice anchors the day's autonomic baseline; the evening practice supports sleep and overnight nervous system recovery. Extended-exhale breathing for five minutes in the morning and a body scan in the evening is a reliable, accessible starting combination for most people.

Layer gradually, just as with supplements. Adding nervous system practices follows the same logic as the supplement protocol from Chapter 12: one addition at a time, observed carefully, before adding the next. If you begin the extended-exhale breathing for a week and notice benefit, then add humming or gargling to your morning routine. The following week, add cold water to the face. Build the practice gradually to a sustainable daily routine rather than front-loading everything at once.

Use the physiological sigh as your immediate-response tool. Keep the physiological sigh available as your first-response tool the moment you notice sympathetic activation—a reaction beginning, an anxious thought escalating, a social situation producing stress. Two to three physiological sighs take fifteen seconds and can meaningfully interrupt the sympathetic cascade before it builds momentum. This is the most accessible acute intervention available and should be practiced until it becomes instinctive.

Connect practices to existing habits. Attaching new practices to existing daily anchors dramatically improves consistency. Humming in the shower. Extended-exhale breathing while the coffee brews. Orienting practice before the first meal of the day. Ear massage during the commute. Body scan after getting into bed. These micro-practices, threaded through existing daily routines, accumulate into meaningful daily practice time without requiring a dedicated block of time that may be difficult to sustain.

Track HRV if possible, but track symptoms regardless. If a wearable device is available, begin recording morning resting HRV alongside your symptom journal. Look for the correlation between high-HRV mornings and lower reactivity days—this connection is typically visible within three to four weeks of consistent practice and provides powerful motivation to continue. If no wearable is available, track morning nervous system state on the same one-to-ten reactivity scale used for symptoms: how activated, tense, or already reactive do you feel before you have done anything that day? This subjective measure tracks well with objective HRV and provides useful trend data.

Seek trauma-informed support when needed. If you recognize that your nervous system dysregulation has significant roots in adverse experience—and for many people with MCAS it does—working with a trauma-informed therapist trained in somatic approaches (Somatic Experiencing, EMDR, sensorimotor psychotherapy) provides a depth of nervous system healing that self-directed practices alone cannot fully achieve. These approaches are not contradictory to the self-practices in this chapter; they are their complement. The self-practices provide daily nervous system maintenance; the therapeutic work addresses the deeper structural roots.

Theresa's five-minute morning practice became ten minutes within a month, then fifteen, then an evening body scan was added, then humming in the shower, then cold water after the shower. Not all at once—one addition at a time, each one observed, each one earned by the stability the previous one had built. Eight months after that first skeptical week, she described her morning body as "a different animal." The hum of alarm had not disappeared entirely—she was realistic about that. But it had dropped to a background whisper that she could meet with curiosity rather than dread, that she could shift with her breath in real time, and that no longer set the entire tone of every day that followed from it.

The nervous system work had not cured her MCAS. But it had given her a body that could receive the rest of her treatment—a foundation stable enough to hold the healing work that had been slipping off her for years.

✦ ✦ ✦

Chapter 14 at a Glance

What to Remember:

- Nervous system regulation is biological treatment for MCAS, not optional self-care. Sympathetic dominance directly primes mast cells through norepinephrine; parasympathetic activation directly suppresses them through the cholinergic anti-inflammatory pathway. Every practice in this chapter changes mast cell behavior through measurable autonomic mechanisms.
- Extended-exhale breathing—inhaling for four counts and exhaling for six to eight—is the simplest, most portable, and most immediately effective vagal intervention available. Five minutes every morning before rising meaningfully shifts the day's autonomic baseline.
- Resonance frequency breathing at five to six breaths per minute (five-second inhale, five-second exhale) produces the maximum HRV benefit and is the gold standard daily autonomic training practice when time allows for ten to twenty minutes.
- The physiological sigh—double inhale through the nose followed by a long complete exhale—is the fastest single-breath acute autonomic downshift available and should be the first-response tool for moments of escalating sympathetic activation or early reaction signs.
- Direct vagal stimulation through humming, gargling, cold water facial immersion, ear vagal massage, and the modified Valsalva breath provides additional parasympathetic activation through the anatomical pathways of the vagus nerve itself, complementing breathwork with varied and accessible daily practices.
- Somatic practices—including body scanning, orienting responses, and somatic awareness training—address the learned association between bodily sensation and threat that perpetuates sympathetic dominance in the absence of current external stressors.

- Sleep optimization in MCAS requires specific attention to histamine's wakefulness-promoting effects, temperature management, light exposure, meal timing, and a consistent wind-down routine that actively signals safety to the nervous system before sleep.
- Consistency matters far more than perfection or duration. Twenty minutes of daily practice, distributed across morning and evening, consistently performed, produces measurable autonomic change within weeks and meaningful mast cell reactivity reduction within months.

Coming Up in the Next Chapters:

With the foundations of healing established—the stabilization strategy of Chapter 12, the low-histamine lifestyle of Chapter 13, and the nervous system regulation practices of Chapter 14—we move into the next segment: Natural Remedies for MCAS. The subsequent chapters are where the deeper therapeutic work begins: the foods, supplements, herbs, essential oils, and gut-healing protocols that build on the stable foundation you have created. Chapter 15 opens with the dietary dimension of active healing—the foods that don't just avoid triggering mast cells but actively work to stabilize them.

CHAPTER 15

Anti-Histamine Foods

Eating Toward Calm: Foods That Actively Support Mast Cell Stability

More Than Avoidance

For most people who discover the low-histamine approach, the first chapter of the dietary story is entirely about subtraction: what to remove, what to avoid, what to put away. That chapter is necessary and important—Chapter 13 covered it thoroughly. But it is only half the story, and for many people it becomes the whole story, which is a significant missed opportunity.

The second chapter of the dietary story is about addition. It is about the foods that do not merely fail to trigger mast cells, but actively work to stabilize them—foods rich in natural compounds that block histamine receptors, suppress mast cell degranulation, reduce the inflammatory signaling that keeps the mast cell system primed, and support the gut and nervous system function that underpins mast cell regulation. These are not exotic therapeutic substances. They are ordinary foods, accessible in any well-stocked grocery store, that carry within them some of the most powerful natural mast-cell-modulating compounds known to science.

This shift—from a diet defined by what it excludes to a diet defined by what it actively provides—changes the relationship with food in ways that matter psychologically as well as physiologically. Instead of approaching every meal as a minefield to be navigated, you begin approaching it as an opportunity to give your immune system something useful. That is a different orientation, and it produces a different experience of eating.

Marcus, whom we met in Chapter 2, described this shift as the moment his dietary approach stopped feeling like punishment and started feeling like medicine. "I stopped thinking about what I couldn't eat," he said, "and started thinking about what I was actually building every time I sat down to a meal." His symptom trajectory improved significantly in the months after that shift—not because his diet changed dramatically, but because his relationship with it did, and because he began consistently including foods that were doing real biological work on his behalf.

✦ ✦ ✦

How Foods Can Stabilize Mast Cells: The Core Mechanisms

Foods influence mast cell behavior through several distinct mechanisms, and understanding these helps you choose strategically rather than simply following a list. The most important mechanisms are natural histamine blocking, mast cell membrane stabilization, anti-inflammatory signaling, and gut and barrier support.[308,309,310]

Natural Histamine Blocking

Certain plant compounds act as natural antihistamines—they compete with histamine for binding at H1 and H2 receptors, reducing the downstream effects of whatever histamine is present without eliminating the histamine itself. Quercetin, the flavonoid found abundantly in onions, apples, and capers, is the most studied and most potent of these natural antihistamines.[311] Luteolin, found in celery, parsley, and chamomile, has similar receptor-blocking properties. Indeed, its effects surpassed cromolyn sodium—a drug used to manage allergies and mastocytosis by stabilizing mast cells and preventing the release of inflammatory substances—in a mast cell-based model of histamine release.[312] These compounds don't just prevent mast cells from releasing histamine, they reduce mast cell intracellular signaling and downstream pro-inflammatory pathways (e.g., NF-κB, cytokines, calcium signaling), thereby diminishing the physiological effects of histamine even when release is not fully suppressed.[313,314]

Mast Cell Membrane Stabilization

Some dietary compounds directly stabilize the mast cell membrane, reducing the probability of degranulation in response to any given trigger. This is the mechanism by which pharmaceutical mast cell stabilizers like cromolyn sodium work, and several dietary compounds operate through analogous pathways. Quercetin again leads the list—it inhibits the release of both histamine and other inflammatory mediators including leukotrienes and prostaglandins by stabilizing the mast cell membrane and interfering with the calcium influx required for degranulation.[315] Omega-3 fatty acids from fatty fish, flaxseed, and walnuts incorporate into mast cell membranes and alter their physical properties in ways that reduce sensitivity to activation triggers.[316]

Anti-Inflammatory Signaling

A third category of dietary influence involves the broader inflammatory environment in which mast cells operate. Pro-inflammatory cytokines—TNF-alpha, IL-6, IL-33—prime mast cells and lower their activation threshold. Dietary compounds that suppress these cytokines through NF-κB inhibition, COX-2 inhibition, and other anti-inflammatory pathways reduce the priming environment and effectively raise the mast cell threshold. Curcumin from turmeric, EGCG from green tea, resveratrol from red grapes and berries, and sulforaphane from cruciferous vegetables all operate primarily through this anti-inflammatory signaling pathway.

Gut and Barrier Support

As established in Chapter 6, the gut is central to MCAS management, and foods that support gut barrier integrity, microbiome health, and DAO enzyme activity indirectly but powerfully support mast cell stability. Prebiotic fibers that feed butyrate-producing bacteria, collagen-supporting nutrients like vitamin C and glycine, and fermentation-compatible foods (when introduced appropriately after stabilization) all contribute to the gut health foundation that reduces the chronic low-grade mast cell activation described in Chapter 6.

> **The Integrated Approach:** *The most powerful anti-histamine diet is not simply a low-histamine diet—it is a diet that simultaneously reduces histamine input, blocks histamine signaling, stabilizes mast cell membranes, reduces inflammatory priming, and supports gut barrier function. Each of these dimensions reinforces the others, and together they produce outcomes that restriction alone cannot achieve.*

✦ ✦ ✦

Foods That Actively Reduce Histamine Load and Mast Cell Reactivity

The following foods have the strongest evidence for mast cell stabilizing or anti-histamine effects and form the nutritional backbone of a therapeutic anti-histamine diet. Most are well-tolerated by the majority of people with MCAS, though individual sensitivities vary and introduction should always be systematic.

Quercetin-Rich Foods: Onions, Apples, and Capers

Quercetin is arguably the most clinically significant natural mast cell stabilizer in the food supply. Research has consistently demonstrated that quercetin inhibits mast cell degranulation, blocks H1 and H2 histamine receptors, suppresses the release of leukotrienes and prostaglandins, and downregulates the expression of pro-inflammatory cytokines through NF-κB inhibition.[317] Quercetin from foods is absorbed into your body and can reach levels that have real biological effects.[318] However, some laboratory studies use much higher amounts than you would normally get from diet alone, so the effects seen in research may sometimes be stronger than what food by itself can provide.

The richest dietary sources of quercetin include red onions (the outer layers contain the highest concentrations), yellow onions, capers (one of the most concentrated food sources available), apples (particularly the skin), red grapes, blueberries, and broccoli. Cooking reduces quercetin content to some degree, but meaningful amounts survive in well-cooked onions and in raw apple skin. For maximum benefit, including raw or lightly cooked onion in daily meals and eating organic apples with their skin provides a consistent dietary quercetin contribution alongside any supplemental quercetin being used therapeutically.

Vitamin C–Rich Foods: Fresh Bell Peppers, Kiwi, and Broccoli

Vitamin C is both a natural antihistamine and a DAO enzyme cofactor.[319] Research has shown that vitamin C directly degrades histamine in the bloodstream through enzymatic and non-enzymatic mechanisms, and that serum histamine levels correlate inversely with vitamin C status—lower vitamin C is reliably associated with higher circulating histamine. Vitamin C also supports collagen synthesis (relevant for the connective tissue dimension of MCAS–hEDS), supports adrenal function, and is one of the most important antioxidants for the oxidative stress that primes mast cells.

The challenge for individuals with MCAS is that many of the highest-vitamin-C fruits—citrus fruits, strawberries, pineapple—are also histamine liberators. The richest low-histamine sources of vitamin C are fresh red and yellow bell peppers (containing more vitamin C per serving than citrus), fresh kiwi (well-tolerated by most people with MCAS), fresh broccoli and cauliflower, fresh parsley, and fresh mango. These sources provide therapeutic vitamin C without the histamine liberation risk of citrus.

Omega-3-Rich Foods: Fresh Fatty Fish, Flaxseed, and Walnuts

Omega-3 fatty acids—specifically EPA and DHA from marine sources, and ALA from plant sources—are among the most broadly anti-inflammatory dietary compounds available, with well-characterized mechanisms relevant to mast cell biology.[320] EPA and DHA compete with arachidonic acid for incorporation into cell membranes, reducing the substrate available for the synthesis of pro-inflammatory leukotrienes and prostaglandins from mast cells.[321] They also incorporate into mast cell membranes themselves, altering membrane fluidity in ways that reduce degranulation sensitivity. Omega-3s additionally support the resolution of inflammation after activation events—shortening the duration and severity of flares rather than merely reducing their frequency.

The critical caveat for those with MCAS is freshness. Fatty fish—salmon, mackerel, sardines, anchovies—are the richest dietary sources of EPA and DHA, but they are also high-risk foods for histamine accumulation if not handled with strict freshness protocols. Fish consumed fresh on the day of purchase or sourced from high-quality frozen-at-sea products are appropriate and beneficial; the same fish from a restaurant display case or a can is a significant trigger. Fresh-ground flaxseed and raw walnuts provide ALA (which converts to EPA and DHA less efficiently but meaningfully in some people) without the freshness risk of fish, and are reliable daily omega-3 sources for people who cannot reliably access very fresh fish.

Luteolin-Rich Foods: Celery, Parsley, and Fresh Herbs

Luteolin, a flavone closely related to quercetin in structure and mechanism, has documented mast cell–stabilizing properties including inhibition of IgE-mediated degranulation, suppression of TNF-alpha and IL-6 release, and blockade of the antigen-specific mast cell activation pathway.[322] It is less studied than quercetin in clinical populations but consistently demonstrates mast cell–stabilizing effects in laboratory research, and its safety profile in food amounts is excellent.

The richest dietary sources are fresh celery (including celery leaves, which are more concentrated than the stalks), fresh parsley, fresh chamomile (as tea—one of the most concentrated and accessible sources), dried oregano and dried thyme (well-tolerated by most if dried spice aging is managed, as discussed in Chapter 13), and artichokes. Including fresh parsley and celery in daily cooking—as flavoring, in salads, or blended into sauces—provides a consistent dietary luteolin contribution with minimal effort.

Magnesium-Rich Foods: Pumpkin Seeds, Dark Leafy Greens, and Legumes

Magnesium is essential for more than three hundred enzymatic reactions in the body, including several directly relevant to mast cell regulation. Magnesium acts as a natural calcium channel blocker—it reduces the intracellular calcium influx that is required to trigger mast cell degranulation.[323] Low magnesium status is associated with increased mast cell reactivity, elevated histamine levels, and increased inflammatory cytokine production. It is also essential for nervous system regulation (supporting the parasympathetic function that suppresses mast cell activation), sleep quality, and adrenal function.

Dietary magnesium is broadly distributed in whole plant foods. The richest low-histamine sources include pumpkin seeds and sunflower seeds, fresh spinach and Swiss chard (note that spinach is a high-histamine food for some people—individual tolerance varies), cooked black beans and lentils (caution for those sensitive to oxalates), dark chocolate (high in magnesium but also a histamine liberator for many—individual assessment needed), avocado (a liberator for some), and whole grains including quinoa and oats (only consume organic as oats concentrate glyphosate). For those with MCAS, consistent dietary magnesium intake combined with supplemental magnesium glycinate (as discussed in Chapter 14 for sleep support) provides the most reliable path to adequate magnesium status.

Vitamin D–Rich Foods and Sunlight

Vitamin D deficiency is documented at elevated rates in mast cell–associated and related inflammatory conditions,[324] and its relevance goes well beyond bone health. Vitamin D receptors are expressed on mast cells, and vitamin D signaling directly suppresses mast cell proliferation, reduces IgE receptor expression on mast cell surfaces, and promotes the regulatory T cell populations that provide immune tolerance.[325] Low vitamin D is associated with increased mast cell reactivity; correcting deficiency reliably improves immune regulation across multiple inflammatory conditions.

Dietary vitamin D sources are limited—fatty fish, egg yolks, and fortified foods provide modest amounts. The most significant dietary contribution to vitamin D status comes from sun-derived synthesis in the skin, but for many people in northern latitudes, at desk jobs, or with significant sun sensitivity (common in MCAS due to mast-cell-mediated UV reactivity), adequate sun exposure is not reliably achievable. Supplemental vitamin D3 is covered in Chapter 16, but emphasizing vitamin D–containing foods—especially egg yolks from pasture-raised chickens, and fresh fatty fish—as part of the therapeutic diet contributes meaningfully to overall status alongside supplementation.

Anti-Inflammatory Polyphenol Foods: Blueberries, Green Tea, and Turmeric

A broad category of polyphenol-rich plant foods provide anti-inflammatory support relevant to mast cell priming through NF-κB inhibition, COX-2 suppression, and antioxidant activity.[326] Blueberries are particularly notable because they are among the richest dietary sources of anthocyanins—potent anti-inflammatory flavonoids—while being reliably well-tolerated by the majority of individuals with MCAS, in contrast to other dark berries that are higher in histamine or more commonly reactive. Fresh or frozen blueberries provide consistent, accessible polyphenol support.

Green tea contains EGCG (epigallocatechin gallate), one of the most extensively researched anti-inflammatory polyphenols, with documented mast cell–

stabilizing effects including inhibition of IgE-mediated activation and suppression of histamine and cytokine release.[327] For those with MCAS, green tea is generally better tolerated than black or fermented teas, which have higher histamine content due to oxidation during processing. Weak to moderate-strength green tea, fresh-brewed and consumed promptly, is well-tolerated by most. Note: green tea does contain some caffeine, which may be a sympathetic nervous system activator for sensitive individuals—individual assessment is warranted.

Turmeric's active compound curcumin inhibits NF-κB more potently than most other dietary anti-inflammatory compounds, reduces histidine decarboxylase enzyme activity (the bacterial enzyme responsible for histamine formation), and has direct mast cell–stabilizing properties in laboratory research.[328] It is poorly absorbed from food sources and supplements without co-administration of piperine (from black pepper, which enhances curcumin bioavailability by up to two thousand percent), turmeric essential oil, fenugreek galactomannan, or a lipid carrier. Including turmeric in cooking with black pepper and a fat source—coconut oil, olive oil, or ghee—meaningfully improves its absorption and anti-inflammatory effect.

✦ ✦ ✦

At a Glance: Foods to Emphasize and Foods to Minimize

The following summarizes the dietary picture from both Chapter 13 and this chapter, providing a practical single reference for the low-histamine, mast-cell-stabilizing dietary approach.

Foods to Emphasize: Mast Cell Stabilizing and Anti-Histamine

- Fresh proteins: chicken, turkey, fresh beef, lamb, fresh fish (same-day or frozen-at-sea)
- Quercetin-rich: red onions, yellow onions, capers, apples (with skin), broccoli, red grapes
- Vitamin C–rich: red and yellow bell peppers, fresh kiwi, fresh broccoli, fresh parsley
- Omega-3–rich: fresh or frozen-at-sea salmon, mackerel, sardines; fresh-ground flaxseed; raw walnuts
- Luteolin-rich: celery, fresh parsley, chamomile tea, fresh thyme and oregano
- Magnesium-rich: pumpkin seeds, sunflower seeds, cooked lentils and beans, quinoa
- Polyphenol-rich: fresh or frozen blueberries, green tea (fresh-brewed), turmeric with black pepper and fat
- Gut-supporting: cooked and cooled potatoes and rice (prebiotic), cooked vegetables, bone broth from fresh bones

- Healthy fats: cold-pressed olive oil, coconut oil, avocado (if tolerated), ghee from grass-fed sources
- Vitamin D: egg yolks from pasture-raised chickens, fresh fatty fish, moderate sun exposure

Foods to Minimize or Avoid During Stabilization

- High-histamine proteins: aged cheeses, cured and processed meats, deli meats, smoked fish, canned fish
- Fermented foods: sauerkraut, kimchi, kombucha, kefir, yogurt, sourdough, miso, soy sauce, tempeh
- High-histamine vegetables: tomatoes, spinach (for some), eggplant, avocado (for some)
- Histamine liberators: strawberries, citrus fruits, pineapple, papaya, egg white, chocolate, alcohol
- DAO-blocking: alcohol in any form, black tea, energy drinks
- Additives: artificial food colors, sulfites, benzoates, MSG—check labels on packaged foods
- Vinegar-based condiments: ketchup, mustard, mayo, most salad dressings, pickles, hot sauce
- Leftovers: cooked proteins stored and reheated carry significantly elevated histamine
- Overripe produce: histamine content increases as fruit and vegetables begin to break down

✦ ✦ ✦

Sample Meal Plans: Putting It Into Practice

The following meal plans illustrate how a low-histamine, mast-cell-stabilizing dietary approach looks in daily practice. These are starting points, not prescriptions—individual tolerance varies, and your personal safe-food list should always take priority over any generic plan. Introduce new foods one at a time during the stabilization phase and observe for forty-eight to seventy-two hours before drawing conclusions about tolerance.

Sample Day One: Simple and Conservative (Stabilization Phase)

Day 1 — Stabilization Phase: Simple, Fresh, Conservative

Breakfast: Plain organic oats cooked in water, topped with fresh blueberries and a tablespoon of fresh-ground flaxseed. Green tea (weak, freshly brewed). Magnesium glycinate supplement with water.

Mid-morning: Apple with skin (quercetin source). Handful of raw pumpkin seeds (magnesium).

Lunch: Fresh chicken breast cooked same day in olive oil with fresh garlic, served with steamed broccoli and cooked white rice. Fresh parsley garnish. Water with a slice of fresh kiwi on the side.

Afternoon snack: Sliced yellow bell pepper (vitamin C) with a small amount of hummus made from freshly cooked chickpeas if tolerated, or plain pumpkin seeds.

Dinner: Fresh salmon fillet (same-day or frozen-at-sea, not canned), baked with olive oil, turmeric, and black pepper. Served with steamed cauliflower and cooked quinoa. Side salad of cucumber, celery, and fresh parsley with olive oil and a squeeze of kiwi juice instead of vinegar dressing.

Evening: Chamomile tea (luteolin source, also supports sleep). Magnesium glycinate. Body scan and extended-exhale breathing practice.

Sample Day Two: More Variety (Stage 2 Support Phase)

Day 2 — Stage 2 Support: Broader Variety, Still Low-Histamine

Breakfast: Scrambled eggs from pasture-raised chickens (vitamin D, choline) in ghee, with fresh spinach (if tolerated) or Swiss chard, served with a slice of fresh-baked bread (not sourdough). Fresh blueberries on the side.

Mid-morning: Freshly brewed green tea. Handful of walnuts (ALA omega-3s).

Lunch: Turkey mince (cooked same day) formed into patties and cooked in coconut oil. Served with roasted sweet potato, steamed green beans, and a generous amount of fresh herbs. Sliced apple with skin for dessert.

Afternoon: Fresh red bell pepper strips with guacamole made from ripe avocado (if tolerated) and lime juice. Alternatively, sliced pear with raw almond butter.

Dinner: Fresh lamb chops (same day) grilled with fresh garlic, thyme, and rosemary. Served with cooked lentils (freshly prepared), steamed broccoli, and a salad of red cabbage, celery, and fresh parsley dressed with olive oil.

Evening: Chamomile or ginger tea. Low-dose quercetin supplement with dinner or at bedtime. Wind-down nervous system routine as per Chapter 14.

Sample Day Three: Family-Friendly and Practical

Day 3 — Practical and Shareable: Low-Histamine Without the Label

Breakfast: Pancakes made with organic oat flour, eggs, coconut milk, and blueberries—naturally low-histamine, no special explanation needed at the family table. Maple syrup (well-tolerated by most). Fresh kiwi slices on the side.

Mid-morning: Apple. Pumpkin seed mix with sunflower seeds.

Lunch: Chicken and vegetable soup made with fresh whole chicken pieces, carrots, celery, onion, zucchini, and fresh herbs in broth—consumed the same day it is made. Crusty fresh bread (not sourdough) or plain rice crackers.

Afternoon: Sliced mango (fresh, not overripe) with coconut yogurt if tolerated, or plain rice crackers with almond butter.

Dinner: Baked fresh white fish fillet (cod, haddock, or sole—mild and typically well-tolerated) with lemon-herb crust made from fresh parsley, olive oil, and crushed garlic. Served with roasted root vegetables (carrots, parsnips, sweet potato) and steamed peas.

Dessert: Baked apple with cinnamon and a drizzle of honey—naturally satisfying, warming, low-histamine.

✦ ✦ ✦

Deeper Dive: The Quercetin and Luteolin Research

For the Science-Minded Reader

Quercetin and luteolin deserve more detailed scientific attention than a general dietary survey allows, because they are the dietary compounds with the strongest mechanistic evidence for direct mast cell stabilization and because understanding their mechanisms helps explain both why they work and how to use them most effectively.

Quercetin's Multi-Target Mechanism

Quercetin's mast cell–stabilizing activity operates through at least four distinct molecular targets, which is part of what makes it so potent and so broadly effective across different MCAS phenotypes.[329,330] First, it inhibits PI3K (phosphoinositide 3-kinase) and downstream signaling cascades required for IgE receptor activation—directly blocking the most common pathway for mast cell degranulation. Second, it reduces intracellular calcium influx through calcium channel modulation; calcium is the essential second messenger for degranulation, and limiting its entry effectively prevents the release of granule contents even when surface receptors are activated. Third, it inhibits the enzyme histidine decarboxylase, reducing de novo histamine synthesis from its amino acid precursor. Fourth, it suppresses NF-κB activation, reducing the transcription of genes encoding histamine receptors, inflammatory cytokines, and mast cell survival factors.

These four mechanisms act synergistically: quercetin doesn't merely reduce a mast cell's tendency to degranulate—it reduces the available histamine pool, blunts the signal that triggers degranulation, limits the calcium influx required to execute it, and reduces the production of the inflammatory proteins that keep the mast cell system primed. This multi-target action is one reason quercetin consistently outperforms more targeted natural antihistamines in both research and clinical observation.

The main limitation of dietary quercetin is bioavailability. Quercetin from food sources is absorbed at rates of around twenty to fifty percent, depending significantly on the food matrix and the presence of fat and other absorption cofactors.[331] The quercetin in onions, which is present in a glycoside form (quercetin glucoside; bound to a sugar molecule), is actually better absorbed than the aglycone (listed as dihydrate; not bonded to a sugar molecule) form found in supplements—one of the few instances where the food form outperforms the supplement. Consuming quercetin-rich foods with a fat source (olive oil dressing on an onion-containing salad, for example) enhances absorption meaningfully.

Luteolin's Complementary Profile

Luteolin shares several of quercetin's mechanisms but has a somewhat different tissue distribution and receptor affinity profile that makes it a valuable complement rather than a simple alternative. Luteolin is notably more active than quercetin at blocking mast cell activation through the stem cell factor (SCF)–Kit receptor pathway—the signaling axis that drives mast cell proliferation and survival and that is dysregulated in many people with MCAS.[332] This makes luteolin particularly relevant for individuals with more proliferative or Kit-pathway-associated mast cell dysfunction.

Luteolin readily crosses the blood-brain barrier and exerts direct anti-inflammatory activity in the central nervous system.[333] For those with MCAS with significant neuropsychiatric symptoms—brain fog, anxiety, cognitive impairment, the neuropsychiatric endotypes discussed in Chapter 9—luteolin's CNS-active profile makes it a particularly valuable addition to both the dietary and supplemental anti-histamine toolkit. This is one reason that combining both dietary quercetin sources and dietary luteolin sources provides broader coverage than either alone.

✦ ✦ ✦

What This Means for You: Building Your Anti-Histamine Diet

Translating the anti-histamine dietary approach into daily practice is less complicated than it might appear. The following principles guide a practical, sustainable implementation.

Build your diet around the emphasize list, not against the avoid list. The most effective approach is to fill your plate primarily with the foods on the emphasize list—fresh proteins, quercetin-rich vegetables, vitamin C–rich produce, omega-3 sources, prebiotic fibers—rather than spending most of your dietary attention on what to avoid. When the plate is already full of genuinely therapeutic food, there is naturally less room for triggering food, and the focus shifts from deprivation to nourishment.

Make quercetin and vitamin C your daily dietary anchors. These two compounds have the most direct evidence for mast cell–stabilizing and antihistamine effects, and they are accessible in everyday foods. Red or yellow onion in some form at most meals, an apple with its skin daily, fresh bell pepper or broccoli at lunch or dinner, and fresh parsley as a garnish or salad base provide a consistent daily quercetin and vitamin C foundation that costs nothing beyond the ordinary grocery budget.

Handle fresh fish confidently with the right protocol. Many people with MCAS avoid fish entirely because of its histamine risk, missing out on the most potent dietary source of EPA and DHA omega-3s available. The risk is real but manageable with strict freshness protocols: buy fresh fish the morning you will eat it, cook it the same day, eat it at that meal, and discard leftovers. Alternatively, purchase individually vacuum-sealed frozen-at-sea portions (salmon, mackerel, sardines) and defrost only what you will use at that meal. Handled this way, fatty fish is both safe and among the most therapeutically valuable foods in the anti-histamine diet.

Introduce turmeric daily with a fat and black pepper. Turmeric's curcumin is poorly absorbed without bioavailability enhancers, but well absorbed when combined with fat and black pepper piperine—a combination that is both easy to achieve and pleasant in everyday cooking. A quarter teaspoon of turmeric with a crack of black pepper in a stir-fry, soup, roasted vegetables, or even scrambled eggs cooked in ghee provides meaningful daily curcumin exposure at a dose that is both safe and beneficial for most people. Golden milk—turmeric, coconut milk, black pepper, and optional honey—is another accessible daily delivery method.

Use the sample meal plans as a rotation template, not a rigid prescription. The three sample days above are not meant to be followed exactly, day after day. They are illustrations of how the principles translate into practical meals. Use them as a starting-point template, substituting your personal safe foods for any items you know you react to, and build a rotation of ten to fifteen meals that you know works for your system. This rotation provides variety and nutritional breadth without requiring daily creative decision-making about what is safe to eat.

Track how specific foods affect you, not how they affect others. Individual responses to foods within the low-histamine and mast-cell-stabilizing categories vary significantly. Some people tolerate avocado without difficulty; others find it a reliable trigger. Some do well with eggs; others react. Use the three-day tracking window from Chapter 13 consistently, and build your personal picture of which specific foods from the emphasize list work reliably for you. Your personal therapeutic diet is a subset of the general guidelines, calibrated to your individual biology.

Marcus's meals, by the time he had fully implemented the anti-histamine dietary approach, looked nothing like the joyless avoidance-based eating he had initially feared. They were colorful, varied, and—by his own account—genuinely delicious. Fresh salmon with roasted vegetables and herbs. Chicken soup made the same morning and eaten at lunch. Blueberry and flaxseed overnight oats. Apple slices with almond butter. Turmeric-spiced lentil soup with fresh parsley and a drizzle of olive oil.

"I eat better now than I did before I was diagnosed," he said, with a mix of amusement and genuine surprise. "I never ate this much color before. I never thought this carefully about what I was actually putting in my body."

The diagnosis had taken something away—the careless ease of eating without thought. But it had given something back: a relationship with food as medicine, and a body that was noticeably, measurably responding to being fed well.

✦ ✦ ✦

Chapter 15 at a Glance

What to Remember:

- The anti-histamine dietary approach is not only about what to remove—it is equally about what to add. Foods rich in quercetin, luteolin, vitamin C, omega-3s, magnesium, and anti-inflammatory polyphenols actively stabilize mast cells, block histamine receptors, and reduce the inflammatory priming that keeps mast cell thresholds low.
- Quercetin is the most potent natural mast cell stabilizer in the food supply, acting through at least four distinct mechanisms: PI3K pathway inhibition, calcium channel modulation, histidine decarboxylase suppression, and NF-κB blockade. Red onions, capers, and apples with skin are the richest accessible dietary sources.
- Vitamin C is both a natural antihistamine—directly degrading histamine in the bloodstream—and a DAO enzyme cofactor. Fresh bell peppers,

kiwi, broccoli, and parsley provide therapeutic vitamin C without the histamine liberation risk of citrus fruits.

- Omega-3 fatty acids from fresh or frozen-at-sea fatty fish, flaxseed, and walnuts stabilize mast cell membranes, reduce leukotriene and prostaglandin synthesis, and support resolution of inflammation after activation events. Freshness handling is critical for fish sources.
- Luteolin from celery, parsley, and chamomile tea complements quercetin's mechanism with superior CNS penetration and stronger Kit-pathway inhibition—making it particularly relevant for neuropsychiatric MCAS presentations.
- Magnesium acts as a natural calcium channel blocker, reducing the calcium influx required for mast cell degranulation. Pumpkin seeds, cooked legumes, and quinoa are reliable low-histamine dietary sources.
- Blueberries, green tea, and turmeric provide polyphenol-based anti-inflammatory support through NF-κB inhibition and antioxidant activity. Turmeric requires fat and black pepper for meaningful bioavailability.
- Building the diet around the emphasize list—rather than organizing it around the avoid list—produces better nutrition, less food anxiety, and a therapeutic relationship with eating that supports nervous system regulation alongside immune stabilization.

Coming Up in Chapter 16:

Food provides a powerful therapeutic foundation, but the natural remedies for MCAS extend well beyond the plate. Chapter 16 covers the supplement protocol: quercetin and luteolin in therapeutic doses that go beyond what diet alone can deliver, vitamin C, DAO enzymes, magnesium, vitamin D, omega-3s, and the gut-healing compounds that repair the intestinal infrastructure on which everything else depends. Each supplement is presented with its mechanism, evidence base, dosing guidance, and practical considerations for introduction in a reactive system.

CHAPTER 16

Supplements for Mast Cell Stabilization

A Practical Guide to the Compounds That Work—and How to Use Them Safely

The Supplement Drawer

Diane opened her kitchen cupboard and began pulling things out, one by one, until they covered half the counter. A bottle of quercetin—opened but mostly untouched, because she'd reacted to it once and never tried it again. Three different probiotics purchased at different stages of her journey, each abandoned after an uncertain response. A large container of magnesium she had been taking in the wrong form for two years. DAO enzymes she used occasionally but wasn't sure about. Vitamin D she'd been told to take but whose dose she'd never verified against her blood levels. And a collection of gut-healing supplements—glutamine, zinc, collagen peptides—half of which she had never introduced systematically enough to know whether they were helping.

"I've spent so much money on this shelf," she said to her practitioner. "I have no idea what's working."

The practitioner's question was direct: "How many of these did you introduce one at a time, with a week of observation between each one?"

The answer, as both of them already knew, was none of them. Diane had introduced supplements the same way most people do—in clusters, during periods of desperation, without a clear method for assessing individual responses. She had accumulated a supplement drawer rather than a supplement protocol.

The difference between those two things matters enormously in MCAS. A supplement protocol is a deliberately sequenced, individually assessed set of compounds—each chosen for a specific mechanistic reason, introduced at an appropriate dose for a reactive system, observed carefully, and adjusted based on response. A supplement drawer is what happens when the protocol is skipped.

This chapter is designed to help you build the protocol—to understand which supplements have the strongest evidence for MCAS management, why each one works, how to use each one safely, and how to combine them into a coherent daily regimen that supports mast cell stabilization from multiple complementary directions.

✦ ✦ ✦

The Golden Rule: One at a Time

Before moving to the individual supplements, the single most important principle deserves repetition from Chapter 12: introduce supplements one at a time, at a low starting dose, with a minimum of five to seven days of observation before adding the next compound. In a highly reactive mast cell system, even beneficial compounds can trigger reactions—not because they are harmful, but because they are new inputs the sensitized immune system is evaluating. When multiple supplements are introduced simultaneously, reactions become unattributable: you cannot know which compound caused them, you cannot make rational decisions about what to continue, and you cannot build the systematic knowledge of your own response profile that is essential for MCAS management.

The corollary to this rule is starting low. The doses listed in this chapter are therapeutic targets—the doses at which most people with MCAS obtain meaningful benefit. They are not starting doses for highly reactive individuals. During the stabilization Phase 1n particular, beginning at a quarter to a half of the target dose and stepping up slowly over one to two weeks gives the reactive system time to adjust to each new compound before it reaches full therapeutic concentration. Reactions to supplements at low doses are informative and manageable; reactions at full doses in an already-reactive system are neither.

> **The Introduction Protocol:** *Introduce one supplement at a low starting dose. Observe for five to seven days, noting any change in symptoms on your daily tracking scale. If well-tolerated, step up toward the target dose over the following week. Once stable at the target dose, introduce the next supplement. This method takes longer than loading everything at once—but it is the only approach that gives you usable information about what is helping and what is not.*

The supplements in this chapter are organized in the order of typical introduction priority: beginning with the compounds most universally well-tolerated and most immediately relevant to mast cell stabilization, then progressing to gut-healing and immune-modulating compounds that build on the initial foundation. Your personal order may differ based on your specific root causes and your practitioner's guidance.

✦ ✦ ✦

The Supplement Profiles

Each supplement is presented in a consistent format so you can quickly locate the information most relevant to your situation—whether that is the right form to buy, the appropriate starting dose, or the cautions specific to your circumstances.

Quercetin | *The Cornerstone Mast Cell Stabilizer*

Form: Quercetin phytosome, liposomal quercetin, or quercetin dihydrate (powder or capsule). Phytosome and liposomal forms offer significantly better bioavailability and are worth the higher cost for highly reactive individuals. Avoid quercetin glycosides labeled as "quercetin" without clarification—they are a different compound.

Dose: Target: 250–500 mg, two to three times daily. Effective range for mast cell stabilization in research studies. Some individuals benefit from up to 1,000 mg per dose under practitioner guidance.

Timing: Twenty to thirty minutes before meals for maximum mast cell stabilization effect at the gut level. Can be shifted to with-meal timing if GI sensitivity occurs.

With Food? Preferred on an empty stomach for mast cell stabilization. If GI upset occurs (uncommon but possible), take with a small amount of fat-containing food—fat enhances quercetin absorption.

Start Low: Begin at 125 mg once daily for the first week. Increase to 125 mg twice daily in week two, then 250 mg twice daily in week three if well tolerated. Some reactive individuals tolerate quercetin better in liposomal form if the standard form causes sensitivity.

Cautions: May reduce absorption of fluoroquinolone antibiotics (ciprofloxacin, levofloxacin)—separate by at least two hours. May potentiate blood-thinning medications. High doses (>3,000 mg/day) not recommended without clinical supervision. Generally very well tolerated at standard doses.

Vitamin C (Buffered) | *Natural Antihistamine and DAO Cofactor*

Form: Buffered vitamin C (calcium ascorbate, magnesium ascorbate, or sodium ascorbate). Avoid plain ascorbic acid during stabilization—its acidity can irritate the gut lining and trigger reactions in very sensitive individuals. *Note: You may be wondering why liposomal vitamin C is not recommended for its superior bioavailability. The reason is that some people with MCAS may react to the ingredients in the liposomal shell vitamin C is enclosed in (soy lecithin, natural flavors, ethanol).*

Dose: Target: 500–1,000 mg, twice daily. Starting during stabilization: 250 mg once daily and step up. Bowel tolerance varies—loose stools indicate the dose exceeds current absorption capacity; reduce to the highest tolerated dose.

Timing: With meals, twice daily. Dividing the dose maintains more consistent serum levels than a single large dose.

With Food? Always with food. Reduces GI sensitivity and improves tolerability. Vitamin C is absorbed through active transport that is more efficient with food present.

Start Low: Start at 250 mg once daily with the largest meal. Increase to 250 mg twice daily after one week if well tolerated, then increase toward target dose at your own pace guided by GI tolerance.

Cautions: High-dose vitamin C (above 2,000 mg/day) may increase urinary oxalate excretion—relevant for those with oxalate sensitivity or kidney stone history. Use buffered forms only. Citrus-derived vitamin C may cause reactions in patients with citrus sensitivity—choose non-citrus-derived sources. Fermented sources (from corn/citrus) may contain trace amounts of mold or high-histamine byproducts that sensitive people cannot tolerate.

DAO Enzyme Supplement | *Supplementing the Gut's Histamine Drain*

Form: Diamine oxidase derived from porcine kidney (most common commercial source) or pea sprouts. Products include Histamine Block (Seeking Health), Histamine Digest (Seeking Health), DAOsin, DAOfood, DAOfood Plus, DAOfood Veg (from pea sprouts), milDAO (pea sprouts), NaturDAO (pea sprouts), and Vegan DAO Enzyme (Solaray; pea sprouts). Verify porcine source is appropriate for your dietary requirements.

Dose: One to two capsules per dose. Most commercial products are standardized to 0.3 mg of DAO activity per capsule. Dose is consistent across brands regardless of stated weight—HDU activity units matter more than milligrams. Some brands contain 1,000,000 HDU, which is very high potency; while others are a low potency 20,000 to 60,000 HDUs.

Timing: Fifteen minutes before any meal that contains histamine-contributing foods. Not a daily supplement—used situationally before histamine-containing meals rather than at every meal.

With Food? Take before meals, not with them. The enzyme must be present in the gut lumen when histamine arrives from the meal. Taking with food delays gastric emptying and may reduce effectiveness.

Start Low: Begin with one capsule before a histamine-relevant meal per day and observe the response over a week before using more frequently. Some people notice immediate improvement; others need several weeks of consistent use.

Cautions: Porcine-derived—not appropriate for those avoiding pork products. DAO supplements reduce histamine from dietary sources but do not address internally produced histamine from gut dysbiosis (SIBO, Candida) or mast cell degranulation. They are a bridge measure, not a substitute for gut healing. Do not take simultaneously with metformin, certain antidepressants, or aspirin, which impair DAO activity.

Magnesium Glycinate | *Natural Calcium Channel Blocker and Nervous System Support*

Form: Magnesium glycinate (also sold as magnesium bisglycinate). This form is the most absorbable and the least likely to cause loose stools of any magnesium form. Avoid magnesium oxide (poor absorption) and magnesium citrate (laxative effect at therapeutic doses). Magnesium malate is an acceptable alternative with additional mitochondrial support properties.

Dose: Target: 200–400 mg elemental magnesium daily. Most glycinate supplements provide 100–200 mg elemental magnesium per capsule—check the elemental magnesium content, not the total compound weight.

Timing: Evening, thirty to sixty minutes before bed. Magnesium's calming effects support both nervous system wind-down and sleep quality at this timing. Can be split between morning and evening if the full dose causes excessive sedation.

With Food? Can be taken with or without food. Taking with a small meal reduces the small risk of GI discomfort at higher doses.

Start Low: Begin at 100 mg elemental magnesium in the evening. Increase to 200 mg after one week if well tolerated. Loose stools are the clearest signal that the dose exceeds current magnesium tolerance—reduce by 50 mg per day.

Cautions: Individuals with kidney disease or kidney insufficiency should consult a physician before supplementing magnesium. May potentiate the effect of magnesium-depleting medications (omeprazole, esomeprazole, tetracycline, furosemide, prednisone, hydrocortisone). Monitor for excessive sedation at higher doses, particularly when combined with other calming supplements.

Luteolin | *CNS-Penetrating Mast Cell Stabilizer*

Form: Luteolin supplements are available as pure luteolin capsules or as combination products with quercetin (luteolin-quercetin complexes). Luteolin from chamomile extract is also available. Look for products from reputable manufacturers with third-party testing. NeuroProtek (a liposomal luteolin-quercetin product) has clinical research behind it specifically for mast cell and neuroinflammatory conditions.

Dose: Target: 100–200 mg daily. Higher doses (up to 400 mg) are used in some clinical protocols under practitioner guidance.

Timing: Before the largest meal of the day. Some practitioners recommend morning administration to support daytime cognitive function given luteolin's CNS-penetrating properties.

With Food? Take with light food or on an empty stomach. Taking with a small amount of fat enhances absorption of this lipophilic flavonoid.

Start Low: Start at 100 mg once daily. Luteolin is generally very well tolerated even in reactive individuals, but the standard introduction protocol applies.

Cautions: May potentiate the effects of cannabidiol (CBD) through shared metabolic pathways (CYP450 enzymes)—reduce CBD dose if combining. Possible mild interactions with certain blood-thinning medications at high doses. Generally considered one of the best-tolerated mast cell supplements available.

Omega-3 Fatty Acids (EPA and DHA) | *Membrane Stabilizer and Resolution Promoter*

Form: Triglyceride-form fish oil or algae-derived omega-3s (the preferred choice for those avoiding fish products). Triglyceride form is significantly better absorbed than ethyl ester form. Look for products tested for oxidation (low TOTOX score) and heavy metals. Enteric-coated capsules reduce fishy reflux. Algae-based DHA/EPA avoids fish entirely and is appropriate for individuals with fish reactions.

Dose: Target: 1,000–2,000 mg combined EPA + DHA daily. Check the label for EPA + DHA content specifically—total fish oil weight is not the relevant number. A typical 1,000 mg fish oil capsule may contain only 300 mg of combined EPA + DHA.

Timing: With the largest meal of the day. Omega-3 absorption requires dietary fat present in the gut—taking on an empty stomach significantly reduces bioavailability.

With Food? Always with a fat-containing meal. Non-negotiable for meaningful absorption.

Start Low: Begin at 500 mg EPA+DHA daily with the main meal. Step to 1,000 mg after one week. Occasionally people with fish sensitivity react to fish-derived omega-3s; algae-based products are the appropriate alternative.

Cautions: At doses above 3,000 mg/day, omega-3s have blood-thinning effects—inform your physician if on anticoagulants. Fish-derived products may cause reactions in those with MCAS and fish protein sensitivity—use algae-based alternatives. Check product freshness: oxidized fish oil smells strongly rancid and should be discarded.

Vitamin D3 (with K2 and preferably magnesium) | *Mast Cell Regulator and Immune Tolerance Promoter*

Form: Vitamin D3 (cholecalciferol) in oil-based softgel capsules or drops—oil-based forms have significantly better absorption than dry tablets. Always pair with vitamin K2 (MK-7 form, 100–200 mcg daily) to direct calcium to bones rather than soft tissues. Combined D3+K2 products are widely available and convenient. Magnesium is also essential for the absorption and metabolism of vitamin D—without it vitamin D remains inactive in the body.

Dose: Maintenance: 1,000–2,000 IU daily for those with adequate levels. Repletion for deficiency: 5,000–10,000 IU daily under blood level monitoring. Optimal 25-OH vitamin D levels for MCAS management are generally considered to be 50–80 ng/mL (125–200 nmol/L)—higher than the conventional sufficiency threshold of 30 ng/mL.

Timing: With the largest meal of the day, ideally containing dietary fat.

With Food? Always with a fat-containing meal for optimal absorption of this fat-soluble vitamin.

Start Low: If blood levels are unknown, begin at 1,000–2,000 IU daily and test levels at three months before adjusting. Do not begin high-dose vitamin D repletion without knowing your baseline level.

Cautions: Test 25-OH vitamin D levels before and during supplementation. High-dose vitamin D without K2 can lead to inappropriate calcium deposition in the cardiovascular system. Hypercalcemia (rare at typical supplemental doses) causes fatigue, nausea, and confusion—signs to watch for at doses above 5,000 IU daily.

Probiotics (Strain-Specific) | *Microbiome Rehabilitation—With Critical Strain Selection*

Form: Multi-strain capsule products containing only histamine-neutral or histamine-degrading strains. As established in Chapter 6, strain selection is critical: avoid any product containing *Lactobacillus casei, Lactobacillus reuteri, Lactobacillus bulgaricus, or Lactobacillus delbrueckii,* which are histamine producers. Recommended strains: *Lactobacillus rhamnosus* GG or ATCC 53103, *Bifidobacterium longum, Bifidobacterium infantis, Lactobacillus salivarius, Lactobacillus plantarum.* Two products to consider are ProBiota HistaminX (Seeking Health) and Low Histamine Probiotics (VitaMonk; more affordable).

Dose: 10–50 billion CFU daily. More is not necessarily better—consistent use of appropriate strains at moderate doses is more important than very high CFU counts.

Timing: Morning, right before breakfast. Take at least two hours away from antibiotics or antifungal medications.

With Food? Can be taken with or without food. Some evidence suggests gastric acid transit is improved with a small amount of food.

Start Low: Begin with a low-dose single-strain product (*Lactobacillus rhamnosus* or *Bifidobacterium longum* alone) before introducing multi-strain combinations. Introduce probiotics in Stage 2 support, not during acute stabilization. Bloating, gas, or increased reactivity suggests either the wrong strain or introduction too early in the healing process.

Cautions: Histamine-producing strains will worsen symptoms regardless of other benefits attributed to them. Read every ingredient on probiotic labels. If GI symptoms worsen after introducing a probiotic, discontinue and reassess before reintroducing a different strain. *Saccharomyces boulardii* (a beneficial yeast) is an alternative well tolerated by many people with MCAS that avoids the histamine-production question altogether.

L-Glutamine | *Gut Barrier Repair—The First Building Block*

Form: Pure L-glutamine powder is the most economical and flexible form. Unflavored powder dissolves easily in water. Capsules are available but require large numbers for therapeutic doses. Avoid flavored products with artificial additives that may trigger mast cells.

Dose: Target: 2,500–5,000 mg daily, divided into two doses. Some gut-healing protocols use up to 10,000 mg during active repair phases under practitioner supervision. *Note: High-dose glutamine (> 5,000 mg/day) can be a powerful tool for sealing a "leaky gut," which helps reduce the overall number of triggers reaching your mast cells. However, because it can convert into an excitatory brain chemical called glutamate, it is vital to start with a smaller amount to ensure it doesn't cause anxiety, insomnia, or a symptom flare.*

Timing: Between meals on an empty stomach for optimal enterocyte uptake. The gut epithelium uses glutamine as a primary fuel source and uptake is most efficient when not competing with a meal.

With Food? Empty stomach preferred. If GI discomfort occurs, a small amount of water or light food is acceptable.

Start Low: Begin at 1,000 mg once daily between meals. Increase to 2,500 mg divided twice daily after one week. L-glutamine is generally very well tolerated but can occasionally worsen symptoms in individuals with significant gut dysbiosis—begin during early Stage 2 support rather than acute stabilization.

Cautions: L-glutamine converts to glutamate in the body; avoid or use with caution in individuals with known glutamate sensitivity, a history of seizures, or severe hepatic encephalopathy. Not appropriate for individuals with a history of liver disease without physician guidance. Very rarely, individuals with MCAS notice an increase in mast cell reactivity—discontinue and reassess if this occurs.

Zinc Carnosine (PepZin GI) | *Gut Lining Repair and Anti-Ulcer Support*

Form: Zinc carnosine (polaprezinc), sold as PepZin GI by several manufacturers, or as a branded supplement. Standard dose product contains 75 mg zinc carnosine (providing approximately 16 mg elemental zinc). This is a chelated form specifically designed for gut mucosal repair—it is not the same as taking zinc and carnosine separately.

Dose: 75 mg zinc carnosine (providing approximately 16 mg elemental zinc) once or twice daily. Most clinical research uses 75 mg twice daily for active gut repair.

Timing: Before meals or at bedtime. Some protocols prefer bedtime administration to support overnight mucosal repair when gut motility is reduced.

With Food? Can be taken with or without food. Taking before a meal allows the compound to coat the gut lining before food-related acid and enzymatic activity begins.

Start Low: Begin once daily at 75 mg. Well tolerated by most individuals. Step to twice daily after two weeks if gut repair support is a priority.

Cautions: Long-term zinc supplementation (beyond three to six months) at doses providing more than 40 mg elemental zinc daily may deplete copper—supplement with 1–

2 mg copper daily if using zinc carnosine long-term. Do not exceed recommended doses. If already taking a zinc-containing multivitamin or other zinc supplement, account for total zinc intake.

Vitamin B6 (Pyridoxal-5-Phosphate / P5P) | *DAO Cofactor, Methylation Support, and Neurotransmitter Production*

Form: Pyridoxal-5-phosphate (P5P) is the active, already-converted form of B6. Avoid pyridoxine hydrochloride (the most common synthetic form in supplements) if MTHFR impairment or poor B6 conversion is suspected. P5P does not require hepatic conversion and is the preferred form for people with MCAS.

Dose: Target: 25–50 mg P5P daily. DAO enzyme support and neurotransmitter synthesis are achieved at these doses. Higher doses (50–200 mg) are used for specific conditions under practitioner guidance.

Timing: With meals. B vitamins are best taken with food to reduce the small risk of nausea.

With Food? Always with food.

Start Low: Begin at 10–25 mg daily. B6 in the P5P form is generally well tolerated. Some individuals with MTHFR variants notice significant improvement in anxiety and mood within days of B6 supplementation.

Cautions: High-dose pyridoxine (above 200 mg/day of the pyridoxine form—not P5P) has been associated with peripheral neuropathy. At P5P doses of 25–50 mg daily, this risk is negligible. P5P supports the conversion of 5-HTP to serotonin—use caution if taking SSRI medications. Pair with magnesium for synergistic DAO enzyme support.

✦ ✦ ✦

Quick Reference: Daily Protocol Summary

The table below consolidates the key practical details for each supplement in one place. Use it as your daily cheat sheet once you have established your personal protocol. Supplements are listed in recommended introduction order.

Supplement	Dose	Timing	With Food?	Key Caution
Quercetin	125–500 mg, 2–3x daily	20–30 min before meals	Empty stomach preferred	May interact with fluoroquinolone antibiotics and blood thinners; start at 125 mg
Vitamin C (buffered)	250–1,000 mg, 2x daily	With meals	With food to reduce GI upset	Use buffered (calcium or magnesium ascorbate), not plain ascorbic acid; reduce if loose stools

Supplement	Dose	Timing	With Food?	Key Caution
DAO Enzyme	1 capsule per meal	15 min before eating	Before histamine-containing meals only	Porcine-derived—not suitable for pork restrictions; does not replace gut healing
Magnesium Glycinate	100–400 mg daily	Evening, 30–60 min before bed	With or without food	Start at 100 mg; loose stools indicate dose is too high; avoid oxide form
Luteolin	100–200 mg daily	Before largest meal	Empty stomach or light food	May potentiate cannabidiol (CBD) effects; very well tolerated overall
Omega-3 (EPA/DHA)	1,000–2,000 mg EPA+DHA daily	With meals	Always with a fat-containing meal	Use enteric-coated if fishy burp is a concern; check freshness/oxidation of product
Vitamin D3	1,000–5,000 IU daily	With largest meal	Always with a fat-containing meal	Pair with vitamin K2 (100–200 mcg). Test levels before high-dose supplementation
Probiotic (selected strains)	Per label	Morning, away from antibiotics	Can be with or without food	Use only histamine-neutral/degrading strains (*L. rhamnosus, B. longum*); avoid *L. casei, L. reuteri*
L-Glutamine	2,500–5,000 mg daily	Away from meals on empty stomach	Empty stomach for gut uptake	Avoid if history of seizures or glutamate sensitivity; start at 1,000 mg
Zinc Carnosine	75 mg (as PepZin GI) daily	Before meals or at bedtime	Can be taken with or without food	Do not exceed 40 mg elemental zinc long-term; supplement copper if using long-term
Vitamin B6 (P5P)	25–50 mg daily	With meals	With food to prevent nausea	Use active P5P form, not pyridoxine; high doses (>200 mg) can cause neuropathy

> **Important:** *This table reflects therapeutic targets for established protocols. Always begin at the lower starting doses described in the individual profiles above and step up gradually. Work with a practitioner familiar with MCAS when managing multiple supplements simultaneously or when taking prescription medications.*

◆ ◆ ◆

Deeper Dive: Building Your Supplement Stack Intelligently

For the Science-Minded Reader

Understanding how the supplements in this chapter work together—and why their combined effect exceeds what any single compound can achieve—helps make supplement choices feel strategic rather than arbitrary.

The Three Layers of the Supplement Protocol

The supplements in this chapter address mast cell stabilization at three distinct biological layers, and a complete protocol includes representation from each.

The first layer is direct mast cell stabilization: compounds that act on the mast cell itself to reduce degranulation probability, block histamine receptor signaling, or suppress mediator release. Quercetin, luteolin, and omega-3 fatty acids are the primary agents at this layer. Together they cover multiple mast cell activation pathways—IgE-mediated, non-IgE receptor-mediated, and membrane-based—providing broader stabilization than any single compound alone.

The second layer is systemic environment modification: compounds that change the biochemical environment in which mast cells operate, reducing the priming signals that keep thresholds chronically low. Vitamin D modulates immune tolerance and mast cell receptor expression. Vitamin C degrades circulating histamine and supports cortisol synthesis. Magnesium reduces the calcium-channel sensitivity that lowers the degranulation threshold. B6 supports both histamine clearance (via DAO cofactor function) and nervous system neurotransmitter balance. Together these compounds create a less inflammatory, less primed environment across the whole body—not just at the mast cell surface.

The third layer is gut and barrier support: compounds that address the chronic subepithelial mast cell activation driven by intestinal permeability, described in Chapter 6. L-glutamine, zinc carnosine, and strain-specific probiotics work at this layer, repairing the gut architecture and microbiome balance that perpetuate chronic low-grade immune activation. DAO enzyme supplements support this layer by improving histamine clearance capacity at the gut level while the underlying gut healing proceeds.

Synergistic Combinations Worth Knowing

Several specific combinations within this protocol have documented synergistic effects that are worth understanding. Quercetin and luteolin together provide broader flavonoid mast cell coverage than either alone; quercetin is more potent at IgE-receptor blockade while luteolin provides superior CNS penetration and

Kit-pathway inhibition. Taking them together, whether in a combined product or separately within a few hours of each other, provides complementary coverage.

Vitamin C and quercetin have a well-documented mutual stabilization effect; vitamin C prevents quercetin oxidation in the gut, extending its activity, while quercetin regenerates oxidized vitamin C back to its active reduced form. Taking both together—as occurs when eating quercetin-rich foods alongside vitamin C–rich foods—amplifies the antihistamine effect of both compounds. This is one reason that the combined dietary and supplemental approach outperforms either alone.

Magnesium and B6 work synergistically for both DAO enzyme activity and nervous system regulation. DAO requires both copper and B6 as cofactors; magnesium supports the neuromuscular calm that allows the parasympathetic nervous system to suppress mast cell activation through the vagal pathway. Together, they address histamine clearance and autonomic regulation as a coupled intervention.

L-glutamine and zinc carnosine together address gut barrier repair through complementary mechanisms: glutamine provides the primary fuel and building block for enterocyte renewal and tight junction protein synthesis, while zinc carnosine coats and stabilizes the mucosal surface and accelerates ulcer and erosion healing. Using both during the gut repair phase of Stage 2 support produces more rapid and more complete barrier restoration than either alone.

◆ ◆ ◆

What This Means for You: Building Your Personal Protocol

Translating the supplement profiles and reference table into a personal daily protocol requires knowing your own priorities—which biological layers most need support given your specific root causes, symptom pattern, and current stage in the stabilization–support–repair–rebuild framework.

Stage 1 (Stabilization): Start with quercetin only. During the stabilization phase, quercetin is the most appropriate single supplement to introduce first. It is the most broadly effective, the most directly relevant to acute mast cell stabilization, and among the best-tolerated natural compounds available. Begin at 125 mg and increase over two to three weeks. Introduce nothing else until quercetin is established and your response is known.

Add vitamin C and magnesium in Stage 1 to 2 transition. Once quercetin is established, buffered vitamin C is typically the second addition. Its synergistic interaction with quercetin makes the combination particularly valuable, and its dual role as antihistamine and DAO cofactor addresses two dimensions simultaneously. Magnesium glycinate follows shortly after—its nervous system and sleep benefits overlap with the neurological and sleep support being built through the Chapter 14 practices, creating a biochemical complement to those practices.

Introduce gut-healing compounds in Stage 2. L-glutamine and zinc carnosine belong in Stage 2 support once the stabilization baseline is established. Their effectiveness depends on an adequately reduced mast cell load—introducing them into an acutely reactive gut may not produce the expected benefit because the inflammatory environment prevents effective mucosal repair. Introduce them after three to four weeks of established stabilization-phase management, one at a time.

Add luteolin, vitamin D, and omega-3s as secondary foundations. These are important long-term compounds rather than acute stabilizers. Vitamin D levels should ideally be tested before supplementation to calibrate the dose. Omega-3s require consistent daily use over weeks to produce membrane incorporation effects—introduce them steadily and commit to them for at least three months before assessing their contribution. Luteolin can be introduced whenever quercetin is well established.

Introduce probiotics last among the primary supplements. Probiotics are not Stage 1 interventions in most cases. A reactive, dysbiotic gut is not ready to be reshaped by new bacterial populations—it needs the initial gut-healing work of L-glutamine and zinc carnosine first. Introduce strain-specific probiotics after four to eight weeks of gut-healing support, with particular attention to strain selection and gradual dose escalation.

Use DAO enzymes situationally rather than daily. DAO enzymes are a practical situational tool—used before meals that carry histamine risk rather than as a daily foundation supplement. This keeps costs manageable, preserves the supplement's practical value for the situations where it is most needed, and avoids the false confidence of relying on DAO supplementation as a substitute for the gut-healing work that will eventually make them less necessary.

A Note on Low-Dose Naltrexone

Among the options that come up repeatedly in MCAS-aware functional medicine and integrative practices, low-dose naltrexone—commonly abbreviated LDN—deserves a brief, honest mention, even though it falls outside the "supplement" category. This is not a natural remedy. It is a pharmaceutical agent, available only by prescription, and any consideration of it belongs in a conversation with a knowledgeable practitioner. But because many individuals with MCAS will encounter it in their research, understanding what it is and why it generates interest is worth addressing directly.

Standard naltrexone (50 mg) is an FDA-approved opioid antagonist used in addiction medicine. At a fraction of that dose—typically between 1.5 and 4.5 mg, taken at bedtime—it appears to exert a distinctly different set of effects on the immune system. This is the off-label application known as low-dose naltrexone, and it has been explored clinically for a range of chronic inflammatory and autoimmune conditions, including fibromyalgia, Crohn's disease, multiple sclerosis, and—more recently—MCAS and related dysautonomia presentations.

How it may help. The proposed mechanisms are still being studied, and LDN should be understood as an emerging clinical tool rather than an established therapy. That said, the current hypotheses are biologically coherent. At low doses, transient opioid receptor blockade appears to trigger a compensatory upregulation of the body's endogenous opioid system, which has downstream anti-inflammatory effects. Of particular relevance to MCAS, LDN has been proposed to modulate microglial and mast cell activity through TLR4 (toll-like receptor 4) antagonism—a mechanism distinct from opioid receptor effects entirely. TLR4 is a pattern recognition receptor expressed on mast cells that, when activated by bacterial components, stress signals, or inflammatory mediators, contributes to mast cell priming. By dampening TLR4 signaling, LDN may help reduce baseline reactivity in sensitized immune cells. Additionally, its effects on reducing neuroinflammation and modulating the central nervous system mast cell burden may explain why some individuals report improvements in brain fog, anxiety, and systemic reactivity.

What the clinical picture looks like. Formal randomized controlled trials specifically in MCAS are lacking as of this writing, and that is an important caveat. What exists is a growing body of case reports, practitioner clinical observations, and mechanistic rationale suggesting benefit in a subset of individuals—particularly those with prominent neurological symptoms, nervous system dysregulation, or refractory reactivity that has not responded adequately to foundational approaches. Some practitioners working with MCAS and hEDS/dysautonomia populations have incorporated LDN into Stage 2 and Stage 3 protocols, observing that it appears best tolerated once some degree of stabilization has already been achieved. Starting too early—in a highly reactive, unstabilized system—may be poorly tolerated.

If you're considering it. LDN requires a prescription and a prescribing provider who understands its off-label use and its nuances in the context of MCAS. Compounding pharmacies typically prepare it, as the low doses are not commercially available in standard formulations. Fillers in compounded preparations matter for sensitive individuals—request filler-free or simple formulations when possible. Begin at the lowest available dose and increase only gradually, as even low-dose naltrexone can produce sleep disturbance or vivid dreams in the initial weeks of use. It is contraindicated in individuals currently using opioid medications.

LDN is not a shortcut and not a replacement for the foundational work this book describes. For some individuals, it may become a useful part of a broader protocol. For others, it may not be appropriate or necessary. What it represents, most usefully, is an example of the expanding toolkit available when foundational stabilization and support have been established—and of the importance of working with practitioners who are both current with emerging evidence and attentive to the specific biology of mast cell reactivity.

Diane's cupboard looked very different eighteen months after that first conversation with her practitioner. Not because she had more supplements—in fact, she had fewer. She had quercetin, magnesium, vitamin C, luteolin, L-glutamine, zinc carnosine, vitamin D3 with K2, and a single strain probiotic she had been taking consistently for eight months. She knew exactly what each one was for. Her practitioner guided her when to introduce each one and what she should notice. She had discarded the supplements that had failed her personal assessment and kept the ones she could trace to specific improvements.

"This is so much simpler," she said. "I know what I'm doing and why."

That—knowing what you are doing and why—is the foundation of an effective supplement protocol. Not more bottles. Better information, better sequencing, and the patience to build knowledge one careful introduction at a time.

✦ ✦ ✦

Chapter 16 at a Glance

What to Remember:

- The golden rule of MCAS supplementation is one compound at a time, starting low, with five to seven days of observation before adding the next. This is not slow—it is the only approach that produces usable information about what is helping.
- Quercetin is the cornerstone mast cell stabilizer: it acts through at least four molecular mechanisms simultaneously and is the appropriate first supplement to introduce during the stabilization phase. Begin at 125 mg and step up gradually.

- Buffered vitamin C (calcium or magnesium ascorbate) directly degrades circulating histamine, supports DAO enzyme function, and has synergistic effects with quercetin. Avoid plain ascorbic acid in reactive individuals.
- DAO enzyme supplements are situational tools—used before histamine-containing meals rather than as daily foundations—that supplement gut histamine clearance capacity while deeper gut healing proceeds. They are a bridge, not a destination.
- Magnesium glycinate at 200–400 mg in the evening supports mast cell regulation (calcium channel blocking), nervous system calming, and sleep quality simultaneously. It is one of the most broadly beneficial supplements in the MCAS protocol.
- The supplement protocol addresses three biological layers: direct mast cell stabilization (quercetin, luteolin, omega-3s), systemic environment modification (vitamin D, vitamin C, magnesium, B6), and gut barrier repair (L-glutamine, zinc carnosine, probiotics). A complete protocol includes representation from all three layers.
- Probiotic strain selection is critical: histamine-producing strains (*L. casei, L. reuteri, L. bulgaricus*) worsen MCAS regardless of their other benefits. Use only histamine-neutral or histamine-degrading strains, introduced after initial gut-healing work is underway.
- The supplement introduction order generally follows: quercetin (Stage 1) → vitamin C + magnesium (Stage 1–2 transition) → L-glutamine + zinc carnosine (Stage 2) → luteolin + vitamin D + omega-3s (Stage 2 ongoing) → probiotics (Stage 2, after gut preparation).

Coming Up in Chapter 17:

Supplements work from the inside—providing concentrated doses of compounds that food cannot deliver in sufficient therapeutic quantities. Herbal medicine works from a different angle: using whole plant preparations that combine multiple active constituents in the ratios nature assembled, often producing effects that isolated compounds cannot fully replicate. Chapter 17 explores the herbal medicines with the strongest evidence for MCAS support—nettles, skullcap, chamomile, and the adaptogenic herbs—covering their mechanisms, forms, dosing, and how they fit into a comprehensive natural MCAS protocol.

CHAPTER 17

Herbal Medicine

Nettles, Skullcap, Adaptogens, and the Plants That Support Mast Cell Calm

The Medicine That Predates the Pharmacy

Long before pharmaceutical antihistamines were synthesized, before mast cells had been named or their role in inflammation understood, people were reaching for stinging nettles when their noses ran and their skin erupted. They were brewing chamomile for nervous stomachs and sleepless nights. They were using skullcaps to quiet the anxious, overactivated mind. They had discovered, through centuries of observation, what modern research is now confirming in molecular detail: certain plants carry within them a remarkable capacity to support the body's healing processes.

Herbal medicine in MCAS is not nostalgia. It is not a rejection of science in favor of tradition. It is the recognition that whole plant preparations—containing hundreds of interacting constituents—sometimes achieve effects that isolated pharmaceutical compounds do not, and do so with a safety and tolerability profile that allows them to be used by even the most reactive individuals. The difference between a pharmaceutical antihistamine and freeze-dried stinging nettle leaf is not that one is real and the other imagined—it is that one blocks a single receptor through a single mechanism, while the other modulates multiple pathways simultaneously through a combination of compounds that evolved together.

That said, herbal medicine in MCAS requires the same disciplined approach as supplement medicine. Herbs are bioactive compounds that can trigger reactions in a sensitized system, and the history of MCAS management is full of people who reacted to "natural" remedies they assumed were automatically safe because they came from plants. The introduction protocol from Chapter 16 applies fully here: one herb at a time, at a low starting dose, with careful observation before adding anything further.

This chapter covers the herbs with the strongest evidence and clinical track record for MCAS support—organized into two groups: the anti-histamine and mast-cell-stabilizing herbs, and the adaptogenic herbs that address the adrenal and nervous system dimensions of chronic mast cell dysregulation.

✦ ✦ ✦

How Herbs Work Differently From Isolated Compounds

Understanding why herbal medicine occupies its own chapter—rather than simply being listed alongside supplements—requires appreciating a concept called the entourage effect: the way that multiple compounds within a whole plant preparation interact synergistically to produce effects that exceed what any single constituent achieves alone.

Chamomile provides a useful illustration. Chamomile's anti-inflammatory and calming effects have been attributed to apigenin, its primary flavonoid—and indeed, isolated apigenin does produce anti-inflammatory and GABA-receptor modulating effects in research models.[334] But chamomile's clinical effects are attributed to the combined activity of multiple compounds—including apigenin, other flavonoids, and volatile oils—rather than a single isolated constituent.[335] The other constituents—bisabolol, matricin, quercetin glycosides, luteolin, and chamazulene—modulate the bioavailability of apigenin, modify its receptor interactions, and contribute independent mechanisms that apigenin alone cannot provide. The plant is, quite literally, greater than the sum of its measurable parts.

This is why standardization in herbal medicine is important but not sufficient. A chamomile extract standardized to apigenin content is a better-controlled product than an unstandardized extract, but it is still a whole-plant preparation whose full activity depends on the complete constituent profile. The standardization marker is a quality indicator, not a description of the complete mechanism.

> **Safety First:** *Herbal medicines are not automatically safe because they are natural. Some herbs interact with medications. Some are contraindicated in pregnancy or specific health conditions. Some products are adulterated with misidentified species or contaminants. Sourcing matters enormously—purchase from reputable manufacturers with third-party testing and clear botanical identification. The cautions in each herb profile below are not exhaustive; always inform your healthcare providers about herbs you are using.*

The herbs in this chapter are divided into two functional categories. The first group—antihistamine and mast-cell-stabilizing herbs—works most directly on the mast cell and histamine pathway. The second group—adaptogens and nervous system modulators—addresses the HPA axis, adrenal function, and autonomic regulation that indirectly but powerfully shape mast cell reactivity through the mechanisms described in Chapters 9 and 10. Both categories have a place in a comprehensive MCAS herbal protocol.

✦ ✦ ✦

Antihistamine and Mast Cell–Stabilizing Herbs

The following herbs have documented antihistamine, anti-inflammatory, or mast cell–stabilizing properties in peer-reviewed research, combined with a clinical track record in MCAS and histamine intolerance populations. Each is presented in the same structured format used in Chapter 16.

Stinging Nettle (*Urtica dioica*) | *Nature's Antihistamine*

Standardization: Freeze-dried leaf is the essential form—not dried or cooked nettle. The freeze-drying process preserves the natural antihistamine compounds (including lectins and histamine-modulating constituents) that are destroyed by heat drying or cooking. Look for products specifically labeled freeze-dried leaf. Standardized extract products are also available, sometimes standardized to plant silica or chlorophyll content as quality markers.

Dose: 300–600 mg of freeze-dried leaf extract, two to three times daily. Some protocols use up to 1,200 mg daily during acute flares. Nettle tea, while pleasant, uses heat-processed nettle and does not deliver the same freeze-dried leaf activity.

Timing: Before meals. Taking nettle before eating may help blunt the histamine load from the meal itself. Spacing doses through the day maintains more consistent antihistamine coverage than a single daily dose.

With Food? Preferred on an empty stomach or twenty minutes before meals for maximum anti-allergic effect. Can be taken with food if GI sensitivity occurs—absorption is only mildly reduced.

Start Low: Begin at 300 mg once daily for the first week. Increase to twice daily in week two. Most individuals find freeze-dried nettle very well tolerated from the beginning, but the standard introduction protocol applies. Occasionally, people with significant histamine burden notice a brief initial worsening—if so, reduce to 150 mg and step up more slowly.

Cautions: Stinging nettle has mild diuretic properties—maintain adequate hydration. May contribute to blood pressure lowering—monitor if on antihypertensive medications. Avoid in significant kidney disease. Ensure the product is freeze-dried leaf specifically; dried nettle has markedly reduced activity and is not an appropriate substitute. Rare allergic reactions to nettle plant proteins are possible in highly sensitive individuals—patch test or begin at a very low dose.

Chinese/Baikal Skullcap (*Scutellaria baicalensis*) | *Baicalin, Neuroinflammation, and Mast Cell Membrane Stabilization*

Standardization: Chinese skullcap (*Scutellaria baicalensis*) is the species with the most extensive MCAS-relevant research—not American skullcap (*Scutellaria lateriflora*), which has a different constituent profile and is primarily used for anxiety. Look for products standardized to baicalin content (the primary active flavonoid), typically 85–95 percent baicalin in concentrated extracts. Third-party testing for adulteration is important—skullcap has been adulterated with germander (Teucrium) in some markets, which is toxic to the liver.

Dose: Take 200–400 mg of standardized skullcap extract, one to two times daily. Baicalin is the primary mast cell–stabilizing constituent, demonstrating inhibition of IgE-mediated degranulation, suppression of TNF-alpha and IL-6, and direct anti-inflammatory effects in the brain.[336] Some practitioners use whole root products at 1,000–3,000 mg daily.

Timing: Morning and/or midday. Skullcap's baicalin has a relatively short half-life—dividing doses provides more consistent coverage. Evening dosing is appropriate for people using it for its calming and neuroinflammatory effects rather than as a primary antihistamine.

With Food? It can be taken with or without food. Taking with food reduces the small risk of GI upset, particularly with higher doses of concentrated extracts.

Start Low: Begin at 200 mg once daily. Skullcap is generally well tolerated, but baicalin can interact with CYP450 drug metabolism—start low if taking multiple medications and observe carefully. Increase to twice daily after one week if well tolerated.

Cautions: CRITICAL: Verify the product is *Scutellaria baicalensis* and has been tested for Teucrium adulteration—adulterated skullcap products have caused hepatotoxicity. Purchase only from reputable manufacturers with botanical verification and third-party testing. Baicalin inhibits certain CYP450 enzymes and may affect metabolism of medications cleared by these pathways—inform your physician and pharmacist. Avoid in pregnancy. Rare reports of mild sedation at higher doses.

Chamomile (*Matricaria chamomilla / Chamaemelum nobile*) | *Gentle, Broad-Spectrum, and Exceptionally Well Tolerated*

Standardization: German chamomile (*Matricaria chamomilla*) and Roman chamomile (*Chamaemelum nobile*) have overlapping but slightly different constituent profiles. German chamomile is more studied and contains higher levels of the anti-inflammatory azulene compound chamazulene; Roman chamomile is slightly sweeter and often preferred for tea. For supplements, look for standardized German chamomile extracts standardized to apigenin content (typically 1.2 percent). Chamomile tea from whole dried flowers is also genuinely therapeutic and highly accessible.

Dose: Tea: one to two teaspoons of dried chamomile flowers per cup, steeped covered for ten minutes to preserve volatile oils, one to three cups daily. Extract: 250–500 mg of standardized extract daily. As a tincture: 3–5 mL of a 1:5 tincture, two to three times daily.

Timing: Evening is the primary clinical timing for chamomile's sleep-supporting and nervous system calming effects. A cup of chamomile tea thirty to sixty minutes before bed is one of the most practical and pleasant additions to an MCAS evening routine. Daytime use for gut calming and anxiety support is also appropriate.

With Food? Tea can be consumed any time. Supplements can be taken with or without food. Taking chamomile tea after meals supports its carminative (gas-relieving) and gut-motility calming effects.

Start Low: Chamomile is among the gentlest herbs used in MCAS, and reactions to therapeutic amounts are uncommon. Begin with a daily cup of chamomile tea before introducing extract supplements, observing for several days. Occasionally, individuals with ragweed allergy react to chamomile—if you have known ragweed sensitivity, introduce very cautiously.

Cautions: Chamomile belongs to the Asteraceae (daisy/ragweed) plant family. Individuals with ragweed allergy or confirmed Asteraceae hypersensitivity should introduce chamomile cautiously or avoid it. High-dose chamomile extract may mildly potentiate blood-thinning medications. Chamomile has mild estrogenic activity—clinically insignificant at typical doses but worth noting for those with estrogen-sensitive conditions. Generally among the safest herbs available for MCAS patients.

Perilla (*Perilla frutescens*) | *Rosmarinic Acid and Leukotriene Suppression*

Standardization: Perilla leaf extract standardized to rosmarinic acid content (typically 5–20 percent rosmarinic acid). Rosmarinic acid is a key active constituent of perilla responsible for much of its antihistamine and anti-inflammatory (including leukotriene-modulating) effects.[337] Some products are available as perilla seed oil (rich in alpha-linolenic acid, an omega-3 precursor), which has a complementary but somewhat different mechanism. Perilla leaf is also available as a culinary herb and is a standard component of Japanese cuisine—the culinary use provides modest dietary rosmarinic acid exposure.

Dose: Take 50–200 mg of standardized perilla extract (rosmarinic acid content) daily. Clinical studies in seasonal allergy have used doses equivalent to approximately 50 mg rosmarinic acid daily with significant effect on histamine and leukotriene levels.[338]

Timing: With meals or before meals. Rosmarinic acid's antihistamine and anti-leukotriene effects appear at relatively low concentrations and are maintained with consistent daily use rather than requiring strategic timing around triggers.

With Food? Can be taken with or without food. With food is slightly preferred for tolerability.

Start Low: Begin at 50 mg daily. Perilla is generally very well tolerated among people with MCAS and is an excellent option for individuals who react to many other supplements, given its gentle profile.

Cautions: Generally very well tolerated with no significant known interactions at therapeutic doses. Rare GI upset at higher doses. Avoid perilla seed oil if allergic to seeds. Rosmarinic acid is also present in rosemary, basil, mint, and sage; people who react to these herbs should introduce perilla cautiously.

Butterbur (*Petasites hybridus*) | *Clinical-Grade Antihistamine Activity — PA-Free Only*

Standardization: This herb requires the most stringent sourcing requirements of any herb in this chapter. Raw butterbur plant contains pyrrolizidine alkaloids (PAs), which are toxic to the liver. Only PA-free certified butterbur extracts are safe for use. The well-studied Tesalin (Ze 339) and Petaforce products are standardized PA-free extracts with clinical trial data behind them. Do not use any butterbur product that is not explicitly certified PA-free by an independent laboratory. Standardized to petasin and isopetasin content (the active anti-inflammatory sesquiterpenes).

Dose: Take 50–75 mg of PA-free standardized extract (standardized to petasin), two times daily. Clinical trials in allergic rhinitis have demonstrated efficacy comparable to cetirizine (a pharmaceutical antihistamine) with fewer side effects at these doses.[339,340] Do not exceed 150 mg daily of standardized extract.

Timing: With meals, twice daily. Splitting the dose morning and evening maintains more consistent antihistamine coverage.

With Food? Always with food. This reduces GI side effects (particularly belching, which is a common minor side effect of butterbur) and may improve bioavailability of the fat-soluble petasin compounds.

Start Low: Begin with one dose daily (50 mg) for the first week before increasing to twice daily. Monitor for GI tolerance—mild belching is common and benign. Butterbur is one of the stronger natural antihistamines, and its effects in reducing both histamine and leukotriene-driven symptoms are often noticeable within one to two weeks.

Cautions: CRITICAL: Only use PA-free certified products. Non-certified butterbur products can cause severe liver damage. Do not use raw or unprocessed butterbur root. Even with PA-free products, avoid in pregnancy, breastfeeding, and in individuals with known ragweed or Asteraceae allergy (same plant family). Discontinue if any signs of liver stress appear (jaundice, dark urine, right upper quadrant pain). Belching is common and benign—if it is distressing, take with a larger meal and divided into two smaller doses.

✦ ✦ ✦

Adaptogens and Nervous System Modulators

Adaptogenic herbs are a distinct category defined by their capacity to help the body adapt to stress—normalizing physiological responses that are dysregulated by chronic stress exposure, without pushing the system uniformly in one direction. Unlike stimulants that push the HPA axis upward or sedatives that push it downward, adaptogens are bidirectional regulators: they help a depleted adrenal system recover capacity, and they help a chronically overactivated stress response find its natural set point.

For those with MCAS, adaptogens address a dimension that antihistamine herbs do not: the chronic HPA axis dysregulation, impaired cortisol response, and sympathetic dominance that keep mast cell thresholds chronically low through the mechanisms described in Chapters 9 and 10. Using adaptogens alongside antihistamine herbs addresses both the mast cell and the nervous system dimensions of MCAS simultaneously.

Adaptogens are Stage 2 herbs—appropriate to introduce once the stabilization baseline from Chapter 12 is established, not during the acute stabilization Phase 1tself. The HPA axis modulation they provide is valuable and important, but introducing them into a highly reactive system before any stability has been achieved can occasionally provoke paradoxical activation in the most sensitive individuals.

Ashwagandha (*Withania somnifera*) | *HPA Axis Restoration and Cortisol Normalization*

Standardization: KSM-66 and Sensoril are the two most clinically studied ashwagandha extract forms, with the most extensive human clinical trial data behind them.[341,342] KSM-66 is a full-spectrum root extract standardized to withanolide content (typically 5 percent); Sensoril (typically 10 percent) uses a different extraction process yielding a higher withanolide percentage from root and leaf. Either is appropriate. Avoid unspecified or generic "ashwagandha powder" products whose withanolide content and extraction quality are unknown.

Dose: KSM-66: 300–600 mg once or twice daily. Sensoril: 125–250 mg twice daily. Clinical studies demonstrating cortisol reduction, HPA axis normalization, and anxiety reduction have primarily used these dose ranges. Effects typically build over four to eight weeks of consistent use.

Timing: Morning and/or evening. Morning dosing supports daytime cortisol pattern normalization; evening dosing supports sleep quality. Many practitioners recommend split dosing for HPA axis support. Avoid taking late evening if it produces any stimulating effects—a minority of people find ashwagandha mildly energizing rather than calming.

With Food? Take with meals. Ashwagandha's withanolides are fat-soluble compounds with better absorption in the presence of dietary fat. GI sensitivity is also reduced with food.

Start Low: Begin at 300 mg once daily with breakfast for two weeks before increasing to twice daily. Ashwagandha is generally well tolerated, but occasional patients with Hashimoto's thyroiditis notice a change in thyroid function—monitor thyroid levels if using ashwagandha with established thyroid autoimmunity. The vast majority of patients tolerate it without issue.

Cautions: Ashwagandha is a member of the nightshade (Solanaceae) family—people with nightshade sensitivity should introduce it very cautiously. Avoid in pregnancy (may stimulate uterine contractions at high doses). Ashwagandha can influence thyroid hormone levels—monitor thyroid function if using for extended periods in Hashimoto's thyroiditis. At high doses, may potentiate sedative medications. Rare cases of liver injury with very high doses have been reported—use within the recommended dose range.

Rhodiola (*Rhodiola rosea*) | *Stress Resilience, Fatigue Recovery, and Sympathetic Modulation*

Standardization: Standardized to rosavins (3 percent) and salidroside (1 percent) content—this dual standardization is the established quality benchmark for *Rhodiola rosea* and distinguishes it from *Rhodiola crenulata*, a related species with a different and less-studied constituent profile. Verify both markers on the product label. Well-studied commercial extracts include SHR-5 (used in multiple clinical trials) and similar standardized products.[343,344]

Dose: Consume 200–400 mg of standardized extract (3 percent rosavins / 1 percent salidroside) once daily. Higher doses can have paradoxically activating or anxiety-provoking effects in some individuals—this is not a case where more is better. Indeed, at least one clinical trial found the lower dose to be more effective for mental performance and fatigue.

Timing: Morning only, taken on waking or shortly after. Rhodiola's energizing and stress-adaptogenic effects are best utilized in the first half of the day. Taking in the afternoon or evening disrupts sleep quality in a meaningful proportion of people.

With Food? Preferred on an empty stomach or thirty minutes before breakfast. Absorption is modestly better in a fasted state.

Start Low: Begin at 100 mg once daily in the morning for the first week. Increase to 200 mg after one week if well tolerated. Some people with MCAS find standard doses mildly overstimulating initially—the lower starting dose allows the system to adjust. If increased anxiety or heart rate is noticed at any dose, reduce to the previous well-tolerated dose.

Cautions: Avoid in individuals with bipolar disorder—Rhodiola's activating effects can precipitate hypomanic episodes. Do not take in the evening—sleep disruption is a reliable consequence of afternoon or evening dosing. At high doses, may interact with antidepressant medications through monoamine oxidase inhibitory activity. Some individuals with significant sympathetic nervous system hyperactivation find Rhodiola initially too activating—in these cases, begin with ashwagandha first and introduce Rhodiola once the nervous system has a more established parasympathetic baseline.

Holy Basil / Tulsi (*Ocimum tenuiflorum*) | *Cortisol Modulation, Anti-Inflammatory, and COX-2 Inhibition*

Standardization: Holy basil extract is available standardized to ursolic acid content (a primary anti-inflammatory triterpenoid) or to total phenolic content. However, the herb is often used in whole-leaf extract form or as a tea (tulsi tea) without specific standardization—this is one of the herbs where high-quality whole-herb preparations have a strong clinical tradition and tea form is genuinely therapeutic. Look for products that clearly specify *Ocimum tenuiflorum* (also called *Ocimum sanctum*) rather than common culinary basil (*Ocimum basilicum*), which is a different species.

Dose: Extract: 300–600 mg daily in divided doses. Tea: one to two cups of tulsi tea daily, using one to two teaspoons of dried herb per cup steeped for five to ten minutes. Tulsi tea is one of the most accessible and pleasant herbal interventions available for those with MCAS—broadly well tolerated and inexpensive.

Timing: With meals or as tea throughout the day. Tulsi tea as a morning ritual and/or afternoon calming practice is a genuinely pleasant integration of herbal medicine into daily life. Unlike Rhodiola, tulsi does not have timing restrictions and can be consumed in the evening without disrupting sleep.

With Food? Capsule or extract: with meals. Tea: any time.

Start Low: Begin with one cup of tulsi tea daily for the first week before introducing capsule or extract forms. Holy basil is generally very well tolerated and is an excellent bridge herb for people who are nervous about introducing more potent adaptogens.

Cautions: Mild blood-sugar-lowering effects—monitor closely if on diabetes medications. Avoid in pregnancy, especially high-dose supplementation. Holy basil has mild anticoagulant properties—inform your physician if on blood-thinning medications.

Turmeric / Curcumin (*Curcuma longa*) | *NF-κB Inhibition and Broad Anti-Inflammatory Action*

Standardization: Standardized curcumin extracts typically contain 95 percent curcuminoids (the three primary active compounds: curcumin, bisdemethoxycurcumin, and demethoxycurcumin). Bioavailability-enhanced forms dramatically improve absorption: BCM-95 and others (turmeric essential oil enhanced), Meriva (phytosomal curcumin), Longvida (lipid-based), CurQfen (curcumin-galactomannan), and CurcuWin (water-soluble) all achieve significantly higher plasma concentrations than standard 95 percent extract. At minimum, pairing with piperine (BioPerine) from black pepper increases curcumin bioavailability by approximately 2,000 percent,[345] although this is less than the improved bioavailability achieved by the aforementioned extracts.

Dose: Standard 95 percent extract with piperine: 500–1,000 mg curcuminoids, one to two times daily. Bioavailability-enhanced forms (BCM-95, Meriva,

Longvida): 200–500 mg curcuminoids daily, achieving equivalent or greater effect at lower doses due to improved absorption. Culinary turmeric provides modest curcumin amounts valuable as a dietary foundation but is insufficient as a sole therapeutic source.

Timing: With the largest meal of the day. Curcumin is fat-soluble and requires dietary fat for absorption. For standard extracts paired with piperine, the meal-timing requirement is strict. For enhanced-bioavailability forms, fat is less critical but still preferred.

With Food? Always with a fat-containing meal—it is non-negotiable for standard extract forms. Even enhanced-bioavailability forms benefit from co-administration with fat.

Start Low: Begin at 500 mg once daily with dinner. It is well-tolerated by most individuals with MCAS even from the start. Some notice GI warmth at higher doses—reduce dose if this occurs. Increase to twice daily after one to two weeks if well tolerated and clinical priority warrants higher dosing.

Cautions: At doses above 1,000 mg daily, curcumin has blood-thinning effects—inform your physician if on anticoagulant medications. May worsen symptomatic gallbladder conditions (gallstones, bile duct obstruction) by stimulating bile flow—avoid or use cautiously if gallbladder disease is present. High doses may reduce iron absorption; avoid taking it with iron supplements or iron-rich meals. It is generally very well tolerated within the recommended dose range.

Reishi Mushroom (*Ganoderma lucidum*) | *Immune Modulation, Th1 Support, and Adaptogenic Balance*

Standardization: Reishi is available as dried mushroom (mycelium or fruiting body), extract powder, or concentrated extract. The most active constituents for immune modulation are beta-glucans (polysaccharides) and triterpenoids (ganoderic acids). Look for products standardized to beta-glucan content (typically 10–30 percent) from the fruiting body rather than mycelium-only products, which may have different constituent profiles. Hot-water-extracted products are preferred for beta-glucan extraction; dual extraction (hot water + alcohol) captures both polysaccharides and triterpenoids.

Dose: Dried mushroom: 1,500–3,000 mg daily. Concentrated extract (10:1): 500–1,000 mg daily. Beta-glucan standardized extract: 250–500 mg of beta-glucans daily. Effects build over six to twelve weeks of consistent use—reishi is not an acute intervention but a long-term immune modulating foundation.

Timing: With meals, once or twice daily. Reishi's immune-modulating effects require consistent daily exposure over weeks to months and are not timing-sensitive in the way that acute antihistamine herbs are.

With Food? Take with food. GI tolerance is improved with food and the polysaccharide constituents are well absorbed in the presence of other dietary compounds.

Start Low: Begin at 500 mg of dried mushroom or 250 mg of concentrated extract once daily. Reishi can occasionally cause an initial detoxification response (skin flushing, increased urination, loose stools) in the first week—reduce the dose if this occurs and increase more gradually. This initial response, if it occurs, typically resolves within one to two weeks.

Cautions: Avoid with immunosuppressant drugs (organ transplant medications, high-dose corticosteroids). Reishi actively modulates immune function in ways that may oppose immunosuppression. At doses above the recommended range, reishi has mild blood-thinning effects—inform your physician if on anticoagulants. May cause dry mouth, throat, or nose in some individuals. GI upset (nausea, loose stools) is possible at higher doses—reduce dose if this occurs.

✦ ✦ ✦

Sourcing Quality: Why It Matters More Than the Research

The gap between the herb described in a clinical trial and the herb in an inexpensive retail bottle can be enormous—and for those with MCAS, that gap has real clinical consequences. A butterbur product without verified PA-free certification is not a cheaper version of a safe product; it is a potentially liver toxic product. A Chinese skullcap product adulterated with germander is not less effective—it is actively harmful. These are not hypothetical risks.

Quality indicators worth prioritizing when sourcing herbal products include: third-party testing by an independent laboratory (NSF International, USP, ConsumerLab, or Eurofins are among the reputable certifiers); clear botanical identification specifying species, plant part used, and extraction ratio; standardization to specific active constituent levels; certificate of analysis available on request; and manufacturing in GMP (Good Manufacturing Practice)-certified facilities. In the United States, the FDA does not require herbal supplement manufacturers to prove efficacy or safety before marketing, making third-party testing the primary consumer protection mechanism.

For individuals with MCAS who experience heightened chemical sensitivity, additional considerations include minimal excipients (fillers and binders). Look for products with few and clearly identified non-active ingredients; absence of common sensitizers like magnesium stearate (some people with MCAS react), shellac, or artificial colorings; and capsule materials (gelatin versus vegetarian cellulose capsules, depending on individual tolerance).

> **Practical Recommendation:** *Purchase from companies that provide a certificate of analysis for each batch and that specify the exact botanical species, plant part, and extraction method on their label. Budget brands with generic labeling and no third-party testing are a false economy in herbal medicine—especially for the high-stakes herbs like butterbur where adulteration has documented consequences.*

✦ ✦ ✦

Quick Reference: Herbal Protocol Summary

The following table provides a consolidated reference for the key practical details of each herb covered in this chapter. Use it alongside the individual profiles for daily protocol management.

Herb	Form / Dose	Timing	With Food?	Key Caution
Stinging Nettle (freeze-dried leaf)	300–600 mg, 2–3x daily	Before meals	Empty stomach preferred	May lower blood pressure; avoid in renal disease. Ensure freeze-dried form—not dried.
Chinese Skullcap (*Scutellaria baicalensis*)	200–400 mg (baicalin extract), 1–2x daily	Morning and/or afternoon	Can be with or without food	Adulteration risk—verify species. Rare hepatotoxicity with adulterated products. Avoid in pregnancy.
Chamomile (German or Roman)	Tea: 1–2 tsp dried/cup. Extract: 250–500 mg daily	Evening; tea at bedtime	Tea anytime; extract with or without food	Avoid if allergic to ragweed or Asteraceae family. Generally very well tolerated.
Ashwagandha (KSM-66 or Sensoril)	300–600 mg standardized extract, 1–2x daily	Morning and/or evening	With food for best absorption and tolerability	Avoid in thyroid autoimmunity without monitoring. Avoid in pregnancy. Nightshade sensitivity possible.
Rhodiola (3% rosavins / 1% salidroside)	200–400 mg, once daily	Morning only	Empty stomach preferred	Avoid in bipolar disorder. May be stimulating—do not take in the evening.
Holy Basil / Tulsi (*Ocimum tenuiflorum*)	300–600 mg extract or 1–2 cups tea daily	Morning or with meals	With or without food; tea any time	May mildly lower blood sugar—monitor if diabetic. Avoid high doses in pregnancy.

Herb	Form / Dose	Timing	With Food?	Key Caution
Perilla (*Perilla frutescens*) leaf	50–200 mg standardized extract (rosmarinic acid)	Before meals	Can be with food	Generally very well tolerated. Rare GI upset at high doses.
Butterbur (*Petasites hybridus*)	50–75 mg standardized (PA-free), 2x daily	With meals	Always with food	MUST be PA-free (pyrrolizidine alkaloid-free) certified. Avoid in pregnancy. Can cause belching.
Turmeric / Curcumin (standardized)	500–1,000 mg curcumin with piperine, 1–2x daily	With meals	Always with fat and black pepper	Avoid at high doses with blood thinners. May worsen gallbladder conditions.
Reishi Mushroom (*Ganoderma lucidum*)	1,500–3,000 mg dried mycelium or 500 mg extract daily	Morning or with meals	With or without food	Avoid with immunosuppressant drugs. Blood-thinning effect at high doses. Mild GI upset possible.

> **Reminder:** *The herbs in this chapter follow the same introduction protocol as the supplements in Chapter 16: one herb at a time, starting at a low dose, with five to seven days of observation. Adaptogens (ashwagandha, rhodiola, holy basil) belong in Stage 2 and beyond—not in acute stabilization. Antihistamine herbs (nettle, chamomile, perilla) may be introduced earlier, during the transition from stabilization to early support.*

✦ ✦ ✦

Deeper Dive: Rosmarinic Acid, Baicalin, and the Flavonoid Network

For the Science-Minded Reader

Two compounds that appear across multiple herbs in this chapter—rosmarinic acid and baicalin—deserve more detailed attention because understanding them reveals the mechanistic coherence of herbal antihistamine medicine.

Rosmarinic Acid: The Shared Active in Multiple Herbs

Rosmarinic acid is a polyphenolic compound found in perilla, rosemary, basil, mint, lemon balm, and sage—the entire mint family (Lamiaceae). Its relevance to MCAS is substantial: rosmarinic acid inhibits both COX-2 and LOX (lipoxygenase) enzymes,[346] the dual pathways responsible for prostaglandin and leukotriene synthesis from mast cells. Simultaneously inhibiting both pathways is something that most pharmaceutical anti-inflammatory drugs do not achieve—non-steroidal anti-inflammatories (NSAIDs) primarily inhibit COX, while leukotrienes proceed unchecked, which is one reason NSAIDs are often insufficient for MCAS symptom management.

Rosmarinic acid also directly inhibits mast cell degranulation through phosphodiesterase inhibition, increasing intracellular cyclic AMP levels that stabilize the mast cell membrane.[347] And it reduces the inflammatory activation of dendritic cells and macrophages, contributing to the restoration of immune tolerance that is disrupted in MCAS. The fact that rosmarinic acid is present across an entire herb family—and is a constituent of many herbs used routinely as culinary spices—means that a diet rich in Lamiaceae family herbs (basil, rosemary, mint, thyme, oregano) provides a consistent dietary rosmarinic acid contribution alongside any therapeutic herbal supplementation.

Baicalin: CNS Mast Cell Stabilization and the Brain Barrier

Baicalin, the primary flavonoid from *Scutellaria baicalensis*, is particularly valuable in MCAS for its capacity to cross the blood-brain barrier—a property that most flavonoids lack due to their high polarity and large molecular size.[348] Once in the CNS, baicalin exerts anti-inflammatory effects directly on the central nervous system, including inhibition of TLR-4-mediated signaling and suppression of NF-κB-driven inflammatory pathways, which are involved in mast cell activation.[349,350] This CNS penetration makes baicalin specifically relevant for the neuropsychiatric endotypes of MCAS described in Chapter 9—brain fog, anxiety, cognitive impairment, and autonomic dysregulation driven by mast cell activity in or near the central nervous system.

Baicalin also demonstrates selective modulation of GABA-A receptors through a binding site distinct from benzodiazepines,[351] producing anxiolytic effects through the same pathway as drugs like diazepam but without the sedation, tolerance, or dependence associated with those medications. For people with MCAS who experience significant anxiety as a component of their presentation—which is the majority, given the nervous system dimension of the condition—this combination of peripheral anti-inflammatory activity and central anxiolytic activity makes *Scutellaria baicalensis* a uniquely valuable herbal option.

Combining Herbal and Supplement Protocols

The herbal medicines in this chapter and the supplements in Chapter 16 are not competing approaches—they are complementary layers of a multi-target therapeutic strategy. Quercetin and freeze-dried nettle together provide broader antihistamine coverage than either alone, because quercetin directly stabilizes mast cell membranes while nettle modulates histamine receptor signaling through additional pathways. Baicalin from skullcap and luteolin from Chapter 16 provide overlapping but distinct CNS anti-inflammatory coverage. Ashwagandha's HPA axis normalization and Chapter 16's magnesium and B6 nervous system support work through different but reinforcing mechanisms to raise the mast cell threshold from the autonomic direction.

The practical implication is that a complete Stage 2 herbal and supplement protocol is not merely additive—it is synergistic. The combination of multiple low-dose interventions each targeting a different vulnerability point in the MCAS biology produces outcomes that any single therapeutic approach, however high the dose, cannot replicate. This is the central logic of integrative MCAS management: not one powerful drug, but many gentle, well-chosen interventions working in concert.

✦ ✦ ✦

What This Means for You: Building Your Herbal Protocol

Integrating herbal medicine into an MCAS protocol is most effective when it is approached as a deliberate addition to an already-established supplement foundation, not as a parallel track started simultaneously.

Begin herbal medicine in early Stage 2, not during stabilization. Most antihistamine herbs are appropriate to introduce during the transition from Stage 1 to Stage 2—once reaction frequency has meaningfully reduced and a dietary baseline is established. Chamomile tea is the gentlest and most appropriate first introduction, both for its mast cell benefits and for the sleep and nervous system support it provides within the evening wind-down routine from Chapter 14. Freeze-dried nettle is typically the second herbal introduction for people with significant histamine reactivity.

Reserve adaptogens for established Stage 2. Ashwagandha, rhodiola, and holy basil belong after the initial gut-healing and mast cell stabilization work is underway—typically after six to eight weeks of stable Stage 2 support. The HPA axis modulation they provide is profoundly valuable, but it is most effective and best tolerated when the system is not in acute inflammatory crisis. Begin with ashwagandha as the most broadly appropriate first adaptogen for MCAS, then add rhodiola or holy basil based on your specific symptom profile—rhodiola for fatigue and low resilience, holy basil for inflammation and cortisol dysregulation; either for stress adaptability.

Treat butterbur as a high-evidence option requiring the highest sourcing standards. Of the herbs in this chapter, butterbur has the most direct clinical trial evidence for antihistamine effects comparable to pharmaceutical antihistamines. For individuals with significant seasonal or environmental reactivity who want a stronger natural antihistamine option, PA-free certified butterbur is a genuinely evidence-based choice—but only from manufacturers with documented third-party PA testing. This is the one herb in this chapter where sourcing is not merely a quality consideration but a safety-critical requirement.

Use chamomile tea as a daily ritual rather than a sporadic supplement. The gap between herbal medicine's potential and its typical clinical outcome is often consistency. Chamomile tea drunk occasionally when symptoms are acute provides modest relief. Chamomile tea drunk every evening as a consistent ritual for weeks and months produces cumulative anti-inflammatory and nervous system calming effects that sporadic use cannot. This is true of most herbal medicine—its effects build through consistent daily exposure to a sustained phytochemical signal, not through episodic high-dose rescue use.

Inform your healthcare providers. Herbal medicines are biologically active and interact with medications, laboratory tests, and surgical procedures in ways that matter clinically. Skullcap affects CYP450 drug metabolism. Ashwagandha influences thyroid function. Butterbur affects liver enzyme testing in some individuals. Your physician, pharmacist, and any specialists involved in your care need to know what herbs you are taking—the same way they need to know what supplements and medications you take.

The woman who first reached for stinging nettles thousands of years ago did not know about histamine receptors or NF-κB or the cholinergic anti-inflammatory pathway. She knew that nettles helped. She was right, and for reasons that took millennia to fully articulate. The work of modern phytopharmacology is not to replace that traditional wisdom with something more sophisticated—it is to confirm, explain, and refine it, so that the plants that have always helped can be used with greater precision and greater safety.

That is the spirit in which this chapter is offered: respect for the intelligence embedded in plant medicine, combined with the specificity that modern people need to use it well.

✦ ✦ ✦

Chapter 17 at a Glance

What to Remember:

- Herbal medicine works through the entourage effect—multiple plant constituents interacting synergistically to produce effects that isolated compounds cannot fully replicate. This is why whole standardized extracts often outperform equivalent doses of isolated active constituents.

- Freeze-dried stinging nettle leaf (not dried or cooked nettle) is the most accessible and broadly well-tolerated antihistamine herb, appropriate to introduce during the Stage 1 to Stage 2 transition. The freeze-drying process is essential—other preparation methods destroy its active compounds.
- Skullcap (*Scutellaria baicalensis*) provides mast cell stabilization through baicalin, a blood-brain-barrier-penetrating flavonoid with particular value for neuropsychiatric MCAS presentations including brain fog, anxiety, and CNS-driven inflammation. Sourcing verification is critical due to adulteration risk.
- Chamomile is the gentlest and most versatile herb in this protocol—appropriate for those with MCAS at nearly every stage of reactivity, valuable for sleep, gut calming, and nervous system support, and accessible as a daily tea rather than requiring supplemental forms.
- Butterbur has the strongest clinical evidence among the herbal antihistamines, with trials demonstrating efficacy comparable to pharmaceutical antihistamines—but must be PA-free certified from a verified manufacturer. Non-certified butterbur is hepatotoxic and should not be used.
- Adaptogens (ashwagandha, rhodiola, holy basil) address the HPA axis and adrenal dimension of MCAS that antihistamine herbs do not. They belong in Stage 2 and beyond—not in acute stabilization—and work best when the system has achieved some initial stability.
- Rosmarinic acid, present across the mint herb family, simultaneously inhibits COX-2 and LOX pathways, providing dual prostaglandin and leukotriene suppression—an anti-inflammatory profile more comprehensive than most pharmaceutical anti-inflammatories achieve.
- Quality sourcing is as important as herb selection third-party testing; botanical verification, standardization to active constituents, and GMP-certified manufacturing are non-negotiable minimum standards, especially for herbs with known adulteration risks (skullcap, butterbur).

Coming Up in Chapter 18:

Herbal medicine works primarily through ingestion and absorption—molecules entering the bloodstream and tissues from within. Essential oils share that ingestion route when used appropriately, and they also offer additional access routes that most oral preparations do not: the olfactory system, which carries aromatic compounds directly to the limbic system, and transdermal absorption through topical application. What makes essential oils particularly compelling from a scientific perspective is that they are not simple fragrances—they are powerful signaling molecules that act through multiple pathways, mechanisms, and cellular and molecular targets simultaneously. A single oil may modulate ion channels, bind G protein-coupled receptors, inhibit inflammatory enzymes, and activate olfactory receptors that communicate directly with the brain, all at once. Chapter 18 explores the evidence-informed use of essential oils in MCAS and POTS support—covering the oils most likely to provide benefit, the safety considerations unique to mast cell–sensitive individuals, and practical protocols for aromatic, topical, and appropriate internal use that minimize the risk of triggering the very reactions they are intended to help.

CHAPTER 18

Essential Oils Support for MCAS

Powerful Signaling Molecules for Mast Cell Calm, POTS Support, and Nervous System Regulation

A Drop That Did What a Capsule Couldn't

Anna had tried almost everything in the functional medicine toolkit by the time her integrative practitioner suggested lavender essential oil. She was skeptical in the particular way that scientifically literate individuals often are about aromatherapy—associating it with candles in spas rather than with anything clinically meaningful. She had already seen real benefit from quercetin, dietary changes, and the nervous system practices from Chapter 14. What could a drop of plant oil possibly add?

Her practitioner explained the mechanism rather than the anecdote: That lavender's linalool modulates GABA-A receptors, activating the same calming pathway as certain anti-anxiety medications but through a different binding site; that inhaled volatile compounds trigger neural signals that reach the limbic system within seconds via the olfactory bulb, while their small, lipid-soluble molecules can readily bypass the blood-brain barrier by traveling directly along the olfactory and trigeminal nerve pathways; and that the same lavender that reduces cortisol in research subjects was also suppressing histamine release from mast cells in cell culture studies. This was not fragrance. This was pharmacology delivered through an unconventional route.

Anna tried it. One drop on a tissue, held near her face for sixty seconds before the meal she most consistently reacted to. Not dramatic. Not transformative in the way that dietary change had been. But noticeable—a measurable softening of the pre-meal anxiety she had normalized, a slightly calmer gut response, a morning that started a register lower than usual. Over weeks of consistent use, that small daily calming effect accumulated into something she described as a shift in her background nervous system state.

Essential oils occupy a distinct therapeutic niche in MCAS management—not only because they are the most highly-concentrated natural solutions available, but because they reach the body through access routes that oral preparations do not use, and because they function as genuinely complex signaling molecules rather than simple fragrances. A single essential oil—contained from a dozen to hundreds of constituents—may simultaneously modulate ion channels in sensory neurons, activate olfactory receptors that feed directly into limbic processing, bind anti-inflammatory receptors on immune cells, and when ingested appropriately, exert antimicrobial or anti-inflammatory effects in the gut. This multi-target activity is what makes them worth including in a thoughtful MCAS protocol—with the clear-eyed recognition that they require more care in application, not less, for mast-cell-sensitive individuals.

✦ ✦ ✦

Understanding Essential Oils in the Context of MCAS

Essential oils are concentrated lipophilic volatile compounds extracted from plant material—flowers, leaves, bark, resin, roots, or fruit peel—primarily through steam distillation or cold pressing. They are not oils in the nutritional sense; they contain no fatty acids. They are complex mixtures of dozens to hundreds of individual chemical constituents, primarily terpenes and terpenoids, phenylpropanoids, and oxygenated compounds including alcohols, esters, aldehydes, ketones, and oxides. It is this chemical complexity that gives essential oils their multi-target biological activity and that distinguishes them from isolated aromatic compounds.

The concentration is the critical factor that separates essential oils from herbal teas and culinary spices. Peppermint essential oil is a highly concentrated source of the plant's volatile compounds, containing much higher levels of active constituents than peppermint tea. This concentration is what makes essential oils both therapeutically potent and requiring of precise, careful dosing—particularly for individuals with MCAS, whose mast cells are primed to respond to chemical signals at concentrations that wouldn't register for most people.

Why MCAS Patients React Differently

The mast-cell-rich environments of the skin and respiratory mucosa are precisely where essential oils make their first contact with the body. Mast cells in the nasal mucosa respond to inhaled volatile compounds through olfactory receptor interactions and through direct chemical stimulation of pattern-recognition pathways. Mast cells in the dermal layer respond to topically applied compounds as they penetrate the skin barrier. For individuals with sensitized mast cells and a chronically full bucket, the same compound that produces a calming response in a healthy person may produce a mast cell reaction in someone with MCAS—not because the oil is inherently harmful, but because their threshold for perceiving any aromatic compound as a potential chemical challenge is dramatically lower.

This is why the approach to essential oils in MCAS differs from general aromatherapy guidance in three critical ways: doses are lower (often by a factor of ten or more), introduction is slower and more systematic, and the monitoring period after each new oil is longer. An individual with MCAS who opens a bottle of undiluted eucalyptus oil and inhales deeply, as many aromatherapy resources might suggest, is not doing aromatherapy incorrectly—they are simply applying guidance designed for a less reactive system. The principles of the bucket theory apply fully here: even a therapeutic oil becomes a trigger when the bucket is already full.

Purity, Sourcing, and the Synthetic Fragrance Problem

For those with MCAS, oil quality is not an aesthetic preference—it is a clinical necessity. Synthetic fragrance compounds, which are chemically distinct from the natural constituents they mimic,[352] are among the most reliably documented mast cell triggers in the everyday environment (discussed in Chapter 13). Many commercial "essential oil" products are adulterated with synthetic extenders, isolated aromatic chemicals, cheaper substitute oils, fatty oils, or entirely synthetic fragrance compounds that bear the name of a plant but share little biochemical relationship with it. These products carry the mast cell trigger risk of synthetic fragrances without the therapeutic benefits of genuine plant chemistry.

Quality indicators for therapeutic-grade essential oils include: gas chromatography/mass spectrometry (GC/MS) testing certificates available per batch—along with a series of additional necessary tests, clearly specified botanical origin (genus, species, chemotype, country of origin, and plant part), third-party purity verification, and extraction method disclosure. For people with MCAS, it is worth the additional cost to source oils with verifiable testing data, since adulterated products are disproportionately likely to trigger reactions.

> **Less Is More:** *In MCAS, the therapeutic window for essential oils is narrower than in healthy populations. The goal is to use the smallest amount that produces a beneficial effect—not to maximize exposure. One drop, well-chosen and appropriately diluted or inhaled, consistently outperforms five drops of the same oil in a reactive system.*

✦ ✦ ✦

Three Methods of Use: Aromatic, Topical, and Internal

Essential oils can be used through three primary routes, each with distinct mechanisms, safety considerations, and appropriate applications for those with MCAS. Understanding all three methods—and when each is appropriate—allows for a more complete and strategically applied essential oil protocol.

Method One: Aromatic Use

Aromatic use is the most accessible, the fastest-acting, and generally the lowest-risk method for individuals with MCAS, and it is usually the appropriate starting point for any new oil. Volatile compounds inhaled through the nose reach the olfactory epithelium—a specialized sensory tissue with direct neural connections to the limbic system, the amygdala, and the hypothalamus—within seconds. This direct limbic access is what makes inhaled essential oils uniquely rapid in their effects on autonomic state, emotional tone, and cortisol response. No other route of administration reaches the brain as quickly.

For individuals with MCAS, two aromatic application methods offer the best control over dose. The personal inhaler (a small cylindrical tube containing a cotton wick saturated with a few drops of oil) allows precise, brief, individual-controlled inhalation without dispersing the oil into a shared space. One to three slow inhalations through the nose produces a measurable physiological response within sixty seconds. The tissue method—one to two drops on a tissue, held near the face at arm's length and brought gradually closer—provides similar control and allows even more intuitive dose adjustment.

Diffusion disperses essential oils into ambient air and is appropriate for home use where the environment is controlled, but requires more care in MCAS. Passive diffusion (evaporation from a room diffuser with minimal heat) at low concentrations—one to three drops per hundred milliliters of water—in a well-ventilated room for brief sessions of twenty to thirty minutes is the appropriate starting approach. Ultrasonic diffusers are preferred over heat diffusers, which can alter volatile compound composition. Reed diffusers and plug-in diffusers that run continuously are generally not appropriate during active stabilization, as they provide an uncontrolled, continuous aromatic exposure that may fill the bucket from the sensory dimension even when the oil is therapeutic.

Method Two: Topical Use

Topical application allows essential oil constituents to penetrate the skin and reach local tissues and the systemic circulation. Transdermal absorption rates vary significantly between compounds and between individuals, but fat-soluble terpene constituents absorb meaningfully through intact skin over thirty to sixty minutes. Topical use is appropriate for localized applications—skin reactions, joint inflammation, abdominal discomfort, chest tension—and for applications where sustained systemic exposure is desired, such as nervous system support through pulse-point application.

Dilution is non-negotiable for people managing MCAS. Undiluted ("neat") application of essential oils is appropriate only in very limited circumstances for healthy individuals—it is not appropriate for those with MCAS, whose dermal mast cells are primed to respond to concentrated chemical exposure. The standard dilution guidelines for sensitive individuals are significantly lower than general aromatherapy recommendations. A one percent dilution—roughly six drops of essential oil per five milliliters (one teaspoon) of carrier oil—is the appropriate starting concentration for a primed mast cell system. Some particularly potent or sensitizing oils warrant a half-percent dilution (one drop per ten milliliters) initially.

Carrier oils for dilution should themselves be low-reactivity choices. Fractionated coconut oil, jojoba oil (technically a liquid wax ester), and sweet almond oil are among the best-tolerated carriers for people with MCAS—light, non-comedogenic, and with minimal aromatic compounds that could add to the trigger load. Patch testing on a small area of inner forearm before broader application is essential for any new oil combination, regardless of prior tolerance to the individual components.

Method Three: Internal Use

Internal use of essential oils—ingestion via capsule, honey, food, or beverage—is the most potent and most pharmacologically direct route of administration and also the route requiring the most guidance and caution. It is not appropriate for every oil, every person, or every situation, but when used appropriately under qualified guidance, it is a legitimate and clinically meaningful therapeutic approach that extends the reach of essential oils beyond what aromatic and topical use alone can achieve.

The primary mechanism distinguishing internal use is direct mucosal and systemic absorption. Oils taken in a veggie capsule with a small amount of carrier oil (food-grade fractionated coconut oil, MCT oil, or olive oil) dissolve in the fat carrier, protecting the gastric mucosa from direct essential oil contact and improving absorption. In this form, the pharmacologically active constituents enter the portal circulation, reach the liver, and distribute systemically—achieving concentrations and tissue exposures that aromatic and topical use do not produce. This is the mechanism through which oregano oil addresses gut pathogens, copaiba's beta-caryophyllene acts on CB2 receptors throughout the body, and frankincense constituents exert anti-inflammatory effects in joints and the nervous system.

> **Critical Safety Note:** *When it comes to taking essential oils internally, it's helpful to have a bit of guidance from someone trained in their use—such as an integrative doctor, a clinical aromatherapist, or a naturopath. This isn't because internal use is automatically unsafe, but because everyone's body and situation are a little different. Things like how much to use, which oils are appropriate, and how they might interact with medications can vary, so having expert input can make the experience more effective and personalized.*
>
> *If you'd like to learn more about best practices for internal use, you can find additional details in the author's books "Medicinal Essential Oils: The Science and Practice of Evidence-based Essential Oil Therapy" and "The Molecular Polypharmacology of Essential Oils: Targets, Pathways, and Mechanisms."*

✦ ✦ ✦

Essential Oil Profiles: MCAS and POTS Support

The following profiles cover the essential oils with the strongest evidence and clinical track record for MCAS and POTS support. They are organized in the consistent card format used in Chapters 16 and 17, with fields specific to essential oil use. Introduction should follow the same one-at-a-time protocol established in Chapter 16: begin with aromatic use of a single oil, observe for several days, and expand gradually.

Lavender (*Lavandula angustifolia*) | *Cornerstone MCAS Oil — GABA Modulation and Histamine Suppression*

Target: MCAS primary; POTS secondary (nervous system calming, sleep support). Lavender oil stabilizes mast cells and reduces the release of histamine.[353] It's also a positive allosteric modulator of gamma2-containing GABA-A receptors,[354] which helps "calm the storm" of an overactive nervous system in POTS, reducing the physical jitters, heart rate spikes, and sleep disruptions caused by excessive adrenaline.

Aromatic Use: Place 1–2 drops on a personal inhaler or tissue; 1–3 drops per 100 mL in a cold-air diffuser for up to thirty minutes. Best timing: evening and before meals.

Topical Use: Use 1–2 percent dilution in fractionated coconut oil. Patch test inner forearm first. Apply to wrists, behind ears, or soles of feet. For skin reactions, dilute 0.5–1 percent and apply to unaffected adjacent skin, not directly to reactive area.

Internal Use: Two drops in a veggie capsule with a fatty oil, with a meal.

Start Here: Begin with aromatic use only: one inhalation from a tissue with one drop, once daily, for five days. If well tolerated, proceed to brief diffusion. Introduce topical use only after aromatic is established and confirmed tolerated.

Cautions: Generally among the best-tolerated essential oils for sensitive individuals. May interact with antifungals and antibiotics.

German Chamomile (*Matricaria chamomilla*) | *Chamazulene, Histamine Suppression, and Skin Calming*

Target: MCAS primary—particularly for skin reactions, flushing, and histamine-driven inflammation.

Aromatic Use: One drop on a tissue or personal inhaler—this oil is very concentrated and potent. Brief inhalation only. The deep blue color (from chamazulene) is a quality indicator of genuine German chamomile.

Topical Use: Use 1 percent dilution. Extremely potent anti-inflammatory for skin—a small amount goes a long way. Patch test mandatory. Applied to flushing areas, reactive skin, or locally inflamed tissue.

Internal Use: Use 1–2 drops in a veggie capsule with a fatty oil, with a meal.

Start Here: Begin with a single brief inhalation from a tissue with one drop. Allow five to seven days before expanding use.

Cautions: Asteraceae family—avoid if allergic to ragweed, chrysanthemum, or daisy. May interact with CYP450 enzymes when used internally. Moderate risk of interaction with aspirin, blood pressure, antiplatelet, anticoagulant, anticholinergic, and cholinergic drugs.

Roman Chamomile (*Chamaemelum nobile*) | *Gentle First-Line MCAS Oil — Vagal Calming and Oxytocin Support*

Target: MCAS primary; POTS secondary. Research shows inhalation significantly increased salivary oxytocin—relevant for vagal calming and parasympathetic support.[355] Gentler than German chamomile and a better introductory oil for sensitive individuals.

Aromatic Use: Place 1–2 drops on personal inhaler. Evening use preferred for sleep support. Brief diffusion (1–2 drops per 100 mL, 20 minutes) is well tolerated by most. The sweet, apple-like scent is among the most pleasant and least likely to be perceived as a threat by a sensitized olfactory system.

Topical Use: Use 1–2 percent dilution. Among the best-tolerated chamomile oils topically. Apply to abdomen for gut calming, wrists and temples for nervous system support, or chest for respiratory symptoms.

Internal Use: Use 1–2 drops in a veggie capsule with carrier oil.

Start Here: This is the recommended first-choice chamomile oil for people with MCAS new to essential oils. Begin with one drop on a tissue, single inhalation, once daily. A logical first oil alongside lavender.

Cautions: Asteraceae family caution (same as German chamomile).

Blue Tansy (*Tanacetum annuum*) | *Targeted Histamine Support – Use With Particular Care*

Target: MCAS—chamazulene, a major constituent of blue tansy oil, is a potent inhibitor of Leukotriene B4 (LTB4) formation.[356] Leukotrienes are inflammatory mediators released by mast cells and white blood cells that are often more powerful than histamine in driving long-term swelling and airway constriction. Primarily useful for cleaning up the inflammatory aftermath following histamine release.

Aromatic Use: Place 1 drop on a tissue. Brief inhalation (1–2 slow breaths). Brief diffusion (1–2 drops per 100 mL, 20 minutes).

Topical Use: Use 1 percent dilution. Patch test mandatory on inner forearm, wait 24 hours before broader use.

Internal Use: Primarily used for skin.

Start Here: Blue tansy is not a first-line introductory oil. Introduce only after lavender and Roman chamomile are established and well tolerated. Use the smallest possible exposure initially—one brief inhalation from a tissue.

Cautions: Asteraceae family caution. Contains camphor—avoid in individuals with epilepsy or seizure history. Do not confuse with common tansy (*Tanacetum vulgare*), which is neurotoxic. May interfere with CYP450 drug-metabolizing enzymes when ingested. The moderate camphor may negatively impact red blood cells and increase the risk of jaundice in children with Glucose-6-phosphate dehydrogenase deficiency (G6PD).

Bergamot (*Citrus bergamia*, FCF) | *POTS Autonomic Support – Sleep, Anxiety, and Blood Pressure*

Target: POTS primary; MCAS secondary (nervous system calming). Research demonstrates bergamot inhalation improved sleep, anxiety, depression, and stress—and was the best intervention in a surgical ICU comparison for sleep quality and anxiety reduction.[357] Relevant for hyperadrenergic stress and autonomic overactivation.

Aromatic Use: Place 1–2 drops on personal inhaler or pillow/tissue inhaler at bedtime. Brief diffusion (1–2 drops per 100 mL, 30 minutes maximum). Best timing: evening and pre-sleep.

Topical Use: FCF (bergapten-free) bergamot only—1 percent dilution; still may be photosensitizing as not all bergapten is removed. Bergapten-free (also labeled as 'BF' or 'furocoumarin-free') is the essential safety requirement for any topical use. Standard bergamot causes severe sensitivity and reactions when exposed to UV rays (sunlight or artificial).

Internal Use: Place 1–2 drops in a veggie capsule with a fatty oil.

Start Here: Begin with a single inhalation from a personal inhaler in the evening. Bergamot's aromatic profile—fresh, citrus-floral—is typically well received even by reactive individuals. Establish aromatic tolerance before any topical use, and verify FCF designation before purchasing for topical application.

Cautions: Must be FCF (bergapten-free) for any topical use—standard bergamot is severely phototoxic and will cause burns with sun exposure. Verify FCF on the label explicitly. Bergamot contains CYP3A4-interacting furanocoumarins even in FCF form at lower levels—inform your physician if on medications metabolized by this enzyme pathway. Moderate risk of interaction with anticholinergic and cholinergic medications.

Copaiba (*Copaifera* spp.) | *CB2 Agonist, Anti-Inflammatory, and Among the Safest for Sensitive Patients*

Target: MCAS + POTS. Beta-caryophyllene, the primary constituent of copaiba (often 50–60 percent of the oil), is a CB2 receptor agonist associated with reduced inflammatory signaling, neuropathic pain reduction, and anti-anxiety effects.[358]

Aromatic Use: Place 1–2 drops in a diffuser or on inhaler. Mild, woody scent is generally well received. No timing restrictions—morning, evening, or as needed.

Topical Use: Use 1–3 percent dilution. Very well tolerated topically. Can be applied over areas of pain, inflammation, or tension. Also appropriate for general systemic anti-inflammatory support applied to large skin surface areas.

Internal Use: Place 1–3 drops in a veggie capsule with carrier oil; it's among the most widely used oils for internal application in integrative practice. Beta-caryophyllene is present in black pepper and other foods—dietary exposure precedent supports its safety profile at therapeutic essential oil doses.

Start Here: Copaiba is an excellent introductory oil for those with MCAS who are new to essential oils or who have had reactions to other oils. Its constituent profile is among the gentlest available. Begin with diffusion and advance to topical, then capsule use when indicated.

Cautions: Very well tolerated overall. Beta-caryophyllene, alpha-humulene, and caryophyllene oxide content may interfere with CYP3A enzyme activity—consult your physician or pharmacist if on medications metabolized by this enzyme pathway.

Frankincense (*Boswellia sacra / carterii / frereana / papyrifera*) | *Anti-Inflammatory, Grounding, and CNS Support*

Target: MCAS + POTS. Anti-inflammatory through multiple pathways and balances immune function;[359,360,361,362] clinical experience shows effects on limbic system, mood, and autonomic state through aromatic use.

Aromatic Use: Place 1–2 drops on personal inhaler or diffuser. The grounding, resinous scent may improve cortisol levels and limbic tone—well suited to the nervous system regulation practices of Chapter 14 as an aromatic accompaniment.

Topical Use: Use 1–2 percent dilution. Patch test first. Well tolerated topically for most people with MCAS. Apply to pulse points, temples, or soles of feet for systemic nervous system support.

Internal Use: Place 1–2 drops in a veggie capsule with carrier oil.

Start Here: Begin with aromatic use as with all new oils. Frankincense is well tolerated by most people with MCAS and is a natural companion to the nervous system regulation practices. Introduce after lavender and Roman chamomile are established.

Cautions: May mildly interact with CYP450 enzymes responsible for metabolizing medications.

Black Pepper (*Piper nigrum*) | *POTS Autonomic Flares and Beta-Caryophyllene Source*

Target: POTS primary (sympathetic modulation); MCAS secondary. Black pepper oil is a potent inhibitor of acetylcholinesterase.[363] This activity helps manage autonomic and immune dysregulation seen in POTS and MCAS. By slowing the breakdown of acetylcholine, parasympathetic (rest and digest) signals are amplified, which can counteract several core symptoms of these conditions. Also a CB2 agonist source alongside copaiba.

Aromatic Use: Place 1–2 drops on a personal inhaler—brief inhalation. The pungent, warming scent can be polarizing; individual tolerance varies. Best used in acute autonomic flares rather than as a continuous background diffusion.

Topical Use: Use 1 percent dilution. A mild warming sensation is a feature of black pepper applied topically—this may be helpful for circulation but can become uncomfortable at higher concentrations or on sensitive skin. Patch test mandatory.

Internal Use: Place 1–2 drops in a capsule with carrier oil.

Start Here: Black pepper is not a first-line introductory oil due to its stimulating and warming nature. Introduce only after milder oils are established. Begin with a single brief aromatic exposure from a tissue.

Cautions: Beta-caryophyllene, alpha-humulene, and caryophyllene oxide content may interfere with CYP3A enzyme activity—consult your physician or pharmacist if on medications metabolized by this enzyme pathway. The stimulating nature of black pepper oil may transiently increase sympathetic tone—use situationally (during autonomic flares) rather than as a continuous daily oil, particularly for patients with hyperadrenergic POTS.

Clary Sage (*Salvia sclarea*) | *Parasympathetic Support and Oxytocin Stimulation*

Target: POTS primary. Inhalation improved mood, reduced cortisol levels, and increased serotonin levels in menopausal women significantly increased salivary oxytocin in clinical research—suggesting vagal and neuroendocrine support relevant to autonomic dysregulation.[364] For someone dealing with autonomic dysregulation, these findings mean that inhalation isn't just relaxing in a psychological sense; it is a physiological intervention. It provides the chemical "permission" for the nervous system to shift out of a hyper-aroused sympathetic state and back into a parasympathetic, restorative state.

Aromatic Use: Place 1–2 drops on personal inhaler. Evening use preferred—clary sage may be sedating in some people.

Topical Use: Use 1–2 percent dilution. Can be applied to abdomen or lower back for menstrual and hormonal support in women with MCAS with estrogen-histamine cycling (discussed in Chapter 10).

Internal Use: It is primarily used topically and aromatically.

Start Here: Begin with brief evening aromatic use. Clary sage is not a first-line introductory oil—introduce after the foundational oils (lavender, Roman chamomile) are established. Particularly relevant for women with MCAS and prominent hormonal cycling of symptoms.

Cautions: Estrogenic-like activity due to sclareol content—theoretically could increase estradiol levels and potentiate the action of estrogen-replacement drugs. Avoid high doses in pregnancy. Avoid with barbiturates as it may increase their seating effects.

✦ ✦ ✦

Oils That May Be More Triggering for People With MCAS

Not all essential oils are appropriate for those with MCAS, and some that have genuine therapeutic properties in healthy populations carry higher sensitization or activation risk in a reactive mast cell system. The following categories warrant particular caution.

- **Phenol-rich oils: oregano, clove, thyme, cinnamon bark** – Phenols including carvacrol, thymol, eugenol, and cinnamaldehyde are among the most bioactive and most potentially irritating essential oil constituents. They have genuine antimicrobial properties (relevant to Chapter 19's gut protocol) but are significant skin sensitizers if not diluted properly, potent mucous membrane irritants, and reliable triggers for mast cell reactions in sensitized individuals likely via MRGPRX2 activation and direct chemical irritation.[365] These oils are not appropriate for general MCAS aromatherapy; their appropriate context is a specific, practitioner-guided gut antimicrobial protocol in encapsulated form.
- **Hot or stimulating oils: eucalyptus, peppermint, camphor** – Menthol (peppermint) and eucalyptol (eucalyptus, rosemary, others) are TRPM8 and TRPV1 channel activators; they stimulate the same sensory receptor pathways that relay temperature and pain signals.[366] For those with MCAS who experience significant neurological sensitization, these oils can trigger reactions through sensory nerve activation (the MRGPRX2-adjacent pathway discussed in Chapter 9).[367] Peppermint is specifically contraindicated in infants and young children for inhalation (it can cause respiratory suppression). For adults with MCAS, introduce with extreme caution and very brief exposure.
- **Synthetic blends and fragrance oils** – Any product that lists "fragrance," "parfum," or "aroma" rather than a specific botanical name is not a genuine essential oil. These are synthetic fragrance compounds—the exact category identified in Chapter 13 as among the most reliable non-dietary mast cell triggers. They provide no therapeutic benefit and carry the full trigger risk of synthetic fragrances.
- **High-ketone oils: sage, hyssop, wormwood** – Certain essential oils contain significant quantities of ketone compounds (thujone, pinocamphone, camphor) that are neurotoxic at higher doses and have provoked seizures in susceptible individuals.[368,369] These are not appropriate for MCAS use.

✦ ✦ ✦

Targeted Applications: Matching Oils to Symptoms

Beyond individual oil selection, understanding how to apply oils strategically to specific symptom patterns helps integrate them into a complete daily protocol.

- **Nervous system support and vagal calming** – Lavender plus Roman chamomile on a personal inhaler, can be used during breathwork practice (Chapter 14) or in the evening wind-down routine. The combination of slow exhale breathing and calming aromatic input creates a compound parasympathetic signal through both respiratory and olfactory pathways simultaneously; this synergy is one of the most practically powerful applications of essential oils in MCAS management.
- **Pre-meal mast cell support** – Use lavender or copaiba on a personal inhaler, two to three slow inhalations, one to two minutes before eating. This brief aromatic exposure supports the parasympathetic state during eating, reducing the sympathetic activation that amplifies food reactions through the nervous system mechanisms described in Chapter 9.
- **Skin reactions and flushing** – Roman chamomile or German chamomile at 0.5–1 percent dilution applied to adjacent unaffected skin (not directly to acutely reactive areas). Lavender at 1 percent dilution can be applied directly to mild hive areas—this is one of the few contexts where slightly higher topical concentration may be appropriate, given lavender's antihistamine properties. Do not apply undiluted oils to reactive skin.
- **Sleep support** – Place bergamot (FCF) plus lavender on a pillow insert, personal inhaler placed near the sleeping area, or passive diffuser. This combination addresses both sleep quality (bergamot's sleep-improvement evidence) and nervous system calming (lavender) without the continuous diffusion that would occur through a room diffuser running all night.
- **POTS autonomic flares** – Use bergamot or black pepper on a personal inhaler during orthostatic symptoms with a brief inhalation (two to three breaths) during the acute cardiovascular stress of positional change or POTS flare.
- **General anti-inflammatory and grounding** – Frankincense + copaiba in diffusion or topical application addresses multiple anti-inflammatory pathways (frankincense, copaiba) and CB2 receptor signaling (copaiba beta-caryophyllene) as a complementary anti-inflammatory aromatic pair suitable for consistent daily background use. They can also be used internally.

✦ ✦ ✦

Quick Reference: Essential Oil Protocol Summary

The table below consolidates the key practical details for each oil covered in this chapter. Due to the number of fields required, the table focuses on the four most clinically critical columns. Refer to the individual oil profiles above for the complete picture.

Essential Oil	Target	Aromatic	Topical	Internal	Key Caution
Lavender	MCAS + POTS	1–2 drops inhaler or 1–3 drops / 100 mL diffuser	1–2% dilution; patch test first	2 drops in capsule with carrier oil	Antifungal drugs and antibiotics
German Chamomile	MCAS	1 drop inhaler; brief sessions	1% dilution; highly concentrated	1–2 drops in capsule with carrier oil	Asteraceae family—avoid if ragweed-allergic; CYP450 interaction
Roman Chamomile	MCAS + POTS	1–2 drops inhaler; evening preferred	1–2% dilution; well tolerated	1–2 drops in capsule with carrier oil	Asteraceae family caution; gentler than German chamomile; good first choice
Blue Tansy	MCAS	1 drop on tissue; very brief	1% dilution; patch test mandatory	Primarily used for skin (topical)	Asteraceae family; epilepsy, seizures, convulsions; G6PD deficiency
Bergamot (FCF)	POTS + MCAS	1–2 drops inhaler; brief diffusion	1% dilution; FCF (bergapten-free)	1–2 drops in capsule with carrier oil	Photosensitizing; anticholinergic/ cholinergic drugs
Copaiba	MCAS + POTS	1–2 drops inhaler or diffuser	1–3% dilution; very well tolerated	1–3 drops in capsule with carrier; among the safest for internal use	Very well tolerated; one of the safest oils for sensitive patients; start here; CYP450 interaction
Frankincense	MCAS + POTS	1–2 drops inhaler or diffuser	1–2% dilution; patch test	1–2 drops in capsule	Well tolerated by most; CYP450 interaction
Black Pepper	POTS + MCAS	1–2 drops inhaler; brief sessions	1% dilution; warming effect	1–2 drops in capsule	Mildly warming; stimulating; CYP3A interaction

Essential Oil	Target	Aromatic	Topical	Internal	Key Caution
Clary Sage	POTS	1–2 drops inhaler	1–2% dilution	Primarily used aromatically and topically	Estrogen-like activity; avoid during pregnancy; barbiturates

> **Introduction Reminder:** *Begin every new essential oil with aromatic use only—one drop on a tissue, one to two brief inhalations, once daily. Observe for two to three days before expanding to diffusion, topical, or any internal use. One oil at a time, following the same protocol logic as Chapters 16 and 17.*

✦ ✦ ✦

Deeper Dive: How Essential Oils Work at the Molecular Level

For the Science-Minded Reader

Essential oils are among the most pharmacologically complex natural substances used in clinical practice, and their multi-target mechanism of action at the cellular and molecular level is what distinguishes them from simple fragrances. Understanding the primary receptor and signaling targets illuminates both their therapeutic potential and the reason for individual variability in response.

Olfactory–Limbic–Autonomic Axis

Smell is unusual among the senses because it reaches emotion- and memory-related brain networks more directly than the classic visual, auditory, and touch pathways. Olfactory neurons in the nose send unmyelinated fibers to the olfactory bulb, which then projects to primary olfactory regions including the piriform cortex, parts of the amygdala, and the entorhinal cortex. This direct anatomical connection is why inhaled essential oils produce measurable changes in autonomic state, heart rate variability, cortisol levels, and emotional tone within seconds—far faster than any oral preparation could achieve systemic effect.[370] For individuals with MCAS, this rapid limbic access makes aromatic essential oils a uniquely fast tool for shifting the nervous system state that determines mast cell threshold.

TRPV1, TRPM8, and Sensory Receptor Modulation

Many essential oil constituents modulate transient receptor potential (TRP) channels—ion channels in sensory neurons that detect temperature, chemical stimuli, pain, and mechanical forces. Menthol from peppermint activates TRPM8 (the cold receptor), producing the familiar cooling sensation.[371] Cinnamaldehyde activates TRPV1 (the heat and pain receptor).[372] Linalool from lavender modulates

TRPA1 (the pain, cold, and itch receptor) in a way that reduces its sensitivity—essentially dampening the pain and sensitization signaling that, through the MRGPRX2 pathway discussed in Chapter 9, can trigger mast cell activation.[373] This is part of the mechanistic explanation for lavender's anti-nociceptive and calming effects—it reduces sensory nerve excitability, which reduces the neuropeptide signals (substance P, CGRP) that activate mast cells through the neurogenic pathway.

Beta-Caryophyllene and CB2 Receptor Signaling

Beta-caryophyllene (BCP), the primary constituent of copaiba and a significant component of black pepper, clove, and several other oils, is the only essential oil constituent identified as a full agonist at cannabinoid CB2 receptors. CB2 receptors are expressed on mast cells, macrophages, and other immune cells, and their activation produces anti-inflammatory, analgesic, and immunomodulatory effects without the psychoactive effects associated with CB1 receptor activation. This makes BCP particularly relevant for MCAS: CB2 agonism directly reduces mast cell mediator release, suppresses NF-κB-driven inflammatory gene expression, and reduces neuropathic pain signaling.[374,375] The fact that BCP achieves this through dietary and aromatic exposure distinguishes it from pharmaceutical CB2 agonists and supports its use as a food-precedented signaling molecule.

The Synergy of Aromatic and Internal Routes

When essential oils are used both aromatically and internally under appropriate guidance, their mechanisms of action are additive and sometimes synergistic in ways that either route alone cannot achieve. Aromatic lavender modulates limbic tone and reduces amygdala-driven sympathetic activation within seconds.[376,377] When taken in a capsule, internal lavender provides a multi-layered approach to calming the nervous system. Rather than just targeting a single receptor, it unselectively inhibits several Voltage-Gated Calcium Channels (VOCCs), specifically the P/Q-type and N-type channels.[378] This inhibition helps dial down the overactive CNS signaling associated with anxiety. The two routes together provide both the rapid limbic onset of aromatic use and the sustained systemic coverage of internal use—a combination that represents the most complete deployment of the oil's pharmacological potential. Essentially, inhalation triggers rapid effects, while ingestion sustains these effects. This layered approach, when clinically indicated, illustrates why essential oils should be understood as multi-pathway signaling molecules rather than single-mechanism interventions.

✦ ✦ ✦

What This Means for You: Building Your Essential Oil Practice

Integrating essential oils into an MCAS protocol is most effective when it is approached as a deliberate, sequenced addition to an already-established foundation—not as a parallel track of casual aromatic experimentation.

Begin with the two most universally tolerated oils: lavender and Roman chamomile. These two oils have the broadest safety profile in sensitive populations, strong evidence for MCAS-relevant mechanisms, and the most pleasant aromatic profiles—making them the lowest-risk, highest-return starting point for most people with MCAS. Begin with lavender, then introduce Roman chamomile one week later using the same aromatic-first protocol.

Integrate aromatic use into your existing practices from Chapter 14. The most natural entry point for essential oils is alongside the nervous system practices already established. One drop of lavender on a tissue used during morning extended-exhale breathing, or Roman chamomile diffused during an evening body scan, layers aromatic benefit onto an already-established practice without requiring new dedicated time. This is not supplemental—it is synergistic.

Build toward targeted applications before considering internal use. The sequence for any person with MCAS approaching essential oils: aromatic → topical → internal. Most people will find substantial benefit at the aromatic and topical stages. Internal use provides a supplementary method to unlock additional benefits that are more systemic in nature.

Treat your collection as a small, curated toolkit rather than a broad collection. The temptation to acquire many oils is understandable but counterproductive for those with MCAS. A small collection of well-chosen, high-quality oils used consistently and skillfully produces better outcomes than a large collection used intermittently and without strategy. Five to seven oils—lavender, Roman chamomile, frankincense, copaiba, bergamot FCF, and one or two targeted additions based on your symptom profile—is a complete and clinically adequate essential oil toolkit for most people with MCAS.

Discuss essential oils with your healthcare team. Like herbs and supplements, essential oils interact with medications through CYP450 pathways, have relevant contraindications in certain health conditions, and warrant disclosure to any provider supervising your care. The integration of aromatic, topical, and internal essential oil use into a medical management plan for MCAS is most safely done transparently and collaboratively.

Anna's morning drop of lavender on a tissue before her most reactive meal did not resolve her MCAS. She would be the first to say so. But it became one of the consistent, low-cost, immediate-access tools in a toolkit that also included her dietary protocol, her supplement regimen, her gut healing work, and the breathwork she did every morning. Together, those tools added up to a life she could live rather than one she was merely surviving. The lavender was one thread in a fabric—and the fabric held.

That is the appropriate frame for essential oils in MCAS: not a single solution, but a meaningful and evidence-informed addition to a comprehensive protocol, applied with the precision and respect that powerful signaling molecules deserve.

✦ ✦ ✦

Chapter 18 at a Glance

What to Remember:

- Essential oils are complex multi-constituent signaling molecules, not simple fragrances. A single oil may simultaneously modulate ion channels, activate olfactory-limbic pathways, bind G protein-coupled receptors, and exert anti-inflammatory effects—making their therapeutic potential meaningfully distinct from isolated aromatic compounds.
- Those with MCAS require lower doses, slower introduction, and more careful observation than general aromatherapy guidelines suggest. The bucket theory applies to aromatic chemical exposure—even therapeutic oils become triggers when the system is already reactive.
- Purity and sourcing are clinical requirements, not preferences. Adulterated or synthetic-fragrance-containing products carry the full trigger risk of synthetic fragrances without the therapeutic benefits of genuine plant chemistry. GC/MS testing documentation is the minimum sourcing standard for MCAS use.
- Aromatic use is always the appropriate starting point—fastest-acting, lowest-risk, and most directly connected to the limbic-autonomic pathway most relevant to MCAS nervous system regulation. Personal inhalers and tissue application provide better dose control than open diffusion.
- Topical use requires dilution around 1 percent for individuals with MCAS—significantly lower than general aromatherapy guidance. Patch testing before any new oil combination is non-negotiable.
- Internal use is a legitimate and pharmacologically meaningful route of administration for appropriate oils using reasonable best practices. Copaiba, lavender, frankincense, and Roman chamomile are among the oils with the most appropriate internal use profiles for MCAS patients.

- The foundational MCAS oil protocol is lavender and Roman chamomile (mast cell stabilization, nervous system calming); copaiba and frankincense (anti-inflammatory, CB2 support); bergamot FCF (POTS and sleep support). Introduce one at a time, aromatically first.
- Phenol-rich oils (oregano, clove, thyme, cinnamon) are not general MCAS aromatherapy oils; their appropriate context is a specific gut antimicrobial protocol (Chapter 19) in encapsulated form under guidance, not daily aromatic use.

Coming Up in Chapter 19:

The gut is both the primary site of histamine production and the primary site of histamine clearance—making gut healing one of the highest-leverage interventions available in MCAS management. Chapter 19 provides the practical gut healing protocol: SIBO management including the evidence-informed role of essential oils as antimicrobial agents, gut lining repair strategies, DAO enzyme production support, and the probiotic guidance that navigates the critical distinction between strains that help and strains that harm.

CHAPTER 19

Gut Healing Protocols

SIBO Management, Gut Lining Repair, DAO Support, and the Probiotic Map

The Factory She Didn't Know Was Running

For three years, Nina had assumed that her MCAS was primarily a skin condition with unfortunate neurological consequences. The hives were the thing she saw. The brain fog was the thing she felt. She ate carefully, she slept carefully, she managed her stress with the practices from Chapter 14. She made real progress. And then progress stopped—hitting a plateau that no dietary adjustment, no supplement tweak, and no additional nervous system work seemed to move.

Her functional medicine practitioner ordered a lactulose breath test. The result was unambiguous: significant hydrogen gas elevation, consistent with small intestinal bacterial overgrowth (SIBO). Alongside it, a stool analysis showed a near-complete absence of *Lactobacillus rhamnosus* and *Bifidobacterium* species, and a high reading for beta-glucuronidase—the bacterial enzyme that recirculates estrogen in the gut, contributing to the estrogen dominance discussed in Chapter 10.

Nina hadn't known that her gut was running a continuous internal histamine factory, independent of everything she ate or didn't eat. While she had been scrupulously avoiding aged cheese and leftovers, billions of bacteria in her small intestine were producing histamine around the clock—absorbed directly into her portal circulation before any DAO enzyme could degrade it. Her bucket hadn't been draining because the tap on the inside was wide open.

Gut healing is not one intervention. It is a protocol—a sequenced set of steps that addresses the overlapping problems of pathogen overgrowth, barrier dysfunction, dysbiosis, and impaired histamine clearance in an order that makes each step more effective and safer than if attempted out of sequence. This chapter provides that protocol in full: how to manage SIBO including the evidence-informed role of essential oils as antimicrobials, how to repair the gut lining, how to support DAO enzyme production, and how to rebuild the microbiome with strains that help rather than harm.

✦ ✦ ✦

Before Starting: The Sequence Matters

Gut healing in MCAS follows the same sequencing logic established in Chapter 12 for the overall recovery framework; interventions must be introduced in the right order, or the ones that should help become additional sources of reaction. The gut healing sequence has four phases that build on each other, and skipping phases consistently produces the frustrated circling pattern that many individuals with gut-driven MCAS know intimately.

The Four-Phase Gut Healing Sequence

Phase 1 — Reduce: Lessen lower dietary inputs that feed pathogen overgrowth and worsen dysbiosis. Begin the low-histamine dietary approach from Chapter 13. Reduce fermentable carbohydrates if SIBO is suspected (temporarily). Dramatically reduce the most significant dietary sources of gut irritation (alcohol, NSAIDs, ultra-processed foods).

Phase 2 — Remove: Address active gut infections—SIBO, *Candida* overgrowth, or other identified pathogens—with targeted antimicrobial agents (pharmaceutical or herbal/essential oil). This is the most medically complex phase and the one that most benefits from practitioner guidance.

Phase 3 — Repair: Restore gut barrier integrity using gut-lining compounds (L-glutamine, zinc carnosine, collagen, aloe vera) and support DAO enzyme activity through nutritional and supplemental means.

Phase 4 — Replenish: Rebuild the gut microbiome with histamine-safe probiotic strains and prebiotic fiber support that feeds beneficial bacteria and promotes butyrate production.

> **Timing Note:** *Phase 2 (removal of pathogens) should not be initiated until Phase 1 dietary foundations are established for at least two to four weeks. Starting antimicrobial protocols in a gut that has not yet reduced its pathogenic feeding substrate (fermentable carbohydrates, sugar, alcohol) produces partial results at best and significant die-off reactions at worst. And Phase 4 probiotics should not be introduced until Phase 2 antimicrobial treatment is complete—probiotics taken during active antimicrobial treatment are largely eliminated alongside the pathogens being targeted—at least by pharmaceuticals; natural solutions, particularly essential oils are at least partly selective and can be taken at least two hours after taking antimicrobial essential oils.*

✦ ✦ ✦

SIBO Management: Clearing the Internal Histamine Factory

SIBO—discussed in its biological detail in Chapter 6—represents one of the most significant and most frequently missed drivers of histamine excess in MCAS. When bacteria establish significant colonies in the small intestine, they convert dietary histidine to histamine continuously, producing a chronic internal histamine burden that no dietary modification can fully address because its source is not the food itself but the bacteria processing it.

SIBO is diagnosed through hydrogen and methane breath testing—typically a lactulose or glucose challenge breath test measuring fermentation gases over a two to three hour collection period. Hydrogen-dominant SIBO involves primarily gram-negative bacteria; methane-dominant SIBO (technically intestinal methanogen overgrowth, or IMO) involves archaea and tends toward constipation-predominant symptoms. Hydrogen sulfide–producing SIBO is the most recently characterized form, associated with diarrhea, fatigue, and a characteristic rotten-egg smell. Each pattern has somewhat different treatment considerations, and accurate diagnosis guides the choice of antimicrobial approach.

Pharmaceutical SIBO Treatment

The most evidence-supported pharmaceutical approach to SIBO is rifaximin—a minimally absorbed antibiotic that acts locally in the gut with minimal systemic absorption or impact on vaginal and urinary microbiomes. For hydrogen-dominant SIBO, rifaximin alone (typically 1,200–1,550 mg daily for fourteen days) produces significant improvement or clearance in clinical trials.[379] For methane-dominant IMO, rifaximin combined with neomycin produces better outcomes than either alone in preliminary studies from methane-positive IBS-C participants, as methanogens require a combined antibiotic approach.[380] Pharmaceutical SIBO treatment is highly effective but requires a prescription, appropriate diagnostic confirmation, and clinical management of die-off reactions—which in MCAS individuals can be significant and require mast cell stabilization support throughout the treatment period. Since rifaximin and neomycin are almost completely non-absorbable—they stay in the intestines—and have a more local action, they don't tend to have the same systemic side effects as other antibiotics.

Herbal Antimicrobial SIBO Treatment

Herbal antimicrobial protocols for SIBO have been studied in clinical trials and show efficacy comparable to rifaximin for hydrogen-dominant SIBO in head-to-head comparisons. The most studied herbal combination protocols use berberine-containing herbs (Oregon grape, goldenseal, or berberine extract), allicin (from garlic-derived allicin preparations), and oregano oil or other antimicrobial herb combinations over four to six weeks. The primary advantage of herbal protocols for those with MCAS is the more gradual die-off response compared to antibiotics, which reduces the severity of the Herxheimer-like mast cell flares that acute bacterial die-off can provoke. The primary disadvantage is a longer treatment course and more variable efficacy for methane-dominant and hydrogen sulfide SIBO.

Herbal SIBO Protocol: Dosing, Timing, and Practical Guidance

The three primary agents in herbal SIBO protocols each have distinct mechanisms and dosing considerations, and they work most effectively in combination rather than individually.

Berberine (400–500 mg, two to three times daily with meals) acts against gram-negative SIBO bacteria and *Candida*—through membrane disruption, mitochondrial disruption, and interference with fungi cell cycle and DNA-related processes—and inhibition of bacterial DNA replication.[381,382,383] It also has documented prokinetic effects—improving the migrating motor complex that sweeps the small intestine between meals—which addresses one of the primary conditions that allows SIBO to establish and recur.[384] Indeed berberine, and 400 mg twice daily has shown efficacy comparable to rifaximin.[385,386] Take with food to reduce GI irritation. Use standardized berberine HCl or berberine sulfate rather than whole herb preparations for more predictable dosing. Important caution: Berberine significantly inhibits CYP3A4 and P-glycoprotein enzymes and can raise serum levels of many medications metabolized by these pathways, including certain antihistamines, antidepressants, and immunosuppressants. Disclose berberine use to your prescribing physician before starting. Avoid in pregnancy.

Allicin (from stabilized allicin preparations, 450–900 mg daily in divided doses) is the primary active compound from garlic. Unlike raw garlic (whose allicin content is highly variable and unstable), stabilized allicin preparations such as Allimax or AlliUltra provide consistent, quantifiable activity. Allicin is particularly active against methane-producing archaea—organisms that are not susceptible to rifaximin alone and that require a combined antimicrobial approach.[387] This makes allicin the key addition when breath testing reveals methane-dominant IMO. Take with meals. Allicin's sulfur compounds can cause GI warmth and noticeable breath odor at higher doses—this signals the preparation is active. Start at 450 mg daily and increase over one week if well tolerated.

Oregano oil herbal extract (200–400 mg standardized extract, two to three times daily with meals) is standardized to carvacrol content (minimum

70 percent) and is available as enteric-coated softgels that reduce upper GI contact. This is the same active compound found in oregano essential oil but delivered in a botanical extract form with a more moderate and defined carvacrol concentration. It can be used in place of or alongside encapsulated oregano essential oil. Take with food always.

✦ ✦ ✦

Essential Oils as Gut Antimicrobials: The Evidence-Based Protocol

Essential oils occupy an important and increasingly evidence-supported role in the herbal antimicrobial approach to SIBO and gut dysbiosis. The phenol-rich and terpenoid-rich oils discussed with caution in Chapter 18 for aromatic and topical use in people with MCAS have their primary therapeutic application here—in encapsulated internal form, where their potent antimicrobial activity can be directed at gut pathogens without triggering respiratory or dermal mast cell reactions.

The key principle for gut antimicrobial essential oil use is containment: encapsulating the oil in a vegetable capsule with a fatty carrier (fractionated coconut oil, MCT oil, or olive oil) carries it through the stomach and into the small intestine where it is absorbed and active. This delivery method is the standard approach in integrative gastroenterology for essential oil-based gut antimicrobial protocols.

> **Protocol Parameters:** *The general essential oil gut antimicrobial protocol: 5 drops total of essential oil per dose (this may be one oil at 5 drops or a blend of multiple oils adding to 5 drops total), in a veggie capsule with a small amount of carrier oil, taken with food, up to three times daily. Take at least two hours away from probiotics to prevent the antimicrobial oils from eliminating the beneficial bacteria you are introducing. Always use therapeutic-grade, GC/MS-verified oils for internal use.*

The following profiles cover the essential oils with the strongest evidence for gut pathogen clearance relevant to SIBO and MCAS-associated gut dysbiosis. Each profile specifies the pathogens targeted, the appropriate dose and capsule method, and the cautions specific to internal use in MCAS patients.

Oregano (*Origanum vulgare*, carvacrol CT) | *Broad-Spectrum Gut Antimicrobial*

Pathogen Targets: *Candida albicans, E. coli, Klebsiella pneumoniae, Enterococcus faecalis, Salmonella, Shigella,* including antibiotic-resistant organisms. Carvacrol and thymol (primary constituents) disrupt bacterial cell membranes and inhibit biofilm formation—relevant to the biofilm-protected SIBO organisms discussed in Chapter 7.[388]

Dose: Put 1–2 drops per dose in a capsule with carrier oil. Start at 1 drop and observe before increasing. Total per dose (combined with other oils) should generally not exceed 5 drops.

Capsule Method: Open a size 0 veggie capsule, add 1–2 drops oregano oil, then fill the rest of the capsule with a fatty oil. Seal and take immediately with food. Do not store filled capsules—prepare fresh for each dose.

Timing: With meals, up to three times daily. At least two hours before or after probiotics. Continue for four to six weeks for SIBO treatment, or as directed by practitioner.

Cautions: Most common complaint is eructation (burping back volatile oils). May cause GI warmth or mild cramping initially. Not appropriate during pregnancy. Avoid in individuals with known oregano or thyme allergy. The strong antimicrobial activity means significant die-off is possible—maintain mast cell stabilization protocol throughout treatment and pace dose increases carefully. Potential drug interactions: aspirin, blood pressure meds, antibiotics/antifungals (almost always increases their effectiveness), and anticholinergic/cholinergic drugs.

Thyme (*Thymus vulgaris*, thymol CT) | *Strong Broad-Spectrum Antimicrobial*

Pathogen Targets: Broad-spectrum: *E. coli, Klebsiella, Enterococcus, S. aureus, Candida, Salmonella*, and several antibiotic-resistant organisms are its targets. Thymol is among the most extensively researched antimicrobial compounds in essential oil science.[389] It is particularly effective against biofilm-forming organisms.

Dose: Use 1–2 drops per dose, typically in combination with oregano or another antimicrobial oil rather than as the sole oil. Strong phenol content and longer half-life warrants conservative dosing.

Capsule Method: Same as oregano: veggie capsule with carrier oil, prepare fresh, take with food. Thyme oil can be combined with oregano (1 drop each) for broader spectrum coverage within the 5-drop total limit.

Timing: Take with meals, up to three times daily, two hours away from probiotics.

Cautions: This is highly potent—among the strongest phenol-containing oils. Avoid in pregnancy. Start at 1 drop and assess tolerance carefully before increasing. The CT (chemotype) matters—thymol chemotype is the antimicrobially active form. Potential drug interactions: aspirin, blood pressure meds, antibiotics/antifungals (almost always increases their effectiveness), and anticholinergic/cholinergic drugs.

Oregano and thyme are often used in combination, as their overlapping but not identical constituent profiles provide broader antimicrobial coverage than either alone. A typical starting capsule for SIBO might contain 1 drop oregano plus 1 drop thyme plus 3 drops of a milder oil (fennel or peppermint) in carrier oil—providing antimicrobial action alongside carminative support for gas and bloating symptoms.

Peppermint (*Mentha piperita*) | *IBS, Gut Motility, and Antispasmodic Support*

Pathogen Targets: Moderate antimicrobial activity; primary therapeutic role is antispasmodic and prokinetic rather than antimicrobial. Widely used in clinical trials for IBS—enteric-coated peppermint oil capsules are supported by multiple meta-analyses for reducing IBS symptoms including pain, bloating, and altered motility.[390] Also supports the gut motility improvement needed to prevent SIBO recurrence.

Dose: Place 1–3 drops in capsule with carrier oil, or use commercial enteric-coated peppermint oil capsules (IBgard, Colpermin) that are specifically designed for small intestine release. Standard enteric-coated dose: 180–225 mg (4–5 drops) per capsule, one to two capsules before meals.

Capsule Method: Enteric-coated commercial products are preferred for IBS/motility applications as they deliver oil specifically to the small intestine. For gut antimicrobial blends: 1–3 drops in a veggie capsule with carrier, as part of a combined antimicrobial protocol.

Timing: Before meals for IBS/motility support. With meals as part of antimicrobial blend. Two hours away from probiotics.

Cautions: May worsen gastroesophageal reflux (GERD) by relaxing the lower esophageal sphincter—use enteric-coated capsules in people with reflux to prevent oil release in the stomach. Potential drug interactions: cyclosporine, other immunosuppressants, fluorouracil, antibiotics/antifungals, drugs metabolized by CYP4A or CYP2C, caffeine, codeine (extreme doses), and midazolam (extreme doses). May increase the risk of jaundice in children with G6PD deficiency. Speak to your provider before use if you have ventricular fibrillation or iron-deficiency or iron-deficiency anemia.

Cinnamon Bark (*Cinnamomum verum*) | *Anti-Candida and Broad-Spectrum Antibacterial*

Pathogen Targets: *Candida albicans* (strong activity), *E. coli, Klebsiella, Salmonella, Shigella, Proteus,* and antibiotic-resistant strains. Cinnamaldehyde disrupts *Candida* cell membrane and biofilm formation.[391] Relevant for gut dysbiosis with a significant *Candida* component alongside bacterial overgrowth.

Dose: 1–2 drops maximum per dose—cinnamon is one of the most potent and potentially irritating gut oils. Always combine with carrier oil and a buffering milder oil (peppermint or fennel). Total dose per capsule should include no more than 2 drops cinnamon.

Capsule Method: Veggie capsule with generous carrier oil (the fatty oil mitigates mucous membrane contact). Combine with 2–3 drops peppermint or fennel to buffer the potency. Prepare fresh each dose. Never take undiluted.

Timing: Take with meals only—never on an empty stomach—once to twice daily maximum due to potency; allow two hours from probiotics.

Cautions: Cinnamaldehyde is a potent mucosal irritant—strict dosing adherence is essential. Do not exceed 2 drops per dose. GI burning, cramping, or heat indicates dose is too high—reduce or discontinue. Avoid in pregnancy. Potential drug interactions: aspirin, blood pressure meds, MAOI antidepressants, cholinergic/anticholinergic meds, and antibiotics (normally increases effectiveness).

Anise (*Pimpinella anisum*) | *Mild Broad-Spectrum Option — Better Tolerated by Reactive Patients*

Pathogen Targets: *E. coli, Pseudomonas aeruginosa, S. aureus, S. pyogenes, Candida albicans* are targets. It's a milder but still clinically relevant antimicrobial, described in the source literature as a good option when the stronger phenol-rich oils are too reactive for the individual. Anethole (primary constituent) provides antimicrobial and carminative activity.

Dose: Use 2–3 drops per dose in capsule with carrier oil. Better tolerated than oregano and thyme for people with significant gut sensitivity or high MCAS reactivity.

Capsule Method: A veggie capsule with carrier oil can be used as the primary antimicrobial oil for more sensitive people or as a foundation with 1 drop of oregano added as tolerance builds.

Timing: Take with meals, up to three times daily, providing two hours from probiotics.

Cautions: Avoid in pregnancy. Potential drug interactions include aspirin, blood pressure meds, diabetes drugs, acetaminophen, caffeine, ibuprofen, benzodiazepines, and barbiturates, and antidepressants (fluoxetine and imipramine). Generally well tolerated at therapeutic doses, but can cause mild GI sensitivity initially—start at 2 drops and observe.

Fennel (*Foeniculum vulgare*, trans-anethole CT) | *Carminative, Digestive Support, and Mild Antimicrobial*

Pathogen Targets: With mild antimicrobial activity against gut-associated pathogens, its primary role is carminative (gas-relieving), antispasmodic, and digestive support. It's often used as a buffering companion oil in antimicrobial blends to reduce the GI intensity of stronger oils and provide simultaneous symptom relief for the bloating and cramping that accompanies SIBO treatment.

Dose: Use 2–3 drops per dose as part of a combined protocol. Can be used as the sole oil for mild digestive support without the antimicrobial intent of the other oils.

Capsule Method: A veggie capsule with carrier, it pairs well with oregano (1 drop), thyme (1 drop), fennel (2 drops), peppermint (1 drop) as a comprehensive SIBO blend within the 5-drop limit.

Timing: Take with meals, up to three times daily, but can be taken more often for acute carminative support (reducing gas and bloating).

Cautions: Avoid in pregnancy. Potential drug interactions: aspirin, blood pressure meds, diabetes drugs, acetaminophen, caffeine, ibuprofen, benzodiazepines, and barbiturates, antidepressants (fluoxetine and imipramine). It's generally well tolerated at therapeutic doses; can cause mild GI sensitivity initially—start at 2 drops and observe.

✦ ✦ ✦

Combining Herbal Protocols With Essential Oils: Synergy and Risk

Herbal antimicrobials and encapsulated essential oils can be used together within a SIBO protocol, and in many cases the combination provides broader pathogen coverage than either alone. Berberine covers gram-negative bacteria and *Candida* through different molecular targets than carvacrol (oregano) or thymol (thyme), meaning they address overlapping but distinct microbial populations simultaneously. Allicin provides specific archaea coverage that neither berberine nor carvacrol-based oils achieve as reliably. A well-designed combined protocol—guided by the specific SIBO subtype identified on breath testing—might include berberine and allicin from the herbal category alongside peppermint and fennel from the essential oil category, with oregano in either or both forms depending on tolerated dose. This layered approach mirrors the published herbal SIBO clinical trials that demonstrated rifaximin-comparable efficacy.

The most significant combined-protocol risk for individuals with MCAS is cumulative die-off burden. When multiple antimicrobial agents are introduced simultaneously, pathogen kill-off can be rapid and extensive, releasing large quantities of bacterial endotoxins into the gut lumen and circulation—a potent and direct mast cell trigger. Starting all herbal and essential oil antimicrobials at full dose on the same day consistently produces the overwhelming Herxheimer-like flares that derail treatment. The solution is sequential introduction: begin with the mildest agents first (peppermint, fennel, anise), establish tolerance over one to two weeks, then introduce berberine, then oregano oil, then allicin. This staggered approach spreads die-off burden across the treatment course and keeps individual flares manageable.

A secondary risk is redundancy without complementarity: using both oregano herbal extract and oregano essential oil adds carvacrol dose but not additional spectrum coverage. In a reactive MCAS gut, doubling the same chemical class adds irritation risk without adding antimicrobial breadth. The most strategic combinations pair agents with distinct mechanisms—berberine (membrane and DNA target), carvacrol/thymol (membrane disruption via a different pathway), allicin (sulfur-based thiol reactivity), and cinnamaldehyde (*Candida*-specific cell wall disruption)—rather than stacking the same class.

> **Practitioner Guidance Strongly Recommended:** *Combining herbal antimicrobials and essential oil antimicrobials into a comprehensive SIBO protocol is medically complex territory. The drug interaction profile of berberine, the potency of phenol-rich essential oils, the MCAS die-off management required, and the need to match protocol design to breath test results all argue strongly for working with a knowledgeable practitioner rather than self-designing a combined protocol from reading alone. The information above equips you to have an informed conversation with your practitioner—not to replace it.*

✦ ✦ ✦

Phase 3: Repairing the Gut Lining

Once antimicrobial treatment is underway or complete, gut barrier repair becomes the primary focus. A damaged gut lining—with widened tight junctions, depleted enterocyte populations, and inadequate mucus layer—is both the consequence of dysbiosis and the mechanism through which dysbiosis perpetuates mast cell activation. Repairing it is not optional for those with MCAS since it is a significant gut component to their condition; it is the step that breaks the cycle.

The gut lining repair protocol draws on the compounds introduced in Chapter 16 (L-glutamine, zinc carnosine) and adds several additional targeted agents appropriate for Phase 3.

L-Glutamine: The Enterocyte Fuel

As established in Chapter 16, L-glutamine is the primary energy substrate for enterocytes—the cells lining the small intestinal wall. Glutamine supplementation directly supports enterocyte renewal and tight junction protein synthesis. During Phase 3, glutamine use continues at the doses established in Chapter 16 (2,500–5,000 mg daily in divided doses between meals) and may be increased toward the higher end of the therapeutic range (up to 10,000 mg daily) for individuals with documented significant intestinal permeability.

Zinc Carnosine: Mucosal Coating and Repair

Zinc carnosine (PepZin GI) has a unique mechanism among gut repair compounds: it adheres to the gastric and intestinal mucosa, forming a sustained protective coating that accelerates healing of ulcerations and erosions,[392] stimulates mucus production, and reduces local inflammation. Clinical trials have demonstrated its effectiveness for gastric ulcer healing, and its use in intestinal permeability repair is supported by functional medicine clinical observation. At the doses from Chapter 16 (75 mg zinc carnosine twice daily), it contributes meaningfully to mucosal repair during Phase 3.

Deglycyrrhizinated Licorice (DGL)

Deglycyrrhizinated licorice (DGL) is licorice root extract from which glycyrrhizinic acid has been removed—the compound responsible for licorice's blood-pressure-elevating effects. What remains is a collection of flavonoids and other constituents that stimulate mucus secretion, support the thickness of the protective mucus layer in the stomach and small intestine, and reduce mucosal inflammation without the hormonal effects of whole licorice.[393] DGL is particularly useful in Phase 3 for individuals with upper GI symptoms—GERD, gastritis, or a sensation of gastric irritation. Standard dose: 380–760 mg of DGL chewable tablets or powder, taken twenty minutes before meals.

Aloe Vera (Inner Leaf, Decolorized)

Aloe vera inner leaf gel contains acemannan—a complex polysaccharide that supports mucosal integrity, mildly promotes positive shifts in the gut microbiome, and has documented anti-inflammatory effects in the gut lining.[394,395,396,397] The critical qualification is decolorized aloe vera: the outer leaf of the aloe plant contains anthraquinones (particularly aloin) that are laxative and potentially carcinogenic at higher doses. Properly processed inner leaf gel that has been decolorized (the anthraquinones removed) is a safe and effective gut healing agent. Dose: 30–60 mL of decolorized aloe vera gel or 200 mg of standardized decolorized aloe extract, twice daily between meals.

Collagen and Bone Broth

Collagen peptides and bone broth provide glycine, proline, and hydroxyproline—the amino acids that are the primary building blocks of the connective tissue proteins that support intestinal wall structure. Glycine in particular is a conditional nutrient for gut health: it is required for the synthesis of collagen, glutathione (the primary antioxidant in gut epithelium), and bile acid conjugation. High-quality bone broth made from fresh bones (not canned or from stored cooked bones) is one of the few foods that directly supports gut barrier repair while remaining low-histamine if prepared properly. Collagen peptide supplements (unflavored, hydrolyzed, from grass-fed bovine sources) at 10–20 grams daily provide a reliable and quantifiable glycine source.

> **The Gut Repair Stack:** *The Phase 3 repair stack for most individuals with MCAS: L-glutamine (2,500–5,000 mg daily), zinc carnosine (75 mg twice daily), DGL (380 mg before meals if upper GI symptoms are present), decolorized aloe vera (30 mL twice daily between meals), and collagen peptides (10–20 g daily). These work synergistically across the three structural layers of gut barrier repair: tight junction protein synthesis (glutamine), mucosal coating (zinc carnosine, DGL), and connective tissue infrastructure (collagen).*

✦ ✦ ✦

Supporting DAO Production and Histamine Clearance

DAO enzyme activity is not simply a genetic constant—it's a dynamic property of gut health that improves as the gut lining heals, as dysbiosis resolves, and as the nutritional cofactors that the enzyme requires become reliably available. Supporting DAO production is therefore both a direct nutritional intervention and an indirect consequence of the broader gut healing protocol.

Nutritional Cofactors for DAO

Diamine oxidase requires specific cofactors to function at full capacity: copper (as a structural component of the enzyme's active site), vitamin B6 in its active P5P form (required for the pyridoxal phosphate-dependent reaction step), and vitamin C (as a reducing agent that protects the enzyme from oxidative inactivation). These are the same cofactors addressed in Chapter 16, but their role in DAO production deserves specific emphasis here. In people with significant gut dysbiosis, chronic stress, or poor diet quality, deficiencies in all three are common and represent a correctable bottleneck in histamine clearance.

Dietary sources of copper include shellfish (oysters are the most concentrated source), liver, nuts and seeds (cashews, sunflower seeds), and dark chocolate (well tolerated in moderate amounts by individuals without cocoa sensitivity). Vitamin C from fresh bell peppers, kiwi, and broccoli (as established in Chapter 15) and P5P from poultry, fish, and potatoes provide the remaining cofactors. Supplemental copper at 1–2 mg daily alongside zinc supplementation (copper and zinc compete for absorption), supplemental P5P at 25–50 mg daily, and buffered vitamin C at 500 mg twice daily address deficiencies reliably across most MCAS patients.

Probiotic Strains That Upregulate DAO

Lactobacillus rhamnosus GG has been specifically shown to modulate gene expression related to allergy-related high-affinity IgE receptor subunits α and γ (FCER1A and FCER1G, respectively) and histamine H4 receptor in gut epithelial cells—one of the few probiotics with direct evidence for diminishing mast cell allergy-related activation due to a high affinity for IgE and histamine receptor genes.[398] This strain's combination of downregulation histamine receptor genes, histamine-safety, and anti-inflammatory gut properties makes it the most important probiotic choice for those with MCAS with significant histamine intolerance. It is the probiotic introduced in Phase 4 of the gut healing protocol, after antimicrobial treatment is complete.

Gut Healing and DAO Enzyme Expression

The enterocytes that produce DAO are concentrated in the villi of the small intestinal epithelium.[399] When these villi are damaged—as they frequently are in active gut dysbiosis, with SIBO-mediated inflammation, and in high-permeability states—DAO expression falls alongside the reduction in functional enterocyte mass.[400,401] Every Phase 3 repair intervention that restores enterocyte health and increases villous surface area simultaneously increases DAO production. This is the mechanistic link between gut healing and histamine tolerance improvement; as the gut lining heals, the patient's own histamine clearance capacity rises, producing the progressive improvement in dietary tolerance that many patients notice six to twelve months into a comprehensive gut healing protocol.

✦ ✦ ✦

Phase 4: Rebuilding the Microbiome — The Probiotic Map

Phase 4 is the most misunderstood phase of gut healing in MCAS—and the most consequential for getting it wrong. The general advice to "take a probiotic" for gut health, while sound in healthy populations, requires critical reinterpretation for those with MCAS. The most widely available commercial probiotic strains include several histamine-producing species that will worsen mast cell reactivity despite their other health benefits. Strain selection is not a detail; it is the determinant of whether probiotics help or harm.

The table below provides a comprehensive reference for probiotic strains in the MCAS context, including both the strains to prioritize and the strains to avoid. This distinction—established biologically in Chapter 6—is summarized here as a practical clinical reference.

Strain	Action	MCAS Safe?	Best For	Notes
L. rhamnosus GG / ATCC 53103	Upregulates DAO; reduces gut inflammation; supports barrier	Yes	Histamine intolerance, gut barrier repair, general MCAS support	Best-studied histamine-safe strain; widely available
L. plantarum (299v or WCFS1)	Degrades biogenic amines; anti-inflammatory; barrier support	Yes	Histamine clearance, IBS-D, gut motility	Does not produce histamine; mild motility support
B. longum (1714 or NCIMB 41676)	Butyrate support; immune tolerance; reduces HPA axis reactivity	Yes	Anxiety/brain-gut axis, immune regulation, stress resilience	Specifically studied for stress-related gut symptoms
B. infantis 35624	Strong anti-inflammatory; reduces TNF-α and IL-6	Yes	Inflammatory gut conditions, IBS, leaky gut	Good tolerability even in reactive individuals
L. salivarius	Histamine-neutral; mild anti-inflammatory	Yes	General microbiome support without histamine risk	Less studied than *rhamnosus* but safe for MCAS

Strain	Action	MCAS Safe?	Best For	Notes
Saccharomyces boulardii	Beneficial yeast; antidiarrheal; anti-Candida; supports barrier	Yes (usually)	Post-antibiotic gut restoration, SIBO recurrence prevention, Candida	Not a bacterium—avoids the histamine-strain issue entirely
L. casei (e.g., Shirota)	General immune support	AVOID	Not appropriate for MCAS	Significant histamine producer—worsens symptoms
L. reuteri	Gut motility, immune support	AVOID	Not appropriate for MCAS	Histamine producer—commonly found in commercial probiotics
L. bulgaricus / L. delbrueckii	Traditional yogurt cultures	AVOID	Not appropriate for MCAS	High histamine producers—found in most yogurt and kefir
L. helveticus	Calcium absorption, protein fermentation	AVOID	Not appropriate for MCAS	Histamine producer—found in many aged cheese cultures

How to Introduce Probiotics in Phase 4

Phase 4 probiotic introduction follows the same one-at-a-time protocol established throughout this book. Begin with a single-strain product containing only *Lactobacillus rhamnosus* (GG or ATCC 53103 specifically) at a moderate dose (5–10 billion CFU daily). Observe for one to two weeks before adding a *Bifidobacterium* species (*longum* or *infantis*). Introduce multi-strain products only after single strains are individually tolerated.

Timing relative to Phase 2 antimicrobial treatment is critical: only introduce probiotics at minimum two hours away from each antimicrobial dose during the essential oil or herbal antimicrobial protocol. Introducing beneficial bacteria into an active antimicrobial environment eliminates them before they can colonize. For pharmaceutical SIBO treatment with rifaximin, probiotics can typically be introduced within one to two days of completing the antibiotic course, when rifaximin's local activity has cleared.

Saccharomyces boulardii is the notable exception to the timing rule; as a yeast rather than a bacterium, it is not killed by antibacterial antimicrobial treatments (though it is eliminated by antifungal agents). It can be used concurrently with bacterial-targeting antimicrobials to support gut integrity and reduce die-off symptom severity during Phase 2 treatment—one of its most clinically useful roles in MCAS gut management.

Prebiotic Fiber: Feeding the Bacteria You Want

Probiotic supplementation alone produces limited microbiome shift without the dietary fiber that feeds and sustains beneficial bacteria. Prebiotic fibers—indigestible plant carbohydrates that selectively feed beneficial microorganisms—are the food supply for the microbiome you are building. The most clinically relevant prebiotic fibers for people with MCAS include partially hydrolyzed guar gum (PHGG), which is both a prebiotic and a motility support agent shown to reduce SIBO recurrence; cooked and cooled potatoes and rice (resistant starch); and soluble fiber from oats, leeks, and asparagus.

A caution for SIBO patients: High amounts of fermentable prebiotic fiber during or immediately after SIBO treatment can temporarily worsen bloating and gas as the now-partial microbial population ferments the fiber. Begin prebiotic fiber introduction gradually—a tablespoon of cooked and cooled potato daily, increasing over two to four weeks—rather than switching abruptly to a high-fiber diet. The gut's tolerance for fermentable fiber will increase as the microbiome normalizes.

✦ ✦ ✦

Deeper Dive: The Gut–Mast Cell Reset

For the Science-Minded Reader

The four-phase gut healing protocol produces its MCAS benefits through several overlapping biological mechanisms that are worth understanding in their mechanistic detail, both because they explain why the sequence matters and because they illuminate the timescales over which improvement should be expected.

The SIBO–Histamine–Mast Cell Cascade

SIBO creates a histamine-excess state through three simultaneous mechanisms. First, histamine-producing bacteria in the small intestine convert dietary histidine to histamine continuously, producing internal histamine regardless of dietary restriction. Second, SIBO-driven mucosal inflammation reduces enterocyte mass and therefore DAO expression, impairing histamine clearance at the same time production increases. Third, lipopolysaccharides (LPS) from gram-negative SIBO bacteria translocate across the inflamed gut barrier, activating subepithelial mast cells through TLR-4 signaling in the pattern described in Chapter 6. These three mechanisms—increased production, impaired clearance, and direct mast cell activation—act simultaneously to produce a mast cell priming state that dietary modification alone cannot resolve. Addressing SIBO without addressing all three mechanisms, or addressing only one at a time, produces partial improvement that plateaus.

Why the Essential Oil Gut Protocol Avoids the Aromatic Trigger Problem

The phenol-rich essential oils that are potential respiratory and dermal mast cell triggers (oregano, thyme, cinnamon) become appropriate therapeutic agents in the encapsulated gut protocol because the route of exposure changes the dose-response relationship entirely. Inhaled carvacrol from oregano reaches olfactory and respiratory mast cells at concentrations that may trigger direct degranulation in people with MCAS. The same carvacrol in a capsule with fatty carrier oil passes through the stomach largely intact (no gastric acid degradation of the fat-soluble oil) and reaches the small intestine where it is absorbed gradually across the epithelium. The mast cells of the respiratory mucosa are never exposed. The gut epithelial mast cells do receive some exposure, but in the presence of fat and food, the concentration and contact time are reduced compared to direct mucosal application. This route-specific pharmacology is why the "avoid phenol-rich oils in MCAS" guidance from Chapter 18 coexists without contradiction with the therapeutic internal use guidance here.

The Microbiome and Mast Cell Threshold: A Delayed but Durable Effect

Microbiome rehabilitation—the establishment of a histamine-degrading, butyrate-producing, anti-inflammatory microbial community through Phase 4 interventions—is the slowest phase of gut healing to produce measurable effect but the most durable. Probiotic colonization requires weeks to months of consistent daily administration to produce meaningful shifts in microbiome composition. Butyrate production from fiber fermentation builds over months as the butyrate-producing population expands. DAO upregulation by *L. rhamnosus* accumulates incrementally with each week of colonization.

The clinical implication is that Phase 4 improvements are on a different timescale from Phase 2 improvements: SIBO clearance often produces dramatic symptom improvement within weeks of completing treatment, while microbiome rehabilitation produces a slower, more gradual expansion of dietary tolerance, reduction in background reactivity, and improvement in gut comfort that people typically first notice at three to six months and may continue to improve for twelve to eighteen months after Phase 4 is initiated. Setting this expectation accurately prevents premature abandonment of a protocol that is working but has not yet reached its full effect.

✦ ✦ ✦

What This Means for You: Building Your Gut Healing Plan

Translating the four-phase gut healing protocol into a personal action plan requires honest assessment of where you are in the sequence and what each phase requires before the next becomes appropriate.

Get tested before treating. SIBO testing, Candida assessment, and stool analysis are not optional luxuries—they are the diagnostic foundation that determines which Phase 2 interventions are appropriate and whether the more aggressive antimicrobials (oregano, thyme, cinnamon combinations) or the milder ones (anise, fennel alone) are warranted. Treating blindly for SIBO when it is not present, or treating hydrogen-dominant SIBO with a protocol designed for methane-dominant IMO, produces unnecessary die-off reactions and limited clinical benefit. Test first.

Maintain mast cell stabilization throughout Phase 2. Die-off reactions—the Herxheimer-like responses produced when pathogens release endotoxins and inflammatory compounds as they are killed—are significant mast cell triggers. During Phase 2 antimicrobial treatment, continue or increase quercetin, vitamin C, and magnesium from Chapter 16, maintain the nervous system practices from Chapter 14, and pace the antimicrobial protocol conservatively (starting at lower doses) to keep die-off reactions manageable. A die-off reaction so severe that it triggers prolonged mast cell flares is a sign that the antimicrobial is being introduced too aggressively for the current system tolerance.

Overlap phases strategically, not simultaneously. Phase 3 repair can begin while Phase 2 antimicrobial treatment is still underway; glutamine, zinc carnosine, and DGL do not interfere with antimicrobial efficacy and provide mucosal protection during a period when the gut lining is under additional stress from pathogen die-off. Phase 4 probiotics, however, should wait until Phase 2 is complete. Aloe vera and collagen can begin in Phase 3 as repair foundations before Phase 2 is finished.

Address SIBO recurrence prevention. SIBO recurs in a significant proportion of people, often because the underlying cause of small intestinal dysmotility—the most common predisposing factor—has not been addressed. Prokinetic agents (partially hydrolyzed guar gum, low-dose naltrexone in some protocols, ginger root, or in pharmaceutical contexts, prucalopride or low-dose erythromycin) support the migrating motor complex—the gut's "housekeeping wave" that clears the small intestine between meals. Supporting gut motility after SIBO treatment is as important as the treatment itself for preventing recurrence, particularly in those with MCAS and dysautonomia-related gut motility impairment.

Be patient with Phase 4 timelines. The three-to-six-month window before Phase 4 produces measurable improvements in dietary tolerance is not a failure; it is the biology of microbiome shift. Track the trend rather than the day-to-day: Is the list of reliably tolerated foods gradually expanding? Is baseline reactivity slowly decreasing? Is sleep improving incrementally? These trend signals indicate the protocol is working even when individual days remain difficult.

Nina's plateau broke eight weeks after starting her SIBO treatment protocol. The internal histamine factory had been running for years—dismantling it took four months of consistent phased work, with practitioner guidance through the die-off reactions that came with Phase 2 and the gradual patience required by Phase 4. By month six, she was eating foods she hadn't tolerated in two years. By month ten, her morning reactivity had dropped to a level she described, with some wonder, as something approaching normal.

The gut had been the hidden key. It wasn't the only key—she still maintained her dietary approach, her nervous system practices, and her supplement regimen. But addressing the gut as a living ecosystem with its own internal contribution to her mast cell burden, rather than simply as a passive conduit for the foods she chose to eat, transformed the trajectory of her recovery in a way that nothing else had matched.

✦ ✦ ✦

Chapter 19 at a Glance

What to Remember:

- Gut healing follows a four-phase sequence: Reduce (dietary and lifestyle foundations), Remove (antimicrobial treatment of SIBO and dysbiosis), Repair (gut lining restoration), Replenish (microbiome rehabilitation with histamine-safe strains). Skipping phases or running them simultaneously reduces effectiveness and increases die-off severity.
- SIBO is a major internal histamine source that dietary restriction cannot address—bacteria in the small intestine produce histamine from dietary histidine continuously, independent of what is eaten. SIBO testing (lactulose or glucose breath test) is the essential diagnostic step before treatment.
- Essential oils in encapsulated internal form are evidence-supported gut antimicrobials for SIBO and gut dysbiosis. The five-drops-per-dose-in-

capsule-with-carrier-oil protocol delivers antimicrobial activity to the small intestine without triggering the respiratory or dermal mast cell reactions associated with aromatic use of phenol-rich oils.

- Oregano and thyme (broad-spectrum, phenol-rich) are the most potent gut antimicrobial oils; peppermint provides motility and antispasmodic support; cinnamon is particularly active against *Candida*; anise and fennel offer milder options with better tolerability for reactive patients. Start at lower doses and increase gradually.
- Gut lining repair (Phase 3) uses L-glutamine, zinc carnosine, DGL, decolorized aloe vera, and collagen peptides – each addressing a different structural layer of barrier integrity. Phase 3 can overlap with Phase 2 antimicrobial treatment but should be established before Phase 4 probiotics are introduced.
- DAO enzyme activity improves as the gut lining heals and as nutritional cofactors (copper, P5P, vitamin C) are optimized. *L. rhamnosus* GG directly influence gut mast cells, making it the most important probiotic choice for histamine intolerance specifically.
- Probiotic strain selection is critical. *L. rhamnosus, B. longum, B. infantis, L. plantarum, L. salivarius*, and *Saccharomyces boulardii* are histamine-safe. *L. casei, L. reuteri, L. bulgaricus*, and *L. helveticus* are histamine producers that worsen MCAS—check every probiotic label for these strains.
- Microbiome rehabilitation effects are on a three-to-twelve-month timescale. SIBO clearance produces faster improvement; probiotic colonization and butyrate-production normalization build gradually. Track trending improvement in dietary tolerance and background reactivity rather than expecting rapid transformation.

Coming Up in Chapter 20:

The gut healing protocol addresses one of the primary internal sources of mast cell burden. The next chapter turns to another: the accumulated toxic load that, when it exceeds the body's clearance capacity, keeps mast cells chronically primed through the mechanisms described in Chapter 8. Chapter 20 covers the practical detoxification support protocol—supporting liver pathways gently and systematically, using binders appropriately, and supporting the sweating, hydration, and lymphatic flow that move toxins out of the body through routes the liver and kidneys cannot accomplish alone.

CHAPTER 20

Detoxification Support

Supporting the Pathways That Clear What Keeps Your Mast Cells Primed

The Bucket With No Drain

Owen had done almost everything right. Over eighteen months of dedicated work, he had cleaned up his diet, rebuilt his gut with Phase 3 and 4 protocols, introduced a carefully sequenced supplement regimen, practiced his breathing exercises with unfailing consistency. He had seen real improvement—his reactions were less frequent, his baseline reactivity was lower, and he had started to feel like himself again in ways he had given up expecting.

And then, around month sixteen, progress stalled. Not catastrophically—he didn't relapse to his worst state—but stubbornly, inexplicably. His bucket kept refilling faster than it should have given everything he was doing to empty it. His morning reactivity crept back up. Foods he had reintroduced began causing trouble again. His practitioner ordered a mycotoxin urine test, an organic acids panel, and a hair tissue mineral analysis.

The results told the story: elevated urinary trichothecene mycotoxins, high urinary glutamate (a marker of impaired detoxification pathway function), and elevated mercury alongside low selenium. His body had been accumulating a toxic burden for years—long before his MCAS diagnosis—and his detoxification systems, already stretched by the demands of a chronically inflamed immune system, were not clearing the backlog fast enough to stop it from draining back into the mast cell activation cycle.

Owen's situation illustrates a pattern that experienced MCAS practitioners recognize frequently. Some patients who do significant work on diet, gut healing, and nervous system regulation can plateau because they have not addressed their accumulated toxic burden. The mast cells are being stabilized and the bucket is being managed more skillfully, but a hidden stream of toxin-driven mast cell activation continues to refill the bucket faster than everything else is emptying it.

Detoxification support is not a dramatic or rapid intervention. Done well, it is gradual, systematic, and profoundly boring—which is exactly how it should be for MCAS patients whose reactive systems treat aggressive detox protocols as assault. But done consistently, it produces a slow, sustained lowering of the background activation level that makes everything else work better. This chapter explains how.

✦ ✦ ✦

What Detoxification Actually Means

The word detoxification has been so thoroughly appropriated by wellness marketing—detox teas, cleanses, fad protocols—that it is worth beginning with what it actually refers to in clinical and biochemical terms.

The body has genuine, sophisticated detoxification systems that operate continuously without any supplemental assistance in healthy individuals living in an ideal environment (one that doesn't exist in the modern world). The liver is the primary detoxification organ, processing fat-soluble toxins—environmental chemicals, medications, hormones, microbial metabolites, and endogenous inflammatory compounds—and converting them into water-soluble forms that can be excreted through bile (and then stool) or through the kidneys (and then urine). The kidneys filter blood continuously, excreting water-soluble waste products. The skin excretes water-soluble compounds through sweat. The lymphatic system collects interstitial fluid and delivers it back to the circulation, carrying toxins and inflammatory debris toward liver and lymph node processing.

These systems work well when the toxic input is modest and the nutritional and metabolic resources required to run them are adequate. They become overwhelmed when toxic input exceeds clearance capacity—from accumulated environmental exposures (the mold, heavy metals, and industrial chemicals of Chapter 8), from the byproducts of gut dysbiosis and chronic infection, or from the inflammatory mediators that MCAS itself produces in excess. When clearance capacity is exceeded, toxins and their reactive metabolites recirculate—re-exposing mast cells and immune cells to provocative compounds that should have been cleared, maintaining the priming state that keeps the mast cell threshold low.

> **The Core Principle:** *Detoxification support in MCAS is not about dramatic purging or miracle cleanses. It is about systematically reducing the toxic input that primes mast cells while ensuring that the body's own clearance pathways have the nutritional resources, drainage support, and physical outlets they need to process and excrete what has accumulated.*

The three pillars of detoxification support map directly to the three major clearance systems most relevant to MCAS: supporting liver Phase 1 and Phase 2 processing pathways; using binders to capture toxins in the gut and prevent their reabsorption; and supporting the sweating, hydration, and lymphatic flow that move toxins out of tissues and toward excretion. Each pillar addresses a different stage of the clearance process, and the most effective approach engages all three.

✦ ✦ ✦

Supporting Liver Pathways: Gently and Systematically

The liver processes toxins in two phases. Phase 1 reactions use cytochrome P450 enzymes to chemically modify fat-soluble toxins—oxidizing, reducing, or hydrolyzing them into more reactive intermediate metabolites. In simpler terms, the body is essentially 'tagging' these toxins with a molecular hook, making them easier for other enzymes to grab onto and neutralize in the next stage. Phase 2 reactions conjugate (attach) these intermediates to carrier molecules—glutathione, glucuronate, sulfate, glycine, or methyl groups—making them water-soluble and ready for excretion. Both phases require specific nutritional cofactors, and both can become bottlenecks when these cofactors are depleted, when genetic variants in the relevant enzymes are present, or when the total toxic load exceeds the pathway's processing capacity.

The critical word in MCAS liver support is gently. Aggressive liver stimulation—high doses of Phase 1 inducers or rapid mobilization of stored toxins—can temporarily increase the concentration of reactive Phase 1 intermediates and recirculating toxins in the bloodstream, triggering mast cell reactions before Phase 2 conjugation can catch up. The goal is to support smooth, continuous processing rather than to force a rapid flood of toxin clearance.

Phase 1 Support: Antioxidants and CYP450 Protection

Phase 1 processing generates reactive oxygen species (ROS) as a byproduct—the same oxidative stress that primes mast cells through the mechanisms described in Chapter 8. Ensuring robust antioxidant status while supporting Phase 1 activity protects both the liver and the mast cell system from the oxidative burden of active detoxification. The most important Phase 1 antioxidant supports are:

- **Vitamin C** – As established in Chapters 15 and 16, vitamin C is both a direct antioxidant and a cofactor for several Phase 1 enzyme reactions. Buffered vitamin C at 500–1,000 mg twice daily provides consistent antioxidant coverage without the citrus-sensitivity risk.
- **Green tea extract (EGCG)** – This is a potent NRF2 activator that upregulates the endogenous antioxidant enzyme system including superoxide dismutase and catalase, providing broader Phase 1 protection

than any single antioxidant compound alone. Take 200–400 mg standardized EGCG daily.

- **Alpha-lipoic acid (ALA)** – A unique fat- and water-soluble antioxidant that can regenerate other antioxidants (vitamin C, vitamin E, glutathione), ALA directly supports mitochondrial function during detoxification. Take 300–600 mg daily with food.
- **S-acetyl glutathione** – This is a highly bioavailable, stable form of glutathione that remains intact through digestion to increase intracellular levels, directly neutralizing Phase 1 reactive oxygen species and stabilizing mast cells. Take 100–300 mg daily on an empty stomach.

Phase 2 Support: The Conjugation Nutrients

Phase 2 conjugation requires a continuous supply of specific nutrients; deficiencies in any of them create bottlenecks that allow reactive Phase 1 intermediates to accumulate. The most clinically important Phase 2 support nutrients in MCAS include:

- **Glutathione precursors** – Glutathione is the most important Phase 2 conjugate — used in glutathione conjugation, the primary pathway for many toxic compounds including heavy metal metabolites and reactive oxygen species. NAC (N-acetylcysteine, 600–1,200 mg daily on an empty stomach) provides cysteine, the rate-limiting precursor for glutathione synthesis. Glycine (from collagen or direct supplementation) and glutamine (from Chapter 16's gut healing protocol) complete the glutathione precursor triad.
- **Sulfur-containing foods** – Cruciferous vegetables (broccoli, cauliflower, Brussels sprouts, kale) and allium family plants (garlic, onion, leek) provide sulforaphane, indole-3-carbinol, and sulfur amino acids that support both glutathione synthesis and the sulfation pathway—one of the primary Phase 2 routes for estrogen, dopamine, and many environmental chemicals. Including these foods daily is a form of liver support that requires no supplementation.
- **B vitamins (especially B2, B6, B12, and folate)** – These vitamins are required for multiple Phase 2 conjugation reactions including methylation (B12 and folate), sulfation (B6), and glucuronidation (B2). The active methylated forms discussed in Chapter 11 (methylcobalamin, methylfolate) are particularly important for individuals with MTHFR variants whose Phase 2 methylation capacity is already reduced.
- **Magnesium** – Magnesium is required as a cofactor for glutathione synthetase—the enzyme that completes glutathione production. The magnesium glycinate already in the Chapter 16 protocol simultaneously supports nervous system regulation, mast cell stabilization, and Phase 2 detoxification.

- **DIM (diindolylmethane) and calcium D-glucarate** – DIM (100–200 mg daily with a meal), derived from the breakdown of indole-3-carbinol in cruciferous vegetables, specifically supports the Phase 2 processing of estrogen through the 2-hydroxyestrone pathway—directing estrogen metabolism toward the less proliferative and less mast-cell-sensitizing metabolites. Calcium D-glucarate (500 mg twice daily) inhibits beta-glucuronidase, the enzyme that uncouples conjugated estrogen and allows it to be reabsorbed from the gut. Together, these two compounds address the estrogen clearance problem described in Chapter 10 directly at the liver and gut level.

Milk Thistle: The Liver's Best-Studied Ally

Silymarin, the standardized extract from milk thistle seed (*Silybum marianum*), is the most extensively studied liver protective botanical. Silymarin acts through several mechanisms simultaneously: It stabilizes hepatocyte (liver) cell membranes against toxic injury, scavenges reactive oxygen species generated during Phase 1 processing, supports glutathione synthesis in liver cells, and modestly stimulates Phase 2 regeneration capacity. It is used clinically for liver protection during toxic exposures, for individuals with elevated liver enzymes, and as a foundational liver support during detoxification protocols.

For people with MCAS, milk thistle is particularly appropriate during periods of active toxic clearance—mold remediation, heavy metal removal, or SIBO die-off—when the liver is processing an above-normal load. Standard dose is 140–420 mg of standardized silymarin daily, taken with meals. More bioavailable forms—like silybin cocrystals or silymarin phospholipid complex—are preferred for greater actives in the bloodstream and improved efficacy when tolerated. Milk thistle is very well tolerated by most who have MCAS, though rare reactions occur in those with Asteraceae family sensitivity.

✦ ✦ ✦

Binders and Drainage Support: Capturing Toxins Before They Recirculate

The liver excretes processed toxins through bile into the intestinal tract, where they are normally carried out with stool. The problem is that many toxic compounds—particularly mycotoxins and some heavy metal metabolites—are subject to enterohepatic recirculation: they are reabsorbed from the gut back into the portal circulation before reaching the colon, returning to the liver for another round of processing. This recirculation loop can significantly extend the body's exposure to toxins long after the original source has been removed.

Binders—substances that capture toxins in the gut lumen and bind them strongly enough to prevent their reabsorption—are the primary tool for interrupting this recirculation. A bound toxin cannot be reabsorbed; it travels with the binder through the intestinal tract and exits with stool. Well-chosen binders can meaningfully accelerate toxin clearance and reduce the recirculation burden on both the liver and the mast cell system.

The most important practical rule for all binders is timing: they must be taken well away from food, supplements, and medications—at minimum two hours before or after anything else—because they bind indiscriminately. A binder taken with a quercetin supplement, a probiotic capsule, or a prescription medication will bind those too, reducing their absorption and negating their intended effect.

Activated Charcoal

Activated charcoal is a highly porous carbon substance with an enormous surface area — one gram has the approximate surface area of three tennis courts—capable of binding a wide range of toxins, inflammatory mediators, and metabolic byproducts through adsorption. It is the most broadly acting of the common binders and is appropriate for general toxin support, die-off symptom management during antimicrobial protocols, and acute mast-cell-reaction support where histamine and inflammatory mediators may be contributing to symptoms.

Dose: Take 500–1,000 mg per dose, taken with a large glass of water at least two hours away from all other supplements, foods, and medications. Daily use should be limited to periods of active detox need rather than continuous long-term supplementation, as extended use interferes with nutrient absorption. Activated charcoal reliably turns stool black—this is expected and harmless. Constipation is possible at higher doses; increase water intake accordingly.

Bentonite Clay

Bentonite clay is a naturally occurring volcanic mineral clay with particular affinity for aflatoxins, ochratoxin A, and other mycotoxins, as well as some heavy metal ions.[402,403,404] It binds toxins through ion exchange and physical adsorption and is one of the most commonly used binders in mold-illness protocols. A distinctive property of bentonite clay relevant to people with MCAS is that it also has mild anti-inflammatory effects in the gut lining itself—one of the few binders that provides some gut healing benefit alongside toxin capture.[405,406]

Dose is one teaspoon of food-grade bentonite clay stirred into a large glass of water daily. Quality matters considerably here—bentonite clay must be food-grade and independently tested for heavy metal contamination, as poor-quality clay products can themselves be sources of lead or arsenic. Redmond Clay and similar USP-grade products are appropriate sources. Take on an empty stomach, at least two hours away from all supplements and medications. Constipation is common—prioritize hydration and consider alternating days rather than daily use if this is problematic.

Modified Citrus Pectin (MCP)

Modified citrus pectin is a form of pectin (soluble dietary fiber from citrus peel) that has been enzymatically reduced to smaller molecular fragments capable of crossing the intestinal wall and entering systemic circulation. This distinguishes MCP from other binders: it works partly in the gut (binding lead, cadmium, and arsenic in the intestinal tract to prevent absorption) and partly systemically (circulating through the bloodstream and binding heavy metals for renal excretion).[407,408,409] It is also a specific antagonist of galectin-3,[410] a pro-inflammatory lectin that drives fibrosis and immune dysregulation and is often elevated in chronic inflammatory conditions including mold illness.

Dose is 5 grams of MCP powder dissolved in water, two to three times daily, taken thirty to sixty minutes before meals for optimal gut-level binding. MCP is generally very well tolerated and is an excellent binder choice for individuals with MCAS who need a gentler option than activated charcoal or who are specifically addressing heavy metal burden and galectin-3-driven inflammation.

Cholestyramine: The Primary Mycotoxin Binder

Cholestyramine is a pharmaceutical bile acid sequestrant that has been used off-label in mold illness treatment for decades,[411] popularized in the United States by the Shoemaker protocol. It binds mycotoxins in the gut with high affinity, significantly reducing their enterohepatic recirculation and accelerating their excretion. Its clinical track record in mold illness is the most extensive of any binder, and for patients with confirmed elevated mycotoxin burden, it is often the most effective first-line binder.

Cholestyramine requires a prescription and should be used under physician supervision. Standard dose in mold illness protocols: one scoop (4 grams) mixed in water, four times daily before meals. The most significant limitation is its impact on fat-soluble nutrient absorption: cholestyramine also binds fat-soluble vitamins (A, D, E, K), bile acids required for fat digestion, and many fat-soluble medications. Long-term use requires supplementation with fat-soluble vitamins and monitoring for deficiency. Many patients alternate cholestyramine with natural binders as their mycotoxin burden reduces, transitioning to MCP or activated charcoal for maintenance.

> **Binder Rotation Note:** *Using the same binder every day indefinitely is less effective than rotating among binders with different binding affinities. Different toxins respond to different binding mechanisms; rotating activated charcoal, bentonite clay, and MCP on different days, or in alternating weeks, provides broader coverage than any single binder alone. Discuss rotation strategy and duration of use with your practitioner based on your specific toxin profile.*

✦ ✦ ✦

Sweating, Hydration, and Lymphatic Flow: Moving Toxins Out

The liver and binders address the processing and intestinal clearance of toxins. A third pathway—arguably the most underutilized in conventional medicine—uses the body's physical movement systems to mobilize toxins out of tissues, move lymphatic fluid through filtering lymph nodes, and excrete water-soluble toxins and heavy metals through the skin. These approaches are not alternatives to liver support and binders; they are synergistic additions that address the clearance problem from a completely different angle.

Sweating and Infrared Sauna

Sweating is a genuine excretory pathway. Sweat contains measurable quantities of heavy metals—particularly lead, cadmium, arsenic, and mercury—as well as some organic chemicals including phthalates and bisphenols.[412,413,414] Studies measuring the composition of sweat in individuals with heavy metal burden have consistently found that sweat excretion contributes meaningfully to heavy metal clearance, particularly for compounds that are less efficiently cleared through urine and bile.

For those with MCAS, the primary practical approach to therapeutic sweating is infrared sauna—specifically near- or mid-infrared sauna rather than conventional high-heat Finnish-style saunas. Infrared saunas produce sweating at lower ambient temperatures (typically 120–140°F versus 180–200°F for conventional saunas) by heating the body's tissue directly through infrared radiation rather than primarily heating the air. This lower-temperature environment is significantly better tolerated by individuals with MCAS with heat sensitivity and is less likely to trigger the temperature-change mast cell reactions described in Chapter 5.

The introduction protocol for people with MCAS is conservative: begin with ten minutes at 120°F, three times per week, and observe for any increase in mast cell reactivity over the following twenty-four to forty-eight hours before extending duration or frequency. Most people can work up to twenty to thirty minute sessions three to five times weekly over four to eight weeks as tolerance develops. Shower with soap immediately after each session to remove toxins that have been excreted through the skin and prevent their reabsorption. Hydrate thoroughly before, during (small sips of electrolyte water during the session), and after.

> **Heat Sensitivity Note:** *Some people with MCAS experience mast cell flares from heat exposure, including infrared sauna. If this occurs consistently, infrared sauna is not an appropriate detox tool for your current phase of treatment; it may become appropriate later as overall mast cell reactivity reduces. Do not persist with a modality that reliably triggers reactions; redirect detox support to binder and liver support pathways instead.*

Hydration: The Foundation of All Excretion

Adequate hydration is the most basic and most frequently neglected requirement for effective toxin clearance. The kidneys require sufficient water volume to dilute and excrete water-soluble toxins, heavy metal metabolites, and the conjugated Phase 2 products from liver processing. The lymphatic system requires adequate fluid volume to maintain flow. The gut requires adequate water to ensure daily stool passage that removes bound toxins before they can be reabsorbed.

The minimum effective hydration for active detox support is two to three liters (67 to 101 ounces) of filtered water daily, front-loaded toward the morning when cortisol and metabolic activity are highest. Filtered water—using a reverse osmosis, activated carbon, or multi-stage filter that removes chlorine, chloramines, fluoride, heavy metals, and PFAS—is specifically appropriate for individuals with MCAS, as unfiltered tap water in many areas contains chemical and hormonal residues that add to the very toxic burden being cleared.

For individuals with MCAS and POTS, plain water without electrolytes can worsen orthostatic symptoms by diluting already-low plasma sodium and volume. These individuals should use electrolyte-supplemented water—sodium, potassium, and magnesium in appropriate balance—rather than plain water as their primary hydration source. The electrolyte guidance from Chapter 22 applies here.

Lymphatic Support: Moving the Fluid That Carries Toxins

The lymphatic system is the body's secondary circulatory network—a one-way system of vessels and lymph nodes that collects interstitial fluid (the fluid surrounding cells throughout the body), filters it through immune-active lymph nodes, and returns it to the venous circulation. Unlike the blood circulation, which is driven by the heart's pumping action, lymphatic flow depends primarily on muscle movement, breathing, and external massage to move fluid through the vessels. A sedentary, shallow-breathing, physically inactive person has significantly impaired lymphatic flow—and therefore significantly impaired tissue-level toxin clearance—compared to an active person, regardless of what supplements they take.

Practical lymphatic support approaches particularly appropriate for people with MCAS include:

- **Dry brushing** – Using a natural-bristle brush on dry skin before showering, with long strokes directed toward the heart, stimulates lymphatic flow in the skin and subcutaneous tissue. Five to ten minutes of dry brushing before a morning shower is an accessible daily practice that costs little time and no money beyond the brush itself. Use light to moderate pressure—aggressive brushing can irritate sensitive MCAS skin
- **Rebounding** – Gentle bouncing on a mini-trampoline (rebounder) is one of the most efficient lymphatic stimulation exercises available, because the alternating acceleration and deceleration of the body's tissues during bouncing provides the mechanical compression and release that drives lymph through the vessels. Even one to two minutes of gentle bouncing several times daily produces measurable lymphatic flow improvement. For people with MCAS that experience significant exercise intolerance or POTS, sitting on the rebounder and bouncing gently from seated is an appropriate modification
- **Diaphragmatic breathing** – The diaphragm acts as a lymphatic pump—its expansion during deep inhalation creates negative pressure that draws lymph upward through the thoracic duct, the main lymphatic vessel emptying into the venous circulation. The extended-exhale breathing practices from Chapter 14 simultaneously support vagal tone, nervous system regulation, and lymphatic drainage—one of many reasons they belong at the center of any MCAS protocol
- **Castor oil packs** – Topical application of cold-pressed castor oil over the liver area (right side of the abdomen, below the lower ribs)—especially with a drop or two of the essential oils mentioned in Chapter 18, covered with a cloth and gentle heat, is a traditional naturopathic approach to stimulating hepatic lymphatic drainage. Research and clinical experience support improved lymphocyte function and local lymphatic circulation with regular castor oil pack use.[415] For individuals with MCAS, begin with room-temperature castor oil without additional heat or essential oils, applying it over the liver area for thirty to sixty minutes at rest, and observe skin tolerance before adding a heat source.
- **Manual lymphatic drainage** – Gentle, specialized massage that follows the anatomical pathways of the lymphatic system, performed by a trained lymphatic massage therapist is a manual lymphatic drainage technique. For people with significant lymphatic congestion—which may manifest as chronic puffiness, facial swelling upon waking, or a sense of tissue heaviness—professional manual lymphatic drainage can provide more direct therapeutic benefit than self-directed practices alone

✦ ✦ ✦

Deeper Dive: Why Detox Fails and How to Avoid the Most Common Mistakes

For the Science-Minded Reader

Detoxification support consistently underperforms clinical expectations in people with MCAS for two reasons that are entirely preventable: Phase 1/2 imbalance and binder misuse. Understanding both prevents the most common errors in detox protocol design.

Phase 1/2 Imbalance: The Reactive Intermediate Problem

Phase 1 processing converts fat-soluble toxins into reactive intermediate metabolites—compounds that are often more chemically reactive than the original toxin and that can directly damage proteins, DNA, and cell membranes if they are not rapidly conjugated in Phase 2. This is why Phase 1 and Phase 2 must be supported in balance: stimulating Phase 1 without ensuring that Phase 2 has adequate conjugation capacity floods the system with reactive intermediates that can worsen inflammation, trigger mast cell reactions, and produce symptoms that are commonly misattributed to detox reactions or Herxheimer responses.

The practical implication is that Phase 2 cofactors—glutathione precursors, B vitamins, magnesium, sulfur-containing foods—should be established for several weeks before any significant Phase 1 stimulation is introduced. This is the same sequencing logic as every other phase of MCAS management: Build the capacity to process before increasing the load. Coffee (a CYP450 Phase 1 inducer), intensive cruciferous vegetable supplementation, and high-dose antioxidant therapies that accelerate Phase 1 should be introduced only after Phase 2 nutritional foundations are confirmed adequate.

The Mobilization-Without-Excretion Mistake

The second common detox failure mode occurs when mobilization of toxins from tissue storage is initiated without ensuring that the excretion pathways are open and functional. Heavy metal chelation without adequate gut binder and kidney support, or aggressive liver stimulation without regular bowel movements, can mobilize toxins into the circulation faster than they can be excreted—temporarily raising circulating toxin levels and triggering mast cell activation from the very compounds the protocol is intended to clear.

This is the mechanistic explanation for why some patients feel significantly worse when beginning detox protocols. They have opened the mobilization tap without opening the excretion drain. The practical solution is simple but requires discipline: Establish bowel regularity first (two to three bowel movements daily is the target during active detox), ensure adequate hydration, introduce binders before or simultaneously with any mobilization intervention, and pace mobilization strategies incrementally rather than all at once.

Testing to Guide the Protocol

Detoxification support in MCAS is most effective when guided by objective testing that identifies the specific toxic burdens present rather than treating generically. The most useful tests for guiding an MCAS detox protocol include urine mycotoxin panel (GPL-MycoTOX or Great Plains Organic Acids Test) for mold exposure assessment, hair tissue mineral analysis (HTMA) or provoked urine testing for heavy metal burden, serum or urine organic acids panel for markers of impaired Phase 1/II function, and plasma or red blood cell fatty acid profile for omega-3/omega-6 balance that affects membrane-based cellular detoxification efficiency. Testing before treatment allows the protocol to be targeted rather than generic, reducing unnecessary interventions and ensuring that the most clinically relevant toxic burdens are prioritized.

✦ ✦ ✦

Quick Reference: Detoxification Support Summary

The table below consolidates the primary detoxification support interventions covered in this chapter, organized for daily protocol planning and quick reference.

Intervention	Category	Dose / Method	Timing	Key Caution
Milk Thistle (silymarin)	Liver support	140–420 mg silymarin daily	With meals	Mild laxative effect at high doses; rare allergy in Asteraceae-sensitive patients
DIM (diindolylmethane)	Estrogen clearance / Phase 2	100–200 mg daily	With a fat-containing meal	Can transiently shift estrogen metabolites—monitor for mood changes; avoid in estrogen-sensitive cancers without oncology guidance
Calcium D-glucarate	Estrogen recirculation / Phase 2	500–1,000 mg daily	With meals	Avoid high doses with hormone medications; monitor bowel tolerance
NAC (N-acetylcysteine)	Glutathione precursor / NRF2	600–1,200 mg daily	Empty stomach 30	Avoid with nitroglycerin; may thin mucus—helpful or

Intervention	Category	Dose / Method	Timing	Key Caution
			min before meals	bothersome depending on patient
Magnesium (glycinate or malate)	Phase 2 conjugation support	200–400 mg daily	Evening preferred	Start low; loose stools indicate excess dose
B vitamins (methylated complex)	Methylation / Phase 2 sulfation	Per label; B2 100–400 mg for MTHFR	With food	Methylfolate may cause activation in sensitive patients—start very low
Activated charcoal	Binder—broad-spectrum	500–1,000 mg per dose	Away from meals, supplements, and medications (minimum 2 hrs)	Binds nutrients and medications—never take near supplements or prescription drugs
Bentonite clay	Binder—mycotoxins, heavy metals	1 tsp in water daily	Away from meals and all supplements (minimum 2 hrs)	Ensure food-grade, heavy-metal-tested source; constipation possible—increase hydration
Modified citrus pectin (MCP)	Binder—heavy metals, galectin-3	5 g, 2–3x daily	Away from meals (30–60 min)	Generally very well tolerated; mild GI upset possible at high doses
Cholestyramine (Rx)	Binder—mycotoxins (primary)	Per prescription	Away from all other medications (minimum 4 hrs)	Prescription only; significantly impairs fat-soluble nutrient absorption long-term—supplement accordingly
Infrared sauna	Sweating / skin excretion	15–30 min sessions, 3–5x/week	Not within 2 hrs of meals; hydrate before and after	Start at lower temps (120°F); MCAS patients may react to heat—begin with 10-min sessions
Dry brushing + lymphatic massage	Lymphatic drainage	5–10 min daily before shower	Morning preferred	Use light pressure only; avoid over inflamed or reactive skin
Hydration (filtered water)	All pathways	Minimum 2–3 L daily	Consistent throughout day; front-load mornings	Add electrolytes if POTS is present; plain water without electrolytes can worsen orthostatic symptoms

> **Sequencing Reminder:** *Establish Phase 2 nutritional support (glutathione precursors, B vitamins, magnesium) and bowel regularity before introducing*

> *binders or mobilization strategies. Binders come before aggressive Phase 1 stimulation. Lymphatic and sweating supports can begin at any stage and produce no mobilization risk—they are safe to introduce early and consistently.*

✦ ✦ ✦

What This Means for You: Building Your Detox Foundation

Detoxification support in MCAS is a long game. The toxic burdens that have accumulated over years do not clear in weeks, and the clearance pathways that have been operating under capacity do not restore overnight. Approaching detox support with the same patient, incremental logic applied throughout this book produces the best outcomes.

Start with what costs nothing and carries no risk. The hydration, dry brushing, diaphragmatic breathing, and light movement that support lymphatic flow are free, low-risk, and appropriate to begin immediately regardless of where you are in the stabilization–support–repair framework. Make adequate filtered water intake, morning dry brushing, and consistent breathing practice part of your daily baseline before adding any supplemental detox support.

Build Phase 2 nutritional foundations before anything else. If you are already taking the supplement protocol from Chapter 16, you have begun Phase 2 support: magnesium, B vitamins (if P5P is included), and vitamin C are all Phase 2 cofactors. Add NAC (600 mg daily, starting low in a reactive system) and DIM (100 mg daily with a fat-containing meal) as the targeted additions that specifically address the glutathione and estrogen clearance dimensions most relevant to MCAS. These two additions, alongside the existing Chapter 16 protocol, constitute a solid Phase 2 foundation for most patients.

Introduce binders during or after Phase 2 and 3 gut healing. Binders are most useful when the gut is functioning well enough to move them through efficiently—constipation reduces their effectiveness by extending transit time and allowing bound toxins to be released before they exit. Ensure the gut healing work of Chapter 19 has improved bowel function before relying on binders as a primary detox tool. Begin with MCP (gentlest) or activated charcoal (broader spectrum, use intermittently during die-off), then add bentonite clay once gut function is reliable. Reserve cholestyramine for confirmed mycotoxin burden under physician guidance.

Introduce infrared sauna cautiously, with heat tolerance testing first. Before committing to a sauna protocol, assess your individual heat tolerance by spending five minutes in a warm (not hot) bath and observing for any mast cell response over the following hour. If well tolerated, begin with ten-minute infrared sessions at the lower temperature range and step up only after multiple sessions confirm tolerance. If heat reliably triggers reactions at your current reactivity level, defer infrared sauna until later in the recovery trajectory.

Match your detox intensity to your current system stability. The same logic that governs every other intervention in this book applies here: a highly reactive system in early stabilization needs gentler, more gradual detox support than a stabilized system in Stage 2 or 3. During stabilization, focus on hydration, lymphatic support, and Phase 2 nutrition. More active interventions—binders, infrared sauna, and targeted mobilization strategies—belong in Stage 2 and beyond, once the mast cell system has sufficient stability to handle the temporary increases in circulating toxin metabolites that active detox produces.

Owen's plateau broke slowly—over four months of consistent Phase 2 nutritional support, binder rotation, and weekly infrared sauna sessions alongside his existing protocol. The improvement wasn't dramatic week to week; it was a gradual, almost imperceptible lowering of his background reactivity that he only recognized clearly when he looked back at his symptom journal from six months earlier. The mycotoxin metabolites in his urine were significantly lower on retesting. His mercury had reduced on HTMA. His morning reactivity had returned to the downward trajectory that the plateau had interrupted.

The toxic burden had been a hidden source of ongoing mast cell priming. Addressing it hadn't been the most exciting part of his recovery—there was nothing dramatic about drinking filtered water, dry brushing his skin, and taking a rotating binder rotation every morning. But it had been real work, aimed at a real problem, and the results were real too.

✦ ✦ ✦

Chapter 20 at a Glance

What to Remember:

- Detoxification support addresses accumulated toxic burden—from mold mycotoxins, heavy metals, industrial chemicals, and gut dysbiosis metabolites—that maintains chronic mast cell priming independently of diet, gut health, or nervous system interventions. People who plateau despite doing other things well often have an unaddressed toxic load that continues to refill the bucket.
- The liver processes toxins in two phases: Phase 1 (CYP450 enzyme modification) generates reactive intermediates, and Phase 2 (conjugation with glutathione, sulfate, glucuronate, or methyl groups) renders them water-soluble for excretion. Both phases require specific nutritional

cofactors; Phase 2 must be supported before Phase 1 is stimulated to prevent reactive intermediate accumulation.

- Key Phase 2 support nutrients: glutathione precursors (NAC, glycine, glutamine), B vitamins (B2, B6, B12, folate—active methylated forms for those with MTHFR), magnesium, DIM and calcium D-glucarate for estrogen clearance, and sulfur-containing cruciferous and allium foods daily.

- Milk thistle (140–420 mg standardized silymarin daily) provides hepatoprotection during periods of increased toxic load—particularly appropriate during mold remediation, antimicrobial die-off, and heavy metal clearance.

- Binders interrupt toxin enterohepatic recirculation by capturing toxins in the gut before they can be reabsorbed. The most useful options for MCAS: activated charcoal (broad-spectrum, intermittent use), bentonite clay (mycotoxins, heavy metals), MCP (heavy metals, galectin-3, gentle daily use), and cholestyramine (prescription, primary mycotoxin binder). All must be taken at least two hours away from all supplements, foods, and medications.

- Sweating through infrared sauna (low-temperature, begin at ten minutes) provides genuine skin-level excretion of heavy metals and organic chemicals. Introduction must be cautious in heat-sensitive individuals.

- Adequate hydration (2–3 liters filtered water daily), lymphatic stimulation (dry brushing, gentle rebounding, diaphragmatic breathing, castor oil packs over the liver), and regular bowel function are the foundation of all excretion pathways and carry no mobilization risk.

- Match detox intensity to system stability: lymphatic and hydration support are appropriate from the beginning; binders belong in Stage 2 after gut healing is underway; infrared sauna and active mobilization strategies belong after mast cell stability is established.

Coming Up in Chapter 21 and Beyond:

With the full natural remedies toolkit of the last chapters now in hand—diet, supplements, herbs, essential oils, gut healing, and detoxification—we turn to one of the most important and most frequently under-addressed dimensions of MCAS: its relationship with POTS. Chapter 21 opens with a deep understanding of POTS physiology and the mast cell mechanisms that drive cardiovascular dysfunction, then moves into the practical natural strategies—hydration, electrolytes, compression, movement, and nervous system retraining—that address both conditions simultaneously.

CHAPTER 21

Understanding POTS Physiology

Blood Volume, Circulation, Autonomic Imbalance, and the Mast Cell Connection

The Morning That Won't Begin

She knows the feeling before she fully wakes. It begins as consciousness surfaces—a heaviness, a faint trembling in the chest, an awareness that today will require more than yesterday's strength to accomplish what yesterday required. She lies there, cataloguing: heart rate, fatigue level, how steady her vision seems. She is not catastrophizing. She is performing a clinical assessment she has run every morning for three years, because what happens in the first thirty seconds after she sits up will determine the shape of her day.

She sits. Her heart lurches. Within fifteen seconds, it is hammering—not racing in the way of fear or excitement, but hammering with a mechanical urgency that has nothing to do with how she feels emotionally. Her vision dims briefly at the edges. She grips the mattress and breathes through it, waiting for her body to do what it cannot quite do: compensate, adjust, redistribute blood upward fast enough that her brain receives adequate supply before the compensatory overdrive begins.

This is POTS at 7 a.m. on a Tuesday. Not a crisis—she has learned that it is rarely a crisis, even when it feels like one. But it is an obstacle, and it is exhausting to navigate the same obstacle at the beginning of every day.

Understanding why this happens—mechanistically, precisely, in the language of physiology rather than of mystery or anxiety—has been one of the most empowering things she has learned. When she understood that her heart was not malfunctioning but compensating, that the compensation was not arbitrary but the direct result of specific, addressable deficits in her circulation, she stopped being afraid of her mornings. She started being strategic about them instead.

The last several chapters of this book were devoted to that strategy. But effective strategy requires a clear understanding of the problem. This chapter provides that understanding: what is happening in the body during a POTS episode, why blood volume and vascular tone are at the center of it, and—critically—how mast cell dysfunction drives and perpetuates this cardiovascular instability from within.

✦ ✦ ✦

What Happens When a Healthy Body Stands Up

To understand POTS, it helps to first appreciate what a well-functioning autonomic nervous system does in the moment of standing—a sequence of events so rapid and seamlessly orchestrated that most people are entirely unaware it is occurring.

When you stand up, gravity immediately pools approximately 500 to 700 milliliters of blood in the lower extremities and abdomen—a substantial fraction of central (thoracic) blood volume that was circulating through the chest and brain while you were lying down.[416] This sudden redistribution reduces the amount of blood returning to the heart (called venous return), which reduces cardiac output, which reduces cerebral blood flow. If left uncompensated, this would produce dizziness, visual changes, and within seconds, unconsciousness.

The body prevents this through a remarkably rapid autonomic reflex. Baroreceptors—pressure-sensitive sensors located in the carotid artery, the aortic arch, and the heart itself—detect the drop in blood pressure that accompanies the reduction in venous return. Within one to two seconds of standing, they transmit this information to the brainstem, which responds by increasing sympathetic nervous system output and reducing parasympathetic tone. The result is a coordinated cascade: blood vessels in the legs and abdomen constrict to drive blood upward; the heart rate increases slightly (typically by ten to fifteen beats per minute) to compensate for the reduced stroke volume; and the adrenal glands release small amounts of epinephrine that further support vascular tone and cardiac output.

This entire sequence unfolds in under thirty seconds and produces no perceptible symptoms in a healthy person. Blood pressure may drop by three to five millimeters of mercury transiently and then normalize. Heart rate increases modestly and then returns toward baseline. The person stands up and continues their morning without a second thought.

> **The Key Comparison:** *In a healthy autonomic system, standing produces a modest, self-correcting cardiovascular adjustment that is invisible to the person experiencing it. In POTS, the same gravitational challenge produces an excessive, prolonged, and symptom-generating compensatory heart rate surge because the normal mechanisms of vascular compensation are inadequate to the task.*

✦ ✦ ✦

What Fails in POTS: The Four Core Deficits

POTS is not a single disease with a single mechanism—it is a clinical syndrome (a collection of symptoms and physiological findings) that can arise from several different underlying deficits, each of which impairs the body's capacity to maintain adequate circulation when upright. Understanding which deficit or combination of deficits is present in any given person is the key to targeting treatment effectively. Four core physiological deficits account for the majority of POTS presentations.

Deficit One: Reduced Plasma Volume

The most consistent physiological finding across POTS populations is reduced circulating blood volume—specifically, reduced plasma volume, the liquid component of blood in which red blood cells are suspended.[417] Studies using radiolabeled red blood cell volume measurement have found that people with POTS have, on average, ten to fifteen percent less plasma volume than healthy controls matched for age, sex, and body weight.[418] This is not a trivial deficit; it means that when standing produces gravitational blood pooling in the lower body, there is simply less total blood available to maintain cerebral and cardiac perfusion.

Reduced plasma volume in POTS has multiple contributing causes. Impaired aldosterone signaling—which normally retains sodium and, with it, water in the vascular compartment—is documented in a significant proportion of individuals with POTS. Increased sympathetic-driven sweating and inadequate fluid replacement can acutely worsen volume depletion. Mast cell mediators, as described in Chapter 3, directly increase vascular permeability, allowing plasma to leak from blood vessels into surrounding tissue and reducing circulating volume. And chronic deconditioning, common in people who have been limiting physical activity due to POTS symptoms, reduces blood volume further through cardiovascular adaptation to reduced demand.

Deficit Two: Impaired Peripheral Vasoconstriction

When blood pools in the lower extremities upon standing, the normal response of blood vessels in the legs and splanchnic (abdominal) circulation is to constrict—squeezing the pooled blood upward and back toward the central circulation. In many people with POTS, this vasoconstriction response is inadequate.[419] Blood vessels that should contract promptly and forcefully remain dilated, and blood continues to pool in the periphery rather than being redistributed toward the heart and brain.

This impaired vasoconstriction can result from reduced sympathetic nervous system drive to peripheral vessels, from dysfunction of the alpha-adrenergic receptors on blood vessel walls that mediate vasoconstriction, from structural abnormalities in blood vessel walls (as seen in hEDS, where collagen deficiency reduces vascular wall stiffness and increases compliance), or from the sustained vasodilatory effect of histamine released by MCAS-activated mast cells. The histamine mechanism is particularly important in the MCAS-POTS population: as discussed in Chapter 3, H1 and H2 receptor activation by histamine produces vasodilation through multiple pathways, working directly against the vasoconstriction that the body needs to maintain orthostatic stability.

Deficit Three: Excessive Sympathetic Activation

Because peripheral vasoconstriction is inadequate, the body compensates by dramatically increasing sympathetic nervous system output—particularly to the heart.[420] The result is the defining clinical finding of POTS: a heart rate increase of thirty or more beats per minute upon standing, often reaching 120 to 140 beats per minute or higher within the first few minutes of upright posture.[421] This tachycardia is not the cause of POTS; it is the heart's desperate attempt to compensate for inadequate venous return by beating faster to maintain cardiac output despite receiving less blood per beat.

The excessive sympathetic activation that drives this tachycardia has systemic consequences that extend well beyond the heart rate. It primes mast cells throughout the body through norepinephrine acting on adrenergic receptors, as established in Chapter 9. It maintains a state of chronic physiological arousal that produces the anxiety, palpitations, and hypervigilance that many of those with POTS experience as psychological symptoms—when in reality these are the direct neurological consequences of an overdriven sympathetic nervous system. And it perpetuates the mast cell activation cycle: sympathetic overdrive activates mast cells, activated mast cells release histamine and other vasodilatory mediators, vasodilation worsens orthostatic instability, and the sympathetic system responds with further overdrive.

Deficit Four: Impaired Cerebral Autoregulation

Healthy brains maintain relatively constant blood flow over a wide range of systemic blood pressures through a process called cerebral autoregulation—the brain's blood vessels dilate when pressure falls and constrict when pressure rises, buffering the brain from the moment-to-moment fluctuations in the general circulation. In a significant proportion of individuals with POTS, this cerebral autoregulation is impaired: the brain's blood vessels fail to dilate adequately in response to the reduced perfusion pressure that accompanies orthostatic stress, allowing cerebral blood flow to fall further than it would in healthy individuals with the same systemic hemodynamic challenge.[422]

This impaired cerebral autoregulation is the most direct explanation for the cognitive symptoms of POTS—the brain fog, difficulty concentrating, word-finding problems, and memory lapses that many people describe as among their most disabling symptoms. These are not psychosomatic; they are the direct consequence of intermittently insufficient oxygen and glucose delivery to the brain whenever postural stress reduces cerebral perfusion beyond the brain's capacity to compensate. Interventions that improve overall blood volume and vascular tone—the core of POTS natural management—improve cerebral autoregulation by reducing the magnitude of the perfusion challenge the brain must buffer.

✦ ✦ ✦

POTS Subtypes: Not All POTS Is the Same

Recognizing that POTS has multiple subtypes with different dominant mechanisms helps explain why some individuals respond well to certain interventions while others do not, and why individualized treatment is more effective than a one-size-fits-all protocol. Three subtypes are most clinically relevant to the MCAS-POTS population.

Neuropathic POTS

The most common POTS subtype, neuropathic POTS involves selective denervation of the peripheral sympathetic nerves that innervate the blood vessels of the lower extremities and splanchnic circulation.[423] When these fibers are damaged or dysfunctional, the vasoconstriction response to standing is impaired specifically in the lower body, while the central sympathetic response (which drives the compensatory tachycardia) is preserved or even enhanced. The result is selective lower-body pooling without adequate vasoconstriction, compensated by excessive heart rate elevation. Neuropathic POTS is associated with small-fiber neuropathy—the same progressive damage to small autonomic nerve fibers documented in both MCAS and hEDS and discussed in Chapter 4. The MCAS-driven neuroinflammation that damages these fibers is a direct contributor to neuropathic POTS in the MCAS population.

Hyperadrenergic POTS

Hyperadrenergic POTS is characterized by disproportionately elevated plasma norepinephrine upon standing—typically above 600 picograms per milliliter when upright—indicating a primary dysregulation of the sympathetic nervous system's control of norepinephrine release rather than a simple compensatory response to inadequate vasoconstriction.[424] Individuals with hyperadrenergic POTS often experience prominent symptoms of sympathetic excess: hypertension (rather than hypotension) when upright, severe palpitations, tremor, anxiety, and headache. They may feel more ill in highly stimulating environments. Hyperadrenergic POTS is particularly relevant to MCAS because the chronically primed mast cell system and chronically elevated sympathetic tone reinforce each other directly through the bidirectional mechanisms described in Chapter 3.

Low-Flow (Hypovolemic) POTS

Low-flow POTS is driven primarily by plasma volume depletion—the reduced blood volume deficit is the dominant mechanism rather than peripheral nerve dysfunction or primary sympathetic dysregulation.[425] These people often have the lowest measured plasma volumes, the most prominent symptoms of dehydration and salt craving, and the most dramatic response to aggressive volume expansion through salt and fluid supplementation. In the MCAS population, mast-cell-mediated vascular permeability is a major driver of the plasma volume depletion, making mast cell stabilization a direct and important component of managing this subtype's volume deficit.

✦ ✦ ✦

The Role of Mast Cells in Vascular Tone: A Deeper Look

Chapter 3 introduced the mechanisms by which mast cell dysfunction drives POTS. This section builds on that foundation with the clinical and mechanistic detail needed to understand why mast cell stabilization is not merely an add-on to POTS management but is often its most important lever.

Histamine's Vascular Effects: Permeability and Vasodilation

Histamine acts on the cardiovascular system through two primary receptor pathways with directly opposing effects on orthostatic stability. H1 receptor activation on vascular smooth muscle and endothelium produces vasodilation—blood vessel widening that decreases peripheral vascular resistance and promotes blood pooling in dependent tissues. H1 activation on endothelial cells simultaneously increases vascular permeability, allowing plasma proteins and fluid to leak from the vascular compartment into surrounding tissue—directly reducing plasma volume. H2 receptor activation on the heart increases heart rate and contractility—a direct driver of the tachycardia that defines POTS.

The combined effect of chronic histamine excess in MCAS is, therefore, precisely the cardiovascular vulnerability profile of POTS: reduced plasma volume (H1-mediated permeability), impaired peripheral vasoconstriction (H1-mediated vasodilation competing with sympathetic vasoconstriction), and tachycardia out of proportion to normal orthostatic compensation (H2-mediated cardiac stimulation). This is not a coincidence of co-occurrence—it is a mechanistic derivation: MCAS creates POTS-like cardiovascular physiology through histamine's direct vascular effects.

Prostaglandins and Vascular Instability

Mast cells release prostaglandin D2 (PGD2) during degranulation—a potent vasodilatory eicosanoid that acts on vascular smooth muscle through DP1 and CRTH2 receptors to produce vasodilation, decreased systemic vascular resistance, and increased capillary permeability.[426] PGD2 is among the mast cell mediators most directly implicated in acute hypotensive MCAS episodes, and elevated urinary PGD2 metabolites (specifically 11β-prostaglandin F2α) are one of the more sensitive laboratory markers of active mast cell degranulation precisely because they track this vascular effect.[427] Individuals who notice that their most severe POTS symptoms coincide with clear mast cell events—flushing, hives, gut cramping—are often experiencing the combined hemodynamic effects of histamine and PGD2 released simultaneously during a degranulation event.

Renin-Angiotensin-Aldosterone System Interactions

The renin-angiotensin-aldosterone system (RAAS) is the body's primary long-term blood volume regulator; it maintains plasma sodium and water content, and therefore plasma volume, through a cascade of hormonal signals from the kidneys, liver, and adrenal glands. Mast cell tryptase, released during degranulation, activates protease-activated receptors (PARs) on vascular endothelium and renal cells that interact with RAAS components, potentially impairing the normal sodium and water retention mechanisms that maintain adequate plasma volume. This provides a mechanistic explanation for the plasma volume depletion seen in many with MCAS-POTS—beyond the acute permeability effects of histamine, chronic mast cell tryptase release may impair the hormonal regulation of volume balance, contributing to the persistent hypovolemia that makes orthostatic tolerance so difficult to maintain.

Mast Cells in the Vasculature Itself

Mast cells are not merely circulating immune cells that happen to affect the vasculature through their chemical mediators; they are resident within the adventitia (outer wall) and perivascular connective tissue of blood vessels throughout the body. In this location, they respond directly to mechanical stimuli including vascular stretch, transmural pressure changes, and blood flow shear stress. The baroreceptor-driven mechanical changes that accompany orthostatic stress—vascular stretch in the lower extremities, wall tension changes in capacitance vessels—are potential direct mast cell activation signals through the mechanosensitive MRGPRX2 pathway described in Chapter 9. This means that the postural change of standing may itself trigger local mast cell activation in peripheral blood vessels, adding a mechanical dimension to the biochemical mast cell–POTS loop.

✦ ✦ ✦

Deeper Dive: The Autonomic Nervous System and the Vascular Circuit

For the Science-Minded Reader

The autonomic dysfunction in POTS can be understood at three distinct levels of the nervous system, each of which presents a different therapeutic target and responds to somewhat different interventions.

Central Autonomic Processing: The Brainstem and Hypothalamus

The nucleus tractus solitarius (NTS) in the brainstem is the primary integrating center for autonomic cardiovascular control—receiving input from baroreceptors, chemoreceptors, and visceral afferents, and coordinating the sympathetic and parasympathetic output that controls heart rate, vascular tone, and blood pressure moment to moment. The hypothalamus modulates NTS activity through descending pathways and serves as the interface between the emotional, hormonal, and autonomic dimensions of cardiovascular regulation. In those with POTS, functional neuroimaging and autonomic reflex testing have documented abnormalities at both brainstem and hypothalamic levels—reduced baroreflex sensitivity, altered resting autonomic tone, and impaired integration of cardiovascular and emotional stress responses.[428]

CNS mast cells—particularly those in the hypothalamus and around the floor of the fourth ventricle near the NTS—are positioned to directly influence central autonomic processing through their mediator release. Histamine released by hypothalamic mast cells modulates NTS activity through H1 and H2 receptors; CRH released during HPA axis activation directly activates these CNS mast cells; and neuroinflammatory cytokines from CNS mast cell degranulation alter the synaptic environment of the central autonomic network. This provides a plausible mechanistic pathway through which systemic MCAS perpetuates central autonomic dysregulation—not merely as a peripheral cardiovascular consequence, but as a direct neurological effect.

Peripheral Autonomic Fibers: The Small-Fiber Neuropathy Connection

The post-ganglionic sympathetic fibers that innervate peripheral blood vessels are small, unmyelinated C-fibers—the same fiber type documented in small-fiber neuropathy, and the same type whose density in skin biopsies is reduced in a meaningful proportion of people with POTS. These fibers release norepinephrine onto blood vessel walls in response to sympathetic activation, mediating the vasoconstriction that maintains orthostatic stability. When they are damaged—by the neuroinflammation driven by mast cell mediators, by the metabolic consequences of chronic oxidative stress, or by autoimmune processes triggered by molecular mimicry—their norepinephrine-mediated vasoconstriction is impaired specifically in the territories they innervate, producing the selective lower-body vascular denervation that characterizes neuropathic POTS.

This explains why interventions that reduce neuroinflammation and protect small-fiber integrity—mast cell stabilization, omega-3 fatty acids, alpha-lipoic acid, vitamin B12, and vagal tone training—have the potential to both prevent further small-fiber damage and, through the nervous system's limited but genuine capacity for regeneration, partially restore peripheral autonomic function over the long term. Recovery from neuropathic POTS is slow—measured in years rather than months—but it is documented in those who achieve sustained mast cell stability and address the underlying drivers of small-fiber injury.

The Baroreflex Arc and Heart Rate Variability

Baroreflex sensitivity—the speed and magnitude of heart rate and blood pressure changes in response to detected pressure changes—is a quantifiable measure of autonomic cardiovascular control and is consistently reduced in those with POTS. Low baroreflex sensitivity means that when blood pressure falls upon standing, the baroreceptors transmit a weaker or slower signal to the brainstem, the compensatory autonomic response is delayed or diminished, and the heart must compensate by maintaining a prolonged and excessive tachycardia rather than rapidly normalizing with a brief, proportionate response.

Heart rate variability (HRV)—discussed in the context of MCAS nervous system management in Chapter 14—is closely related to baroreflex sensitivity. Both reflect the flexibility and responsiveness of the autonomic nervous system, and both are improved by the same interventions: consistent vagal tone training, aerobic conditioning within tolerance, adequate sleep, and reduced chronic sympathetic activation. The HRV monitoring and biofeedback approach described in Chapter 14 is therefore directly relevant to POTS physiology; improving HRV through these practices directly improves the autonomic control of cardiovascular function, including the speed and appropriateness of the orthostatic compensation response.

✦ ✦ ✦

What This Means for You: Understanding Your POTS

The physiology in this chapter is not merely academic—it directly informs the treatment priorities described in Chapter 22. Before turning to those strategies, this section translates the key physiological concepts into self-knowledge that will make your management approach more targeted and more effective.

Identify your dominant deficit. Does your POTS present primarily with very low blood pressure and prominent volume depletion symptoms (intense thirst, salt craving, dramatic improvement with IV saline)? Then hypovolemic low-flow POTS is likely dominant, and aggressive volume expansion is your highest priority. Does it present with hypertension when upright, prominent palpitations, and severe anxiety? Then hyperadrenergic POTS is more prominent, and interventions that reduce sympathetic tone—nervous system regulation, mast cell stabilization—take priority over simple volume expansion. Does it present with clear neuropathic features (lower extremity weakness or discomfort, a skin biopsy showing reduced small-fiber density)? Then neuropathic POTS is the dominant mechanism, and anti-neuroinflammatory strategies are central. Many individuals have overlapping subtypes, but identifying the most prominent one sharpens treatment prioritization.

Track the MCAS-POTS relationship in your symptom journal. Note whether orthostatic symptoms worsen on days when other MCAS markers are elevated—more flushing, more gut symptoms, more skin reactivity. If there is a consistent pattern, it confirms that mast cell mediator activity is directly driving your POTS physiology on those days, and that mast cell stabilization is one of the highest-leverage interventions for your cardiovascular symptoms specifically.

Understand that cardiovascular symptoms are not anxiety—and vice versa. The racing heart, the flushing, the sense of impending doom during a POTS episode are physiological responses generated by an overdriven sympathetic nervous system. They feel exactly like anxiety because they use the same neurological machinery. This does not mean they are psychological. It does mean that nervous system regulation practices—the breathing techniques and vagal exercises from Chapter 14—directly address the physiological state producing these symptoms, not merely the emotional experience of them.

Know the role of deconditioning in the cycle. Reduced physical activity in response to POTS symptoms leads to cardiovascular deconditioning, which reduces plasma volume and cardiac fitness, which worsens POTS symptoms. This is the cycle that can make POTS feel like it is inexorably progressing when it is actually being maintained by inactivity. Breaking this cycle through carefully paced, appropriately designed exercise—the subject of Chapter 23—is one of the most important structural interventions available for POTS, but it must be approached with the nuance that exercise is also a potential mast cell trigger in the MCAS population.

Appreciate the timescale of structural improvement. Volume expansion through salt and fluid works within hours. Nervous system regulation practices improve HRV within weeks. Reducing mast cell-driven small-fiber neuroinflammation and beginning to restore peripheral vascular innervation takes months to years of consistent intervention. This timescale mismatch is a major source of discouragement for people with POTS who feel immediate symptomatic relief from some interventions but incomplete resolution overall. The acute interventions manage day-to-day symptoms; the deeper interventions restructure the physiology. Both are necessary, and patience with the deeper timeline is essential.

The woman from the beginning of this chapter—the one who runs her morning clinical assessment before her feet hit the floor—has learned something important about her body: it is not fragile, and it is not incompetent. It is managing an extraordinarily difficult circulatory challenge with the tools available to it, doing its best with an autonomic system that has been dysregulated by a combination of mast cell inflammation, volume depletion, and small-fiber damage. It is not failing. It is compensating—imperfectly, exhaustingly, but persistently.

Understanding this has changed not just her strategy but her relationship with her symptoms. She is no longer fighting her body. She is working with the physiology to give it what it needs: more volume, better vascular tone, reduced mast cell activation, a nervous system that can access its parasympathetic brake, and the gradual reconditioning that will allow her cardiovascular system to rebuild the capacity it has lost. Chapter 22 is where that work begins in practical detail.

✦ ✦ ✦

Chapter 21 at a Glance

What to Remember:

- When a healthy person stands up, baroreceptors detect the blood pressure drop from gravitational pooling and trigger rapid sympathetic activation that constricts peripheral blood vessels and modestly increases heart rate. The entire compensation occurs in under thirty seconds and produces no perceptible symptoms.

- In POTS, this orthostatic compensation fails—producing a heart rate increase of thirty or more beats per minute upon standing because peripheral vasoconstriction is inadequate to maintain venous return without cardiac overdrive.
- Four core physiological deficits underlie POTS: reduced plasma volume, impaired peripheral vasoconstriction, excessive sympathetic activation, and impaired cerebral autoregulation. Different people have different dominant deficits, which should guide treatment prioritization.
- Three POTS subtypes—neuropathic (impaired peripheral autonomic innervation), hyperadrenergic (primary sympathetic dysregulation with elevated norepinephrine), and hypovolemic/low-flow (plasma volume depletion dominant)—have somewhat different mechanisms and treatment emphases.
- Mast cell dysfunction drives POTS physiology through multiple mechanisms: H1 receptor-mediated vasodilation and vascular permeability (worsening pooling and volume depletion), H2 receptor-mediated cardiac stimulation (contributing to tachycardia), prostaglandin D2 release (additional vasodilation during degranulation events), and tryptase-mediated impairment of RAAS volume regulation.
- Mast cells resident in blood vessel walls may be directly activated by the mechanical forces of orthostatic postural change through MRGPRX2 receptor signaling—creating a loop in which standing itself triggers mast cell activation that worsens the cardiovascular physiology of POTS.
- Small-fiber neuropathy—driven by MCAS-related neuroinflammation and documented in a significant proportion of people with POTS—impairs the sympathetic innervation of peripheral blood vessels, producing the selective lower-body vascular denervation that characterizes neuropathic POTS. Anti-neuroinflammatory interventions can limit further damage and support gradual recovery over months to years.
- Heart rate variability (HRV) directly reflects autonomic cardiovascular control and baroreflex sensitivity. The HRV-building practices from Chapter 14 directly improve the neurological infrastructure of orthostatic compensation—connecting the nervous system practices to the cardiovascular improvement goals found later in the book.

Coming Up in Chapter 22:

With a clear understanding of the physiology driving POTS, we turn to the practical natural strategies that address each of its core deficits. Chapter 22 covers the evidence-informed foundations of natural POTS management: hydration and electrolyte protocols calibrated to individual subtype and POTS severity, compression strategies that physically support venous return, and the nervous system retraining approaches that target the autonomic dysregulation at POTS's cardiovascular root. These strategies are complementary—not alternatives to—the mast cell stabilization work throughout this book, and together they form the most complete natural approach to POTS management available.

CHAPTER 22

Natural Strategies for POTS

Hydration, Electrolytes, Compression, and Nervous System Retraining

The Difference a Morning Protocol Makes

Tom had been living with POTS for two years when he finally found a cardiologist who sat down with him and explained—plainly, without condescension—exactly what his body needed and why. The conversation lasted forty minutes. By the end of it, Tom understood three things he had not understood before: that his blood vessels were failing to constrict adequately when he stood up; that his circulating blood volume was lower than it should be; and that his heart, far from being the problem, was doing its heroic best to compensate for both.

He left with a plan that cost almost nothing and required no prescriptions: a specific electrolyte drink to begin every morning before getting out of bed, compression stockings to put on before standing, and a set of breathing exercises to practice daily. Not dramatic. Not complicated. But within three weeks, his standing heart rate had dropped by an average of eighteen beats per minute. His morning fog had lifted noticeably. He was making it through work days that had previously required him to leave early.

Natural strategies for POTS are not a replacement for medical care, and they are not a guarantee of full resolution. But for many people with POTS, particularly those in whom mast cell dysfunction is a contributing driver, they produce real, measurable, often substantial improvement when applied consistently and intelligently. This chapter translates the physiology of Chapter 21 into the practical strategies that address each of POTS's core deficits: volume expansion through hydration and electrolytes, mechanical support for venous return through compression, and autonomic retraining through targeted nervous system practices and movement.

* * *

Hydration and Electrolytes: Filling the Volume Deficit

The most immediately effective natural intervention for most individuals with POTS is also one of the simplest: increasing circulating blood volume through strategic fluid and electrolyte intake. As established in Chapter 21, reduced plasma volume is one of the most consistent findings in POTS—and it is a deficit that can be meaningfully and rapidly addressed without medication.

The critical word is strategic. Drinking large volumes of plain water alone does not reliably increase plasma volume in those with POTS—it is excreted relatively rapidly by the kidneys, which have no particular reason to retain it without the osmotic signal of sodium. To expand plasma volume, fluid intake must be paired with adequate sodium intake. Sodium draws water into the vascular compartment and retains it there, expanding the liquid volume that the heart can work with and that the venous system has available to compensate for gravitational pooling.

The Sodium and Fluid Target

Most POTS management guidelines recommend significantly higher sodium intake than standard dietary advice suggests—typically three to five grams of sodium daily (roughly seven to twelve grams of salt, or table salt), alongside two to three liters of fluid. These targets are substantially higher than the general population recommendation of approximately 2.3 grams of sodium daily and represent a deliberate therapeutic elevation to address the volume deficit specific to POTS.

These targets should be discussed with a physician, particularly for anyone with a history of high blood pressure, heart failure, or kidney disease—conditions in which elevated sodium intake requires clinical supervision. For the majority of people with POTS without these comorbidities, however, therapeutic sodium and fluid intake is safe and produces rapid symptomatic benefit. Blood pressure typically does not rise in individuals with POTS with volume depletion because the additional sodium and fluid is filling a deficit, not overloading an already-adequate system.

> **The Morning Protocol:** *Drinking 500 mL (roughly 16 ounces) of electrolyte-containing fluid before getting out of bed is one of the highest-impact morning practices for POTS. Doing this while still lying down gives the fluid time to begin expanding plasma volume before the gravitational challenge of standing begins. Many people with POTS find this single habit reduces their morning symptoms dramatically.*

Electrolyte Sources: What Works and What to Watch

Plain water is insufficient—the fluid must contain electrolytes, particularly sodium, to produce meaningful plasma volume expansion. Several approaches work well for different patients and budgets:

- **Electrolyte powders and drinks** – Commercially available electrolyte products range from minimally processed options to pharmaceutical-grade oral rehydration solutions. For those with MCAS, reading ingredient labels carefully matters: some products contain artificial colors, citric acid, or flavoring compounds that can trigger reactions. Plain or mildly flavored options are safer starting points.
- **Homemade electrolyte solution** – One quarter teaspoon of sea salt or Himalayan salt, a small pinch of cream of tartar (potassium), a squeeze of fresh lemon or lime (small amounts are typically tolerated), and water provides a low-cost, clean-ingredient electrolyte drink that most with MCAS can prepare without triggering reactions.
- **Salt capsules or salt sticks** – For those who find flavored drinks triggering, plain sodium chloride capsules with plain water provide the essential sodium without any additional ingredients.
- **Salty foods at breakfast** – Olives, a sodium-containing broth, or eggs with liberal salt seasoning can contribute to morning sodium intake through food rather than supplementation—an approach that integrates naturally into the low-histamine meal plan from Chapter 13.

Magnesium: The Often-Missing Electrolyte

Magnesium is as important as sodium in POTS management, but for different reasons. While sodium expands plasma volume, magnesium supports vascular tone regulation, nervous system function, and the regulation of heart rate variability. Low magnesium is associated with increased cardiac excitability—worsening the tendency toward tachycardia—and with impaired blood vessel relaxation and contraction cycling.[429] The magnesium glycinate from Chapter 16's supplement protocol serves both mast cell stabilization and POTS vascular support simultaneously, making it one of the most efficient supplements in the combined MCAS-POTS protocol.

Potassium deserves mention here as well; high sodium intake increases urinary potassium loss, and adequate potassium is necessary to balance the sodium-potassium pump that maintains normal cellular membrane potential throughout the cardiovascular system. Potassium-rich low-histamine foods—cooked potatoes, cooked lentils, and bananas (if tolerated)—or a modest potassium supplement (99 mg daily, the standard over-the-counter maximum) helps maintain this balance during therapeutic sodium intake.

✦ ✦ ✦

Compression: Giving Gravity a Counterforce

If sodium and fluid fill the tank, compression is the mechanical intervention that keeps the blood in the tank when you stand up. Compression garments apply graduated external pressure to the legs and abdomen—highest at the feet, progressively lower toward the waist—that physically counteracts the gravitational pooling of blood in the lower extremities. They are one of the most immediately effective and evidence-supported non-pharmacological interventions for POTS.

The mechanism is straightforward: by squeezing the veins in the legs and abdomen, compression garments reduce the volume of blood that can pool there when upright, increasing the amount that remains available in the central circulation for cardiac output and cerebral perfusion. Studies of compression in those with POTS consistently demonstrate reduced standing heart rate and improved orthostatic tolerance—not by fixing the underlying autonomic dysfunction, but by mechanically reducing the severity of the gravitational challenge the impaired autonomic system must compensate for.[430]

Choosing Compression That Works

The most important parameter in compression garment selection for POTS is coverage: compression that extends to the thighs and ideally to the waist provides substantially more benefit than knee-high stockings alone, because it also compresses the large venous reservoir of the thighs and the splanchnic (abdominal) circulation—where a significant proportion of blood pooling occurs in POTS. Studies comparing knee-high, thigh-high, and waist-level (abdominal binder plus thigh-high) compression consistently find that higher coverage produces better orthostatic tolerance.[431]

Compression level is measured in millimeters of mercury (mmHg). For POTS management, at least 20–30 mmHg at the ankle is typically needed to produce meaningful benefit—this is the range labeled as medical-grade or class II compression in most countries. Over-the-counter "support stockings" at 8–15 mmHg are generally insufficient. Prescription-grade compression (30–40 mmHg) provides additional benefit for more severely affected patients.

Practical Compression Guidance for POTS

Put on compression garments before standing up in the morning—ideally while still lying in bed, before any orthostatic stress begins.

Thigh-high or waist-high coverage is significantly more effective than knee-high alone for most individuals with POTS.

An abdominal binder or high-waisted compression leggings that compress the abdomen adds measurable benefit beyond leg compression alone, particularly for patients with significant splanchnic pooling.

Medical-grade 20–30 mmHg compression is the minimum effective level; 30–40 mmHg provides greater benefit for more severely affected patients.

Many people with MCAS find compression fabric itself a trigger if the fabric contains synthetic dyes or nickel-containing elastic. Look for products labeled latex-free and uncolored, or test tolerability on a small skin area before full use.

Compression garments are not comfortable for everyone—particularly in warm weather, and particularly for those with skin sensitivity. Cooling the skin before putting them on, choosing seamless and uncolored products when possible, and accepting that some discomfort is a reasonable trade-off for significantly improved orthostatic tolerance are all part of the practical learning curve. Some people find that alternating between garments on cooler days and managing without on very hot or highly reactive days is the most sustainable approach.

✦ ✦ ✦

Nervous System Retraining: The Longer Game

Hydration and compression address POTS's immediate, hour-to-hour symptom burden—they are the acute management tools. Nervous system retraining is the longer-term strategy: the work of gradually shifting the autonomic nervous system's set point toward greater flexibility, better baroreflex sensitivity, and a less chronically overdrive sympathetic state. It is slower to show results but ultimately more transformative, because it addresses the underlying dysregulation rather than only compensating for its consequences.

The connection between nervous system retraining and POTS is direct and mechanistically clear. Heart rate variability (HRV)—the direct measure of autonomic flexibility described in Chapters 14 and 21—reflects the health of the baroreflex arc that governs orthostatic compensation. Every intervention that improves HRV improves the baroreflex. Every improvement in the baroreflex makes the body's response to postural change more appropriate—reducing the magnitude and duration of the compensatory tachycardia, improving the speed of peripheral vasoconstriction, and reducing the cognitive and cardiovascular symptoms that result from inadequate compensation.

The Breathing Practices Revisited for POTS

The extended-exhale breathing and resonance frequency breathing described in Chapter 14 have specific and documented effects on cardiovascular autonomic function that are directly relevant to POTS. Resonance frequency breathing at five to six breaths per minute—the heart rate variability training approach—produces the largest measurable improvements in baroreflex sensitivity of any non-pharmacological intervention studied in human subjects. A consistent practice of fifteen to twenty minutes of resonance frequency breathing daily produces measurable HRV improvement within four to six weeks in most people, with progressive gains continuing over months of sustained practice.

For those with POTS specifically, morning breathing practice before rising has an additional strategic value: it raises vagal tone before the orthostatic challenge of standing begins, essentially pre-loading parasympathetic capacity into the cardiovascular system at the moment it will face its greatest daily test. The five-minute extended-exhale practice while still lying in bed—combined with the electrolyte drink consumed before rising—constitutes a morning pre-standing protocol that addresses both the volume deficit and the autonomic deficit before the first step is taken.

Posture Strategies and Counter Maneuvers

Certain physical maneuvers can acutely reduce POTS symptoms by physically reducing venous pooling or increasing venous return without drugs or compression garments. These counter maneuvers are well-studied in orthostatic intolerance research and represent a practical toolkit for managing symptoms in real-time situations.

- **Leg crossing** – Standing with legs crossed and squeezing the thigh muscles compresses the large veins of the thighs, actively driving blood upward into the central circulation. Studies show leg crossing during standing reduces the heart rate surge of orthostatic stress in individuals with POTS—a significant acute improvement achievable in any public setting without any equipment.[432]
- **Muscle pumping** – Repeatedly tensing and releasing the calf and thigh muscles while standing activates the skeletal muscle pump—the mechanism by which walking drives venous blood upward against gravity. Even small, repetitive movements (rising on the toes, clenching the thighs, shifting weight from foot to foot) can meaningfully reduce pooling during prolonged standing.
- **Physical elevation of the head of the bed** – Head-up sleeping (elevating the head of the bed) has been used as a non-pharmacologic strategy in orthostatic intolerance to reduce nocturnal diuresis and

support blood volume regulation, with some evidence suggesting it may improve orthostatic tolerance, although data in POTS are limited.[433]

- **Squatting or sitting promptly** – When presyncope symptoms begin (vision darkening, hearing changes, severe dizziness), immediately squatting or sitting—rather than waiting to see if the feeling passes—interrupts the hemodynamic cascade before it progresses. Early intervention is dramatically more effective than waiting; sitting promptly reduces recovery time from minutes to seconds in most cases.

The Role of Mast Cell Stabilization in Nervous System Retraining

One of the most important and most frequently missed insights in POTS nervous system retraining is that mast cell stabilization is not separate from autonomic retraining—it enables it. A nervous system that is continuously being activated by mast cell–released histamine, CRH, and sympathomimetic mediators cannot effectively shift toward parasympathetic dominance through any amount of breathwork or biofeedback. The autonomic set point is being driven upward from the immune system faster than any retraining practice can drive it down.

This is why the combined MCAS-POTS protocol produces better cardiovascular outcomes than either the POTS-specific or MCAS-specific components pursued independently. As mast cell reactivity decreases—through the dietary, supplement, gut healing, and detoxification work mentioned earlier—the nervous system has increasing room to respond to retraining efforts. The baroreflex improves because the neuroinflammatory noise impairing it is quieter; HRV rises as sympathetic override from mast cell mediators falls; morning tachycardia decreases as histamine-driven vasodilation reduces.

People who begin HRV biofeedback practice while still at peak mast cell reactivity often find limited gains. The same people who then address their MCAS through the protocols in this book and return to HRV biofeedback practice several months will likely experience dramatically faster improvement—sometimes within weeks rather than months—because the underlying condition driving their autonomic dysfunction has been reduced enough that retraining can finally produce its intended effect.

✦ ✦ ✦

Deeper Dive: The Science Behind Salt, Compression, and Baroreflex Training

For the Science-Minded Reader

The three core natural POTS strategies—volume expansion, compression, and nervous system retraining—each have a growing body of clinical trial evidence behind them, and understanding that evidence helps calibrate expectations and confirms that these are genuine therapeutic interventions rather than anecdotal approaches.

The Evidence for High-Volume, High-Sodium Hydration

The Vanderbilt University Autonomic Dysfunction Center, one of the leading academic POTS research centers in the world, has conducted extensive studies on blood volume and sodium in POTS. Their work has consistently demonstrated that plasma volume is reduced by an average of ten to fifteen percent in those with POTS compared to healthy controls; that acute saline infusion (equivalent to IV fluid expansion) significantly reduces heart rate and improves orthostatic tolerance within hours; and that sustained high-sodium diet (five grams daily) combined with adequate fluid intake produces meaningful improvement in orthostatic symptoms and quality of life over weeks of consistent use.[434] The therapeutic sodium target used in this chapter directly reflects the doses validated in these studies.

The renin-angiotensin-aldosterone axis response to therapeutic sodium intake in POTS is also documented: many people with POTS show elevated plasma renin activity and reduced aldosterone—indicating the kidneys are already straining to retain sodium. High sodium intake in these individuals normalizes this ratio toward the target range rather than driving it into excess, supporting the safety of therapeutic sodium for this population.[435,436]

Compression: What the Research Actually Shows

A systematic review and related studies have found that compression garments—particularly those providing abdominal and thigh compression (e.g., waist-high, 20–40 mmHg)—can reduce standing heart rate and improve orthostatic symptoms in patients with orthostatic intolerance, including POTS, although the magnitude of effect varies across studies.[437,438] The addition of abdominal compression to leg compression produced incremental benefit beyond leg compression alone, consistent with the physiological role of the splanchnic reservoir in POTS. The practical implication is that people who are using only knee-high stockings and finding limited benefit should consider upgrading to thigh-high or waist-level coverage before concluding that compression does not work for them.

Heart Rate Variability Biofeedback: The Evidence Base

HRV biofeedback—using real-time heart rate variability feedback to guide resonance frequency breathing practice—has been studied in multiple randomized controlled trials in populations with overlapping biology to POTS: chronic fatigue syndrome, fibromyalgia, anxiety disorders, and dysautonomia.[439] Consistent findings across these trials include significant improvement in HRV and baroreflex sensitivity within four to eight weeks of daily practice, reduction in symptom burden measured by validated quality-of-life questionnaires, and improvement maintained at six-month follow-up when practice is sustained. The effect sizes are clinically meaningful—not just statistically significant—and comparable to those achieved by pharmacological autonomic modulators in some comparison studies.

The mechanism is neuroplastic; consistent practice trains the baroreflex arc through repeated activation, progressively improving the speed and sensitivity of the cardiovascular compensation response. Like any conditioning process, gains accumulate over months rather than weeks—patients who discontinue after two weeks miss the gains that typically emerge at four to six weeks and continue building with sustained practice.

✦ ✦ ✦

Exploring BPC-157 in hEDS and POTS

BPC-157 is a lab-made peptide originally found in stomach proteins, and it's gained attention for its possible role in healing soft tissues like tendons and ligaments. For people with hypermobile Ehlers-Danlos syndrome (hEDS), this is interesting because many symptoms—joint instability, frequent sprains, slow healing, and chronic pain—are tied to fragile connective tissue.

In animal studies, BPC-157 appears to support tissue repair by increasing blood flow, helping cells involved in healing (like fibroblasts) work more effectively, and improving how collagen is formed and organized.[440] Because of this, some people with hEDS report that it helps them recover faster from injuries, feel more stable, or have less lingering pain. It may also support gut lining health, which can matter since digestive issues are common in EDS.

For POTS (which often overlaps with hEDS), the potential benefits are more indirect. Early research suggests BPC-157 may help protect blood vessels, support circulation, and reduce inflammation.[441] Some users report improvements in energy, dizziness, or "brain fog," possibly related to better blood flow or gut health. However, these effects are based mostly on animal research and personal reports—not solid clinical trials.

It's important to keep expectations realistic. BPC-157 does not fix the underlying genetic cause of hEDS or directly treat autonomic dysfunction in POTS. At best, it may offer supportive, symptom-level improvements—and even those vary widely from person to person.

There are also practical concerns: it's not FDA-approved, quality can vary, and long-term safety isn't well studied. If you're considering it, it's best to talk with a knowledgeable healthcare provider and continue prioritizing proven strategies like physical therapy, hydration, compression, and appropriate medications.

BPC-157: Oral and Injectable Protocols

Oral Protocol

The oral route is the appropriate starting point for most individuals with MCAS, as it acts directly on the gut lining where repair is most needed. Standard dosing is 250–500 mcg twice daily. Begin at 250 mcg, observe for five to seven days, then increase to 500 mcg if well tolerated.

Take on an empty stomach—at least thirty minutes before eating or two hours after a meal. Gastric acid and digestive enzymes present during active digestion degrade the peptide before it can act on the gut lining. Morning dosing before breakfast and evening dosing before bed is the most practical structure. A typical course is eight to twelve weeks.

Injectable Protocol

Injection delivers BPC-157 systemically, making it more appropriate when broader tissue-level effects are the goal—particularly for connective tissue healing in the hEDS–MCAS overlap, or when gut repair has been partially established and deeper systemic support is the next step.

Standard dosing is 250–500 mcg subcutaneously, once daily. Inject into the fatty layer beneath the skin—not into muscle—using a 27–29 gauge half-inch insulin syringe. Timing relative to meals is not clinically significant for injectable administration.

Preferred injection sites, in order of practical ease:

- **Abdomen**—two to three inches from the navel, alternating sides with each dose
- **Outer thigh**—lateral upper thigh, pinching a small skin fold before injecting
- **Flank**—soft tissue at the sides of the lower back

Rotate sites systematically to prevent localized tissue irritation. Allow refrigerated solution to reach room temperature before injecting, and discard each syringe after single use.

MCAS-Specific Considerations

Introduce BPC-157 as a single new variable—not alongside other new supplements—and observe for five to seven days before evaluating response. Most individuals with MCAS tolerate it well. Mild digestive changes in the first week of oral use are occasionally reported and typically self-resolve; if they persist, reduce to 125 mcg BID and rebuild slowly.

> **Key Takeaway.** *BPC-157 is a targeted adjunct tool, most appropriately introduced in the Support or Repair stages of recovery—not during initial stabilization. It works alongside the foundational protocol, not in place of it.*

✦ ✦ ✦

What This Means for You: Your Daily POTS Management Plan

Combining the three strategies in this chapter into a practical daily routine transforms abstract physiological principles into a manageable set of habits. The following framework represents a sustainable starting point that most POTS patients can adapt to their own schedules and circumstances.

Before rising each morning: Drink 500 mL of electrolyte fluid while still lying down. Do five minutes of extended-exhale breathing (four counts in, eight counts out). Put on compression garments before sitting up. This three-part morning pre-standing protocol addresses volume, autonomic tone, and mechanical support before the first orthostatic challenge of the day.

First fifteen minutes upright: Move slowly. Sit on the edge of the bed for thirty to sixty seconds before fully standing. Use the leg-crossing or muscle-pumping counter maneuvers during any prolonged standing. Sit or lean against a wall when waiting in lines, at counters, or in any situation where prolonged static standing is unavoidable.

Throughout the day: Continue electrolyte fluid intake toward the two-to-three-liter daily target. Eat regular, moderate-sized meals rather than large meals—large meals divert blood toward the gut for digestion, temporarily worsening orthostatic tolerance through a mechanism called postprandial hypotension. A moderate salt intake at each meal (rather than a single large bolus) sustains plasma volume more consistently than morning-only sodium loading.

Daily HRV practice: Do fifteen to twenty minutes of resonance frequency breathing (five counts in, five counts out), either in the morning as part of the waking routine or during the midday period when energy is typically highest. HRV monitoring with a compatible wearable provides objective feedback and tracking. Even people who begin with poor HRV consistently see measurable trend improvement at four to six weeks of daily practice.

Evening: Elevate the head of the bed by fifteen to twenty degrees using bed risers rather than extra pillows (which do not maintain spinal alignment and reduce the kidney-position benefit). Continue evening breathwork and the Chapter 14 wind-down routine. Take the evening magnesium glycinate dose, which supports both overnight nervous system recovery and morning vascular tone.

Track your response: Note your standing heart rate before and after implementing these strategies using a simple home pulse oximeter or smartwatch. Note morning symptom severity on your daily tracking scale. Most individuals see measurable heart rate reduction and symptom improvement within two to four weeks of consistent implementation, which provides the motivation to maintain these habits through the longer trajectory of nervous system retraining.

Tom's forty-minute conversation with his cardiologist gave him a framework that cost him almost nothing and improved his life substantially within the month. The electrolyte drink, the compression stockings, the morning breathing—none of it was remarkable individually. Together, consistently applied, it added up to mornings that were manageable rather than formidable, workdays that were complete rather than truncated, and a sense that his body was something he could work with rather than something that was happening to him.

That shift—from passive sufferer to active manager of a physiology you understand—is what this chapter is ultimately about. The strategies are straightforward. The consistency is the harder part. But the rewards of that consistency are real, documented, and available to most people willing to commit to them.

✦ ✦ ✦

Chapter 22 at a Glance

What to Remember:

- Volume expansion through therapeutic sodium and fluid intake is the most immediately effective natural POTS intervention. Target three to five grams of sodium and two to three liters of fluid daily. Sodium without adequate fluid is insufficient; fluid without sodium is excreted too rapidly to expand plasma volume.
- The morning pre-standing protocol—electrolyte drink consumed lying down, five minutes of breathing practice, compression garments applied before rising—addresses volume, autonomic tone, and mechanical support before the first orthostatic challenge of the day. This single habit change produces measurable morning improvement for many POTS patients within days.

- Compression garments reduce standing heart rate by mechanically counteracting venous pooling. Thigh-high or waist-level coverage (20–30 mmHg or higher) is significantly more effective than knee-high stockings alone. Put them on before standing, ideally while still lying in bed.
- Elevating the head of the bed by fifteen to twenty degrees using bed risers—not extra pillows—reduces overnight fluid loss through the kidneys, preserving the plasma volume that determines morning orthostatic tolerance.
- Physical counter maneuvers—leg crossing, muscle pumping (toe raises, thigh squeezes), and prompt sitting at the first sign of presyncope—provide real-time symptom management in public settings without any equipment.
- Resonance frequency breathing (five counts in, five counts out, fifteen to twenty minutes daily) improves baroreflex sensitivity and HRV within four to eight weeks of consistent practice, progressively improving the autonomic infrastructure of orthostatic compensation over months.
- Mast cell stabilization enables nervous system retraining. A nervous system continuously driven by histamine, CRH, and other mast cell mediators cannot effectively shift toward parasympathetic balance through breathwork alone. Reducing MCAS reactivity through the protocols in the earlier chapters creates the physiological space in which autonomic retraining produces its full benefit.
- The natural POTS strategy is a daily practice, not a one-time intervention. Consistency over weeks to months produces structural autonomic improvement; individual days of implementation produce acute symptom management. Both are real, valuable, and complementary.
- BPC-157 is an experimental peptide with encouraging animal research suggesting it may support tissue repair, vascular health, and inflammation, but in hEDS and POTS its benefits remain unproven, likely indirect, and highly variable—making it a potential adjunct at best, not a substitute for established therapies.

Coming Up in Chapter 23:

Exercise is one of the most powerful long-term interventions available for POTS—it increases plasma volume, improves vascular tone, rebuilds cardiac fitness, and progressively retrains the cardiovascular system's orthostatic response. But exercise is also a significant mast cell trigger and a reliable cause of post-exertional crashes in people with MCAS-POTS. Chapter 23 navigates this tension with the specific pacing strategies, recumbent exercise protocols, and gradual reconditioning approaches that make exercise genuinely therapeutic rather than destabilizing for this population.

CHAPTER 23

Exercise Without Crashing

Pacing, Recumbent Training, and Gradual Reconditioning for MCAS-POTS

The Exercise Trap

Every person with POTS has heard the advice . . . from cardiologists, from physiotherapists, from well-meaning friends who discovered a YouTube video: exercise. It will help. Studies show it works. You need to build your cardiovascular fitness.

They are not wrong. Exercise is one of the most powerful long-term interventions available for POTS. The studies really do show it works. But what the advice routinely fails to specify is how—and for someone navigating MCAS alongside POTS, the how matters enormously.

Maya tried running. Twice around the block, heart rate spiking to 170 beats per minute, and she spent the following two days in bed with a mast cell flare that left her worse than she had been before she laced up her shoes. She tried yoga. The heated studio was a disaster. She tried a gentle class at the gym and reacted to someone's cologne before she had finished warming up. She concluded that exercise made her worse, that her condition was incompatible with physical activity, and she stopped trying.

The conclusion was understandable and wrong. The problem was not exercise. The problem was applying exercise protocols designed for healthy people—or even for people with POTS without significant MCAS—to a system that could not handle upright exertion, thermal stress, sympathetic surge, or chemical triggers. The right approach exists. It is specific, it is graduated, and it begins where Maya's body actually was rather than where a general recommendation assumed it should be.

This chapter describes that approach in full.

✦ ✦ ✦

The Dual Nature of Exercise in MCAS-POTS

Exercise is genuinely therapeutic for POTS through mechanisms that are well-established. Regular aerobic conditioning increases plasma volume—one of the primary deficits of POTS—through adaptations in aldosterone regulation and red blood cell mass. It increases the strength of the heart's left ventricle, allowing more blood to be pumped per beat so that the compensatory heart rate increase upon standing can be smaller. It increases the tone and reflexivity of peripheral blood vessels, improving the vasoconstriction response to orthostatic stress. And it progressively retrains the autonomic nervous system toward greater flexibility and better baroreflex sensitivity—the same benefit achieved through HRV biofeedback but through cardiovascular conditioning rather than breathing practice alone.

Exercise is also, for individuals with MCAS-POTS, a reliable mast cell trigger through multiple mechanisms. The sympathetic nervous system surge that accompanies exertion activates mast cells through adrenergic receptors. Core body temperature rises during exercise, stimulating thermal mast cell activation. Physical exertion produces mechanical forces on mast-cell-dense tissues. And the post-exertional increase in prostaglandins and cytokines that is normal after any significant exercise represents a brief but real increase in systemic inflammatory mediator load. Any of these mechanisms alone might be manageable; together, in a sensitized system, they can produce post-exertional crashes that last hours to days.

> **The Resolution:** *The solution is not to avoid exercise—it is to find the intensity, duration, position, and environmental conditions under which the therapeutic benefits of movement exceed the mast cell activation costs. For most people with MCAS-POTS, this window exists. Finding it requires starting lower, progressing slower, and controlling the exercise environment more carefully than standard guidance assumes.*

✦ ✦ ✦

Pacing: Understanding Your Envelope

Pacing is not resting more. It is managing the total energy and physiological demand of each day within a range that the body can recover from overnight, preventing the accumulation of physiological debt that produces crashes. In MCAS-POTS, the crash is not just fatigue—it is a mast cell flare triggered by exceeding the system's tolerance threshold, which then takes hours to days to resolve rather than the overnight recovery that ordinary tiredness requires.

The concept of an energy envelope—the range of activity within which the body can function without triggering a post-exertional deterioration—is central to pacing. The goal is to consistently stay within the envelope, not to push against its edges in the hope that willpower will expand it. The envelope expands naturally and gradually as reconditioning proceeds. Pushing through the envelope's limits slows its expansion, because post-exertional crashes impair the cardiovascular adaptations that would otherwise build capacity.

Heart Rate as a Pacing Guide

Heart rate monitoring during activity is the most reliable objective tool for staying within the aerobic envelope in POTS. The standard guidance for post-exertional malaise prevention uses a heart rate ceiling during activity—typically calculated as 60 percent of maximum heart rate (220 minus age, multiplied by 0.6) or, in the Workwell Foundation approach for ME/CFS and POTS specifically, the anaerobic threshold heart rate minus fifteen beats per minute.

For most individuals with MCAS-POTS in the early stages of reconditioning, this ceiling is lower than feels intuitive—often in the 90 to 110 beats per minute range for adults in their thirties and forties. Activities that seem gentle by conventional standards may already exceed this ceiling. The discipline of staying at or below the ceiling, even when it means stopping a walk significantly shorter than intended, is what prevents the boom-bust cycle that characterizes so many failed exercise attempts in this population.

A practical tool: wear a continuous heart rate monitor during all activities and practice stopping any activity when heart rate approaches the ceiling—not after it has been exceeded for ten minutes. The ceiling is a prevention boundary, not a reaction boundary. Crossing it briefly may produce no immediate symptoms but can still trigger the delayed post-exertional response that appears six to twenty-four hours later.

HRV as a Daily Readiness Check

Morning heart rate variability provides a daily readiness indicator that tells you, before the day begins, whether your autonomic nervous system is recovered enough to tolerate planned exercise. A HRV reading at or above your personal baseline suggests adequate recovery; a reading significantly below baseline suggests the system is already under physiological stress and planned exercise intensity should be reduced or the session postponed. This is not a reason to avoid all movement on low-HRV days—gentle walking and basic mobility work are appropriate regardless—but it is a signal not to push toward the upper edge of your envelope when the system is already depleted.

✦ ✦ ✦

Recumbent Exercises: Starting Where the Body Can

The defining principle of POTS exercise protocols is that upright exercise is both the most beneficial long-term training stimulus and the most triggering short-term challenge. The standard solution, well-established in POTS research and clinical practice, is to begin cardiovascular training in a recumbent or semi-recumbent position—eliminating or dramatically reducing the orthostatic component of exercise while still providing the cardiovascular stimulus needed to begin building plasma volume and cardiac fitness.[442]

Recumbent exercise works because lying down eliminates gravitational blood pooling in the legs. The heart receives adequate venous return without compensatory tachycardia, the mast cell–activating sympathetic surge of orthostatic stress is removed, and the cardiovascular system can be challenged through work intensity rather than through the compounding physiological insult of upright posture. As fitness builds over months of consistent recumbent training, the cardiovascular adaptations—increased plasma volume, improved cardiac output per beat, better vascular tone—translate directly into improved orthostatic tolerance when the patient eventually transitions to upright exercise.

Phase One: Recumbent Foundations (Weeks 1–8)

Phase 1 Recumbent Protocol — Starting Weeks

Exercise with recumbent cycling or rowing, 5–10 minutes at very low resistance, heart rate target 60–70 percent maximum. Aim for three to four sessions per week on non-consecutive days.

Swimming or pool walking: If pool access is available, horizontal positions in water eliminate orthostatic challenge while providing cardiovascular stimulus. The natural compression of water also supports venous return.

Floor-based strengthening: Do supine or prone movements—glute bridges, supine marching, clam shells, prone hip extensions. This builds the lower-body and core strength that supports vascular pump function when eventually upright.

Duration ceiling: Do only 10–15 minutes of aerobic activity maximum per session in the first two weeks. Increase by no more than one to two minutes per week only if no post-exertional response has occurred.

Pre-session: Consume electrolytes, ensure compression garments are on, and check morning HRV. Post-session: Rest horizontally for 10–15 minutes to allow cardiovascular recovery before resuming upright activity.

Phase Two: Building Duration and Adding Semi-Upright (Weeks 8–20)

Once ten to fifteen minutes of recumbent cycling or rowing is consistently well-tolerated without post-exertional response over four consecutive weeks, the protocol can expand in two dimensions: longer sessions of recumbent activity (targeting twenty to thirty minutes by the end of Phase Two), and the introduction of semi-upright activities that begin to add a modest orthostatic component.

Phase 2 Additions—Months 2–5

Recumbent session duration: Progress toward 20–30 minutes at light-to-moderate intensity. Increase by two minutes per week only if the previous week produced no post-exertional response.

Semi-upright introduction: Stationary cycling on a traditional upright bike at low resistance and low heart rate can be introduced. Begin with 5 minutes and treat it as a new Phase 1—the orthostatic component makes it more physiologically demanding than recumbent cycling despite identical work output.

Gentle yoga or Pilates: Do floor-based and wall-supported poses; avoid prolonged standing sequences or inversions that produce rapid positional changes until Phase 3.

Walking: Begin with 5-minute flat walks at a comfortable conversational pace, immediately after completing a recumbent session (not as a standalone—the cardiovascular preparation of recumbent exercise first makes brief upright walking significantly better tolerated).

Phase Three: Gradual Reconditioning to Upright Exercise (Months 5+)

Phase Three begins when twenty to thirty minutes of semi-upright stationary cycling is consistently tolerated without post-exertional response over four consecutive weeks. The goal shifts to progressively replacing recumbent sessions with upright activities, increasing total exercise volume, and beginning the cardiovascular reconditioning that produces the greatest long-term POTS improvement.

The transition to upright exercise is not a clean handoff—it is a gradual substitution. Each week, one recumbent session is replaced by an upright session of equivalent duration, while the remaining sessions stay recumbent. Walking duration is extended by two to three minutes per week, guided by heart rate monitoring. Swimming transitions from horizontal pool walking to lap swimming as tolerance allows. The heart rate ceiling remains the governing boundary throughout. Phase Three is not about abandoning the pacing discipline, but about applying it to progressively more demanding activities.

> **The Twenty-Week Frame:** *Most people with MCAS-POTS who follow a conservative, well-paced reconditioning protocol reach meaningful upright exercise tolerance—consistent thirty-minute walks, light cycling classes, gentle aerobic activity—within five to eight months of starting Phase One. The temptation to accelerate this timeline is understandable but consistently counterproductive. Post-exertional crashes reset the reconditioning progress and can extend the total recovery timeline by weeks. Slow and steady genuinely wins this particular race.*

✦ ✦ ✦

Managing Mast Cell Reactions During Exercise

For people in whom mast cell activation during exercise is a significant issue, several specific strategies reduce the trigger burden while preserving the cardiovascular benefit.

- **Control the environment** – Exercise in a cool, unscented, low-humidity environment whenever possible. Home exercise equipment eliminates gym fragrance triggers and allows temperature control. If exercising outside, early morning when temperatures are lowest is usually better tolerated than midday or afternoon.
- **Pre-exercise mast cell support** – Taking quercetin thirty minutes before exercise reduces mast cell activation during the session for many individuals. Some practitioners also recommend a DAO enzyme supplement before exercise sessions to support histamine clearance during the exertion-related histamine release.
- **Hydrate before, during, and after** – Dehydration is a significant exercise trigger in POTS-MCAS. Beginning each session fully hydrated and maintaining electrolyte intake during sessions lasting more than twenty minutes reduces both cardiovascular and mast cell stress.
- **Cool down completely** – The cardiovascular system's return to resting state after exercise is itself a period of autonomic volatility and residual mast cell activation. A dedicated ten-minute cool-down period—gentle movement, then supine rest with legs elevated—reduces the post-exercise mast cell activation window significantly
- **Track exercise reactions systematically** – Note your resting heart rate and any symptoms in the twenty-four hours following each session. A consistent pattern of post-exercise reactions—even mild ones—signals that the current session intensity or duration exceeds your current tolerance ceiling. The appropriate response is stepping back one week in the protocol, not pushing through.

✦ ✦ ✦

Deeper Dive: The Evidence Behind Recumbent Reconditioning

For the Science-Minded Reader

The foundation for recumbent-first exercise protocols in POTS comes from two landmark studies from the Vanderbilt Autonomic Dysfunction Center. A 2010 study demonstrated that a structured three-month exercise program combining recumbent cycling, rowing, and swimming produced significant improvements in peak oxygen consumption (VO2 max), plasma volume, and left ventricular mass in people with POTS—cardiovascular adaptations that directly translate to improved orthostatic tolerance.[443] Crucially, the study noted that standard upright exercise was poorly tolerated by these patients and that the recumbent approach was essential to achieving compliance and preventing dropout.

A subsequent study replicated and extended these findings, demonstrating that the cardiovascular adaptations achieved through three to six months of recumbent reconditioning persisted at one-year follow-up in patients who maintained their exercise program.[444] Individuals who discontinued exercise relapsed toward their baseline within three to six months—confirming that exercise in POTS is an ongoing practice rather than a course of treatment with a defined endpoint.

For the MCAS dimension specifically, the evidence is primarily clinical observation rather than randomized controlled trials, but the mechanistic rationale is well-supported. Reducing the sympathetic surge, thermal stress, and orthostatic insult of upright exercise through recumbent training eliminates three of the primary exercise-triggered mast cell activation pathways simultaneously. The improvement in plasma volume through recumbent reconditioning directly reduces the histamine-driven vascular permeability that depletes volume—creating a virtuous cycle in which better conditioning reduces mast cell activity and reduced mast cell activity improves the physiological parameters that make conditioning possible.

◆ ◆ ◆

What This Means for You: Starting Where You Are

The most important first step in MCAS-POTS exercise is a realistic and honest assessment of where you currently are—not where you think you should be, not where you were before the illness, but where your body is right now.

If you are currently bedbound or severely deconditioned, Phase One of the recumbent protocol may need to begin with passive or very gentle active range-of-motion exercises while lying down—ankle circles, gentle hip flexion, arm raises—before any cardiovascular component is introduced. Even this modest movement begins the process of maintaining muscle mass, supporting joint health, and signaling to the cardiovascular system that demand is present. Duration begins at five minutes and increases by thirty seconds per week.

If you can tolerate ten to fifteen minutes of gentle movement without post-exertional response, you are ready for Phase One as described above. Begin with recumbent cycling or pool walking if accessible. Three sessions per week on non-consecutive days, capped at your current comfortable duration. Do not increase duration or intensity in the same week—choose one variable at a time.

If you are already doing some activity but consistently crashing afterward, the most likely cause is exceeding your aerobic threshold. Purchase or access a heart rate monitor before continuing, identify your personal ceiling (60 percent of maximum heart rate is a conservative starting estimate), and reduce current session intensity and duration until you are consistently below that ceiling. Yes, this will feel too easy. That is correct. That is the point.

If you are progressing well through reconditioning and feeling ready to advance, the four-consecutive-weeks rule is your governor. Four weeks at a given level without post-exertional response, verified by symptom tracking, is the signal to advance. One crash resets the count to zero. This is not punitive—it is the biologically appropriate signal that the system is not yet adapted to the current demand.

Maya, whose failed exercise attempts opened this chapter, eventually found her way to a knowledgeable physical therapist who understood POTS and MCAS. She began with eight minutes of gentle recumbent cycling three times a week, at a resistance so low it felt almost pointless. She hated the slowness of it. But she did not crash. And the following week she added two more minutes. And the week after that, two more. Seven months later she was cycling for twenty-five minutes, had added two short daily walks, and had not had a significant post-exertional crash in eleven weeks.

It's slow, but it works. That is the honest promise of this approach. Not fast. Not dramatic. But real progress, accumulated carefully over time, in a direction that holds.

✦ ✦ ✦

Chapter 23 at a Glance

What to Remember:

- Exercise is both essential and potentially triggering in MCAS-POTS; it produces cardiovascular adaptations that directly improve POTS physiology, but upright exertion, thermal stress, and sympathetic surge are reliable mast cell activators. The resolution is not avoidance but finding the right intensity, position, and environment.

- Pacing means staying within the energy envelope—the activity range the body can recover from overnight. Pushing beyond the envelope slows reconditioning by triggering post-exertional crashes that impair the cardiovascular adaptations you are trying to build.
- Heart rate ceiling (60 percent of maximum heart rate as a conservative starting estimate) is the primary pacing tool. Stopping activity when heart rate *approaches* the ceiling—not after it has been exceeded—prevents the delayed post-exertional response that appears six to twenty-four hours later.
- Morning HRV provides a daily readiness indicator: at or above personal baseline suggests the system is recovered and exercise is appropriate; significantly below baseline signals the system is under stress and intensity should be reduced.
- Phase One: Do five to fifteen minutes of recumbent cardiovascular exercise (cycling, rowing, pool walking) three to four times per week, plus floor-based strength work, for a minimum of eight weeks with consistent tolerance before advancing.
- Phase Two: Extend recumbent sessions to twenty to thirty minutes and introduce brief semi-upright activity (stationary cycling, short walks immediately after recumbent exercise) over months two through five, governed by the four-consecutive-weeks-without-crash advancement rule.
- Phase Three: Progressively substitute upright activity for recumbent sessions while maintaining heart rate monitoring and pacing discipline. Most of those with MCAS-POTS reach meaningful upright exercise tolerance within five to eight months of consistent Phase One entry.
- Pre-exercise quercetin, environmental control (cool and unscented), electrolyte hydration, a dedicated ten-minute cool-down, and systematic symptom tracking after each session reduce mast cell activation costs while preserving cardiovascular benefit.

Coming Up in the Next Section:

The last several chapters have provided the complete natural remedies toolkit for MCAS and POTS. The next section turns to the integrative work of building a personalized protocol: identifying your own dominant root causes through functional testing and pattern recognition, creating a step-by-step plan that sequences the right interventions in the right order for your specific biology, and navigating the inevitable challenges of setbacks, flares, and the moments when healing feels impossibly slow. Chapter 24 begins this work with the practical guide to root cause identification.

CHAPTER 24

Identifying Your Root Causes

Testing, Pattern Recognition, and Building Your Personal Map

The Map, Not the Territory

By this point in the book, you have a thorough understanding of the full landscape of MCAS root causes: gut dysfunction, chronic infections, environmental toxins, nervous system dysregulation, hormonal imbalance, and genetic predispositions. You have a complete toolkit of natural interventions. What you may not yet have is clarity about which of these causes are most active in your own body.

That clarity matters enormously. Applying the full protocol universally—treating every possible root cause with equal intensity regardless of whether it is actually present—is expensive, exhausting, and counterproductive. The person who pursues aggressive mold clearance when mold is not their driver, or who commits months to an antimicrobial SIBO protocol when their gut is not the primary problem, is wasting resources and tolerance capacity that could be directed where they would actually produce results.

Identifying your root causes is the work of this chapter. It is not a single test or a single conversation. It is a process of pattern recognition—observing your symptoms, your history, your response to interventions—combined with targeted testing that confirms or rules out specific drivers. The goal is a personal map: a clear picture of which root causes are most active in your case and in what order they deserve attention.

✦ ✦ ✦

Start With Your History: Pattern Recognition Before Testing

The most powerful diagnostic tool in MCAS root cause investigation is not a laboratory panel; it is a carefully observed personal history. Before ordering a single test, your symptom timeline and life history contain information that no lab can provide: When did symptoms begin, what preceded them, and what patterns connect specific exposures or circumstances to symptom flares?

Several historical patterns strongly point toward specific root causes and should be identified before determining testing priorities.

- **Onset after a clear infectious event** – Symptoms that began or dramatically worsened after a tick bite, a prolonged viral illness (particularly EBV mononucleosis), a severe gastroenteritis, or a COVID infection strongly implicate chronic infection or post-infectious immune dysregulation as a primary driver.
- **Symptoms that are location-dependent** – Feeling significantly better on vacation, away from work, or in a different home—and reliably worse upon returning—is the most important signal that environmental mold or chemical exposure is a significant driver. Many individuals report feeling this pattern for years without connecting it to their environment.
- **Menstrual cycle tracking of symptoms** – Reliable worsening in the premenstrual week and improvement at the start of menstruation implicates the estrogen-histamine axis described in Chapter 10 as a primary hormonal driver.
- **Gut symptoms preceding systemic reactivity** – A history of IBS, chronic bloating, or loose stools alongside or preceding the development of systemic MCAS symptoms suggests gut dysbiosis or SIBO as a significant contributing driver.
- **Family pattern of similar presentations** – Multiple family members with overlapping symptoms, particularly across generations, points toward genetic and epigenetic contributors including MTHFR variants, HαT, or the shared environmental and infectious exposures that cluster in family units.
- **Gradual worsening over years with no clear trigger** – Slow, incremental accumulation of reactivity over months to years without an identifiable precipitating event often indicates a progressive toxic burden or chronic low-grade dysbiosis that crossed a threshold rather than an acute precipitating event.

> **Before You Test:** *Write out your symptom timeline before your first testing appointment. When did symptoms begin? What was happening in your life in the six months before onset? Where were you living and working? What illnesses, injuries, or significant life events preceded the worst periods? This narrative is irreplaceable clinical information that guides everything that follows.*

✦ ✦ ✦

Testing Options: What to Test, When, and Why

Functional and conventional testing in MCAS root cause investigation serves two purposes: to confirm suspected drivers that the history already suggests, and to identify hidden drivers that the history alone cannot reveal. Testing should be targeted and sequential—beginning with the tests most likely to be positive based on your history, not ordered comprehensively all at once.

The reference table below covers the most clinically relevant tests for MCAS root cause investigation, organized to support targeted ordering rather than a blanket panel approach.

Test	Category	What It Reveals	Notes / Timing
Serum tryptase + mast cell mediator panel (histamine, PGD2, heparin)	MCAS confirmation	Baseline mast cell burden; elevated mediators support MCAS diagnosis	Draw baseline and ideally during or within 1–2 hrs of a reaction
24-hour urine histamine and methylhistamine	MCAS / histamine load	Total daily histamine production and clearance; more sensitive than serum tryptase alone	Collect during symptomatic period for highest sensitivity
Lactulose / glucose breath test	SIBO	Hydrogen-vs methane-dominant bacterial overgrowth in small intestine	Perform after 24-hr dietary prep; results guide antimicrobial protocol choice
Comprehensive stool analysis (GI-MAP or similar)	Gut microbiome / dysbiosis	Pathogen load, microbiome composition, DAO-relevant organisms, leaky gut markers	Guides probiotic strain selection and targeted antimicrobial choices
Urine mycotoxin panel (GPL-MycoTOX)	Mold / mycotoxin exposure	Identifies specific mycotoxins present; confirms mold illness as a driver	Collect first-morning urine; repeat after sauna or provocation if initial is low
Hair tissue mineral analysis (HTMA)	Heavy metals / mineral status	Long-term tissue mineral and toxic metal accumulation; identifies mercury, lead, cadmium	More accurate for chronic burden than serum levels; inexpensive screening tool
EBV reactivation panel (VCA IgG/IgM, EA IgG)	Viral reactivation	Distinguishes past exposure from active reactivation driving immune dysregulation	EBV EA IgG elevated = active reactivation; VCA IgM elevated = recent primary infection
HLA-DR typing	Mold susceptibility genetics	Identifies ~25% of population with impaired mycotoxin clearance capacity	Useful when mold exposure is suspected but symptom burden seems disproportionate

Test	Category	What It Reveals	Notes / Timing
Comprehensive thyroid panel (TSH, fT4, fT3, rT3, TPO Ab, Tg Ab)	Thyroid / autoimmunity	Full thyroid status including conversion efficiency and autoimmune component	TSH alone misses Hashimoto's and conversion problems; request full panel
Salivary cortisol x4 (diurnal curve)	HPA axis / adrenal function	Cortisol pattern across the day; identifies dysregulation, not just deficiency	Four-point collection (waking, noon, afternoon, evening) is more informative than single AM serum draw
MTHFR C677T / A1298C genotyping	Methylation genetics	Identifies impaired methylation capacity affecting histamine clearance and detoxification	Available through consumer genomics or clinical lab; guides B-vitamin protocol
DAO enzyme activity (plasma)	DAO genetic / functional	Functional DAO enzyme capacity; complements AOC1 genetic testing	Low DAO activity + dietary histamine = significant driver; guides DAO supplementation priority

How to Prioritize Testing

Not every test in this table is appropriate for every person, and the order matters. The following clinical reasoning guides sequencing:

- **Confirm MCAS first** – Before attributing a complex symptom picture to any specific root cause, confirming that mast cell dysfunction is present and active (serum tryptase, 24-hour urine histamine, and ideally a mediator panel drawn during a symptomatic period) establishes the diagnostic context for everything else.
- **Test the gut early** – Because gut dysfunction is both extremely common in MCAS and directly addressable, SIBO breath testing and comprehensive stool analysis should be among the first functional tests pursued—particularly in individuals with significant GI symptoms, bloating, or a history of IBS.
- **Test for mold when location-dependence is present** – Urine mycotoxin testing and HLA-DR typing are most informative when the history includes location-dependent symptoms or known water-damaged building exposure; ordering these without this history context produces lower-yield results.
- **Thyroid and hormonal testing are often missed** – Many people have been evaluated by specialists who tested TSH alone. A full thyroid panel including antibodies, full sex hormone assessment timed to the menstrual cycle, and a diurnal cortisol profile are often revealing in individuals whose symptoms include fatigue, menstrual cycle variation, or unexplained mood symptoms.

✦ ✦ ✦

Symptom Tracking and Pattern Recognition

Testing reveals what is present. Symptom tracking reveals what matters most to you day to day—and often identifies patterns that guide testing priorities more powerfully than any general checklist.

A useful MCAS symptom tracker captures four dimensions daily: overall reactivity on a one-to-ten scale, specific symptoms and severity, potential triggers or exposures, and any interventions used. Reviewing this data weekly rather than daily allows trend patterns to emerge that daily observation misses. The patterns most worth looking for include:

- **Cyclical timing** – Symptoms that worsen on a predictable schedule—weekly, monthly, or seasonally—suggest cyclical drivers. Monthly cycling implicates hormones; seasonal variation may implicate environmental allergens, light changes affecting the HPA axis, or recurring infections.
- **Environmental clustering** – Noting specific locations, times of day, or settings consistently associated with symptom worsening narrows the environmental exposure investigation considerably.
- **Food-reaction inconsistency** – If the same food triggers reactions sometimes but not others, this is strong evidence for the bucket theory at work—the food itself is not the primary driver, and identifying what else is filling the bucket on high-reaction days is more useful than eliminating the food entirely.
- **Response to interventions** – Systematic tracking of which interventions reliably improve your baseline versus which produce no discernible effect is itself root cause information. If quercetin alone produces significant improvement, mast cell stabilization is likely a high-leverage target. If it produces only modest improvement despite consistent use, a significant unchosen root cause is still active.

The Appendix contains a structured symptom tracker template designed specifically for MCAS pattern recognition. Using it consistently for four to six weeks before a practitioner appointment maximizes the clinical value of that consultation—you arrive with objective data rather than recollection.

✦ ✦ ✦

Deeper Dive: Functional vs. Conventional Testing

For the Science-Minded Reader

A consistent frustration among those with MCAS is that standard medical workups—comprehensive blood panels, normal reference ranges, specialist evaluations—

frequently return unremarkable results despite clearly abnormal physiology. Understanding the difference between conventional and functional laboratory reference standards helps explain this gap and guides effective use of testing.

Conventional laboratory medicine establishes reference ranges from large population samples, defining "normal" as the range in which the middle ninety-five percent of sampled individuals fall. This approach works well for detecting overt disease—severely elevated TSH, markedly low red blood cell count, clearly abnormal liver enzymes—but systematically misses functional impairment that falls within the bottom or top five percent of normal. A TSH of 3.8 mIU/L is within the conventional normal range; a person with Hashimoto's thyroiditis, symptoms of hypothyroidism, and high TPO antibodies whose TSH is 3.8 will be told their thyroid is normal. A cortisol of 8 mcg/dL at 8 a.m. is technically within range; a person whose HPA axis is depleted and whose morning cortisol should be three times higher will be told their adrenal function is normal.

Functional medicine laboratories use tighter reference ranges derived from research on optimal physiological function rather than population averages, and they assess patterns (such as the diurnal cortisol curve) rather than single-point measurements. For MCAS root cause investigation, this distinction matters because many of the drivers described in this book—subclinical thyroid dysfunction, mild cortisol dysregulation, borderline DAO activity—fall in the gap between clearly abnormal and clearly normal. Accessing this gap requires testing that is designed to find it.

Working with a practitioner who understands both conventional and functional laboratory interpretation—typically a functional medicine physician, naturopathic doctor, or integrative practitioner—provides the most complete picture. When this is not accessible, patient advocacy organizations and online communities familiar with MCAS often maintain practitioner referral resources that can help identify qualified clinicians in your region.

✦ ✦ ✦

What This Means for You: Building Your Root Cause Map

Step 1: Write your timeline before your next appointment. Document symptom onset, major life events in the preceding six to twelve months, location history, infection history, and any clear patterns you have already noticed. This narrative takes thirty minutes to write and saves hours of diagnostic time.

Step 2: Identify your top two or three likely drivers based on history. Using the pattern recognition signals in this chapter, identify which root cause categories your history most strongly implicates. These are your first testing priorities—not a comprehensive panel, but the targeted tests most likely to confirm or rule out your most probable drivers.

Step 3: Order tests with a practitioner who will interpret them functionally. Many of the tests in the reference table—mycotoxin panels, comprehensive stool analysis, diurnal cortisol curves—are not routinely ordered in conventional settings. A functional medicine or integrative practitioner is most likely to order them appropriately, interpret them in clinical context, and act on results that fall in the functional-but-not-pathological range.

Step 4: Use symptom tracking data to guide test interpretation. When test results return, compare them against the patterns you have observed in your symptom journal. A test that is mildly abnormal in a person with a strong clinical pattern matching that driver is more actionable than the same mildly abnormal result in a person with no corresponding symptom pattern. Clinical context always governs test interpretation.

Step 5: Build a prioritized driver list, not an exhaustive one. The goal is not to identify every possible contributing factor—it is to identify the two or three drivers most likely to produce significant improvement when addressed. Begin with those. As they are treated and reassessed, the next tier of drivers becomes clearer. Root cause investigation in MCAS is iterative, not definitive.

The map you build through this process is not a fixed document. It evolves as you learn more about your own biology, as interventions reveal new information through their responses, and as circumstances change. But having a map—even an incomplete one—is infinitely more useful than navigating without one. It is the difference between treating MCAS as a mysterious and capricious condition and approaching it as a solvable, if complex, biological puzzle.

That shift in relationship with your own illness—from bewilderment to informed strategy—is what this chapter is designed to support.

✦ ✦ ✦

Chapter 24 at a Glance

What to Remember:

- Identifying your personal root causes before designing your protocol prevents wasted effort on interventions targeting drivers that are not active in your case. A targeted, informed approach consistently outperforms the comprehensive-but-untargeted one.
- Personal history is the first and most powerful diagnostic tool: symptom onset timing, location-dependent patterns, menstrual cycle tracking, gut

symptom history, family patterns, and the nature of the precipitating event (if any) all point toward specific root cause categories before a single test is ordered.

- The most clinically useful first tests for most MCAS are mast cell mediator confirmation (24-hour urine histamine/methylhistamine), SIBO breath testing, and comprehensive stool analysis. Additional tests are selected based on history signals—mycotoxin testing when location-dependence is present, viral panels when infectious onset is clear, genetic testing when family patterns are strong.
- Functional laboratory medicine uses tighter, optimally-derived reference ranges that detect the subclinical dysfunction most relevant to MCAS—the gap between clearly pathological and fully optimal that conventional ranges systematically miss.
- Symptom tracking for four to six weeks before a practitioner consultation provides objective pattern data that is irreplaceable for root cause investigation. The Appendix contains a structured template.
- Root cause investigation is iterative: Identify the top two or three most likely drivers, test and address them, then reassess. The picture clarifies progressively through action and observation, not through exhaustive upfront testing.

Coming Up in Chapter 25:

With your root causes identified and prioritized, the next step is assembling them into a coherent, sequenced action plan. Chapter 25 translates the Stabilize–Support–Repair–Rebuild framework into a concrete personal protocol—showing how to order interventions by stage, avoid the most common sequencing mistakes, and build a sustainable plan that progresses without overwhelming a still-reactive system.

CHAPTER 25

Creating a Step-by-Step Plan

Stabilize → Support → Repair → Rebuild: Turning Knowledge Into a Livable Daily Practice

The Distance Between Knowing and Doing

Kamila had read everything she could find about MCAS. She had a notebook filled with research summaries, a browser folder organized by topic, and a working understanding of histamine receptors, mast cell mediators, and gut microbiome composition that would have impressed many clinicians. What she did not have—what all this knowledge had somehow not produced—was a clear sense of what to do on Monday morning.

The gap between knowing and doing is one of the most common and most frustrating experiences in complex chronic illness. The information exists. The interventions are described. But assembling them into a coherent, prioritized sequence that is manageable by a person who is still sick—still reactive, still fatigued, still carrying the cognitive load of the condition itself—is genuinely difficult work that knowledge alone cannot accomplish.

This chapter bridges that gap. It takes the four-stage framework introduced in Chapter 12 and makes it concrete: what to do first, what comes next, how long to expect each stage to take, and how to recognize when you are ready to advance. It also names the most common sequencing mistakes and shows you how to avoid them—because in MCAS, doing the right things in the wrong order is almost as unproductive as doing the wrong things entirely.

✦ ✦ ✦

The Four Stages in Practice

The Stabilize–Support–Repair–Rebuild framework introduced in Chapter 12 is the organizing architecture of your personal protocol. It answers the question that every MCAS patient eventually asks: I have all these things I need to do—where do I begin?

The framework answers it clearly: you begin at the beginning. Not at the most exciting intervention. Not at the one your practitioner mentions first. Not at the one that sounds most powerful or most directly targeted at your worst symptom. You begin with stabilization—and you stay there until the four markers of readiness described in Chapter 12 are met.

The table below summarizes all four stages with their timelines, primary focus, key interventions, and the signs that indicate readiness to advance. Use it as a planning reference alongside the individual chapter protocols.

Stage	Timeline	Primary Focus	Key Interventions	Signs Ready to Advance
1 — Stabilize	Weeks 1–12	Calm the reactive system; establish a healing baseline	Low-histamine diet; quercetin (start 125 mg); fragrance removal; sleep consistency; nervous system practices begin	Fewer reactions per week; reliable safe zone identified; sleep meaningfully improved; less brain fog on good days
2 — Support	Months 3–8	Repair foundations: gut barrier, nervous system, nutritional repletion, hormonal balance	Vitamin C + magnesium added; L-glutamine + zinc carnosine; targeted probiotics; HRV biofeedback practice; Phase 1 exercise begins	Gut symptoms stabilizing; dietary tolerance expanding slowly; HRV trending upward; tolerate 2–3 supplements without reaction
3 — Repair	Months 6–24+	Address identified root causes systematically	SIBO treatment; mold/mycotoxin clearance; heavy metal protocol; viral reactivation management; Phase 2–3 exercise; hormonal correction	System stable enough to tolerate die-off; bucket level consistently lower; can push boundaries occasionally without prolonged crash
4 — Rebuild	Month 12 onward	Expand tolerance; reintroduce; establish long-term sustainable life	Gradual food reintroduction; social and exercise expansion; reduce supplement burden; maintain gains without managing everything daily	Life is expanding, not contracting; reactions are exceptions rather than the rule; sustained progress over 3+ months

> **How to Use This Table:** *Find the stage that best describes where you are right now—not where you think you should be, but where your body actually is based on your current symptom burden and stability. That is your starting point. The table's readiness criteria, not elapsed time alone, determine when you advance.*

✦ ✦ ✦

What Each Stage Actually Looks Like Day to Day

Stage 1: Stabilize (Weeks 1–12)

Stage 1 is the stage that most motivated, knowledge-equipped individuals find hardest to respect. The temptation to do more is constant—you have identified your root causes, you know what needs addressing, and doing nothing but simplifying your diet and starting a single supplement feels inadequate.

It is not inadequate. It is precisely calibrated. During Stage 1, the mast cell system is in a state of high priming, and every new input—every new compound, every new protocol—is being processed by immune cells whose threshold is critically low. The goal is not passivity; it is targeted restraint. The interventions that are appropriate in Stage 1 are the ones that lower the activation level without introducing anything that could raise it.

A typical Stage 1 week looks like this: eating from a small rotation of known safe foods, prepared fresh at every meal. Taking one supplement—quercetin, starting at 125 mg—and nothing else new. Doing ten minutes of extended-exhale breathing each morning. Sleeping and waking at consistent times. Removing the most significant environmental chemical triggers from the immediate living space. Tracking symptoms daily. Nothing dramatic. Nothing expensive. Just the consistent, boring work of giving the system consistent low-trigger conditions and watching the bucket level drop.

Stage 2: Support (Months 3–8)

Stage 2 begins when Stage 1's four readiness markers are met: reactions are less frequent and less severe, a reliable safe zone has been identified, sleep has meaningfully improved, and cognitive function is returning on good days. The system has enough margin to receive new inputs without immediately reacting to them.

Stage 2 is when the foundational interventions are built out. The supplement protocol grows from one compound to several, introduced one at a time on the schedule from Chapter 16. Gut healing begins in earnest—L-glutamine and zinc carnosine added to the protocol after quercetin and vitamin C are established. Nervous system regulation practices deepen and become daily non-negotiables. Phase 1 recumbent exercise is introduced. Hormonal assessment and initial corrections happen here. Dietary variety begins cautiously expanding as the safe zone is tested and widened.

A Stage 2 month looks like steady, incremental building. One new thing per week at most. Everything tracked. Reactions used as information rather than catastrophe. The bucket is lower than it was in Stage 1, but it still fills. The difference is that it now has more room before it overflows, and it takes longer to refill after it has been managed down.

Stage 3: Repair (Months 6–24+)

Stage 3 is when the root cause treatments that were identified in Chapter 24 are pursued directly and systematically. SIBO treatment begins. If mycotoxins are confirmed, the remediation and binder protocol from Chapter 20 is implemented fully. Viral reactivation protocols are initiated. Heavy metal clearance begins. Hormonal corrections are made.

This is the longest and most variable stage because root cause complexity varies enormously between individuals. Someone with a single well-defined driver—hydrogen-dominant SIBO, confirmed by breath test, no mold, no heavy metals—may complete Stage 3 in four to six months. Someone with SIBO plus mold illness plus EBV reactivation plus hormonal dysregulation may spend two years in Stage 3, addressing each driver in order of clinical priority—usually mold illness first, followed by SIBO, then EBV, and last, hormones.

The critical discipline of Stage 3 is maintaining the Stage 1 and 2 foundations as a safety net throughout. Quercetin, dietary management, and nervous system practices are not abandoned because you are now doing more sophisticated work—they are the floor that makes it possible to do that work without constant destabilization.

Stage 4: Rebuild (Month 12 Onward)

Stage 4 begins before Stage 3 ends; dietary expansion and social reengagement start incrementally throughout the later stages of Stage 3 rather than waiting for a clean endpoint. The defining feature of Stage 4 is that the orientation shifts from managing illness to building life. Foods are reintroduced one at a time and observed carefully. Activities and social engagements that had been reduced are tested and gradually reclaimed. The supplement protocol is reviewed and reduced as systems recover—not because supplements are bad, but because a healing body needs fewer external supports over time.

Stage 4 is not a finish line. It is a different relationship with the body—one characterized by ongoing awareness and self-knowledge rather than the acute management of Stage 1. Most people who reach stable Stage 4 describe not a return to their pre-illness baseline but something more informed and more intentional—

a life built around what actually supports their wellbeing rather than one that simply ignores it.

✦ ✦ ✦

Avoiding the Most Common Sequencing Mistakes

MCAS management has a predictable set of errors that appear repeatedly across different people, different practitioners, and different resource levels. Knowing them before you encounter them makes them avoidable. The table below summarizes the six most consistently damaging mistakes and their solutions.

Common Mistake	Why It Happens	What to Do Instead
Jumping to Stage 3 root cause treatment before Stage 1 is established	Diagnosis is validating and triggers urgency to fix everything at once	Confirm your healing baseline (4 markers from Ch. 12) before introducing antimicrobials, binders, or chelation
Introducing multiple supplements simultaneously	Enthusiasm or fear drives loading up; it also mirrors how conventional medications are prescribed	One supplement at a time, 5–7 days of observation, then add the next. This is the only way to know what is helping
Abandoning an intervention after 2–3 weeks because it isn't working	The timescale expectations of MCAS recovery differ from acute illness; people expect faster results	Know the expected timeline before starting: gut healing 3–6 months, HRV improvement 4–8 weeks, microbiome shift 3–6 months
Increasing restriction rather than expanding tolerance	Each new reaction prompts eliminating another food or activity; over time, the world shrinks	Use reactions as bucket-filling data, not as permanent prohibitions. The goal is raising the threshold, not eliminating every trigger
Neglecting the nervous system dimension while pursuing physical interventions	The science of supplements and protocols is tangible; the science of breathwork feels soft or secondary	Nervous system regulation is a direct biological intervention—not optional. Allocate real daily time to it from Stage 1 onward
Pursuing aggressive detox or die-off without managing mast cell activation	Practitioners or protocols recommend aggressive antimicrobials/chelation without accounting for MCAS reactivity	Maintain full mast cell stabilization protocol throughout any die-off period; pace dose increases slowly; have an exit plan

One additional mistake deserves special mention because it is both common and deeply understandable: comparing your timeline to someone else's. Online MCAS communities are full of people who seem to have recovered faster, who are further along, whose protocols look different, whose practitioners are doing something you have not tried. The variation is real—different root cause profiles, different genetic vulnerabilities, different bodies at different starting points produce genuinely different timelines. Someone else's faster progress does not mean your slower progress is failure. It means you have different biology. Honor your biology rather than resenting it.

✦ ✦ ✦

Building Your Week: A Practical Structure

Translating the stage framework into a weekly routine makes it livable. The following structure is a template for Stage 2—the stage when the most daily elements are in motion simultaneously. Earlier and later stages require simpler versions of this structure.

- **Morning anchor (before rising)** – Drink an electrolyte drink if POTS is present, followed by five minutes of extended-exhale breathing; use compression garments if POTS-MCAS; take quercetin twenty minutes before breakfast.
- **Breakfast** – Consume fresh protein from the low-histamine protocol; take vitamin C with food; take magnesium glycinate in the evening—not morning—unless splitting the dose.
- **Midday** – This is the largest meal of the day with fat-containing foods that support absorption of omega-3s and vitamin D—DAO enzyme if the meal contains any higher-histamine foods; collect ten minutes of HRV biofeedback practice if not done in the morning.
- **Movement** – Do Phase 1 or 2 exercise on non-consecutive days three to four times per week; on non-exercise days, a short walk or gentle yoga is appropriate.
- **Evening** – Consume chamomile tea or similar calming herbal tea; take magnesium glycinate thirty to sixty minutes before bed; perform a body scan or orienting practice; develop a consistent sleep time.
- **Weekly review** – Take fifteen minutes reviewing your symptom journal: what was the trend this week compared to last? Any clear patterns? Any reactions to investigate? One item to adjust based on observation?

> **The 80 Percent Rule:** *Consistency at 80 percent is more therapeutic than perfection attempted and abandoned. Missing a morning supplement, skipping a breathwork session, eating something off-protocol once—these are ordinary human events, not failures. What matters is the overall trend of consistent practice, not unblemished compliance. Perfectionism in MCAS management tends to produce anxiety that fills the bucket faster than the missed intervention emptied it.*

✦ ✦ ✦

Deeper Dive: Why Sequencing Is Not Just Preference

For the Science-Minded Reader

The sequencing principle in MCAS—stabilize before repair—is not a clinical preference or a conservative caution. It is a biological necessity grounded in three specific mechanisms that Chapter 12 introduced and that are worth reviewing here with the full context of the book behind them.

First, the priming state of mast cells determines their response to new inputs. A mast cell population operating at sixty percent of its activation threshold responds to novel compounds—herbal antimicrobials, new probiotics, mobilized toxin metabolites—as potential threats because their pattern recognition receptors are sensitized and their degranulation threshold is low. The same compound introduced to mast cells operating at twenty percent of threshold is processed as a neutral or beneficial input rather than as an attack signal. Stabilization is the biological work of moving from sixty percent to twenty percent—and that work cannot be shortcut.

Second, gut barrier integrity determines how treatments are absorbed. When intestinal permeability is high—as it characteristically is in active MCAS—supplement proteins and herbal compounds enter the subepithelial immune environment in partially digested forms that directly activate gut mast cells. The partial gut barrier healing of Stage 2 genuinely changes how the same supplement is absorbed in Stage 3. This is the mechanistic explanation for the clinical observation that compounds tolerated poorly in the reactive phase become well tolerated after months of foundational work.

Third, the autonomic nervous system context determines treatment response. A chronically sympathetically dominant nervous system amplifies adverse reactions to interventions that produce temporary discomfort—die-off, detox symptoms, exercise-induced fatigue—because these discomforts are processed in a context of heightened threat sensitivity. The vagal tone built through the nervous system practices of Stage 1 and 2 measurably shifts the autonomic context in which Stage 3 treatments are received, reducing the probability of reactions and improving the system's capacity to tolerate and integrate therapeutic challenge. Skipping the autonomic preparation does not just miss a nice-to-have; it removes the biological conditions under which root cause treatment is most effective.

✦ ✦ ✦

What This Means for You: Building Your Personal Protocol

The most useful final action in this chapter is building your own version of the stage table—a personalized protocol document that reflects your specific root causes, your current stage, and the next three concrete steps you will take.

Identify your current stage honestly. Using the readiness criteria from Chapter 12 and the stage descriptions in this chapter, locate yourself in the framework. If you are unsure, default to Stage 1. The cost of starting more conservatively than necessary is a few weeks of slower progress. The cost of starting at a more advanced stage than you are ready for is potentially months of setback.

Name your next three actions, not your full plan. Trying to design a comprehensive twelve-month protocol on day one is both premature (you do not yet know how your system will respond to early interventions) and overwhelming. Name your next three concrete actions in sequence. For most people in Stage 1, these are dietary simplification plus quercetin introduction plus one nervous system practice. That is the whole plan for week one. Week two follows from how week one went.

Set realistic reassessment points. Build in regular review moments rather than evaluating progress day to day. A four-week check-in asks: Is overall reactivity lower than it was four weeks ago? A twelve-week check-in asks: Have the Stage 1 readiness markers been met? A six-month check-in asks: Is Stage 2 established well enough to begin targeted root cause work? These are the timeframe questions. Daily symptom tracking answers the trend question. Both are needed; neither replaces the other.

Hold the plan lightly and the direction firmly. The specific interventions in your protocol will change as you learn more about your own biology, as root cause testing returns results, and as your system's response guides adjustments. The direction—stabilize, support, repair, rebuild, in that order—does not change. The specific path through those stages belongs to you and your body. Navigate it with both structure and flexibility.

Kamila printed the stage table and put it on her refrigerator. She drew a small circle around Stage 1 and wrote the date. She made a short list: low-histamine meals, quercetin at 125 mg, morning breathing, fragrance-free dish soap. That was Monday's plan. Not the whole protocol. Not the root cause treatments she already knew she needed. Just Monday.

Three months later the circle was around Stage 2. Six months after that she was in early Stage 3, working through a SIBO protocol with her functional medicine practitioner, tolerated in a way her system could not have managed a year earlier. The knowledge had not changed. The sequence had.

✦ ✦ ✦

Chapter 25 at a Glance

What to Remember:

- The Stabilize–Support–Repair–Rebuild framework is the architecture of your personal protocol. Every intervention belongs to a stage, and its effectiveness depends on the stage's foundations being in place before it is introduced.
- Stage 1 (weeks 1–12) focuses exclusively on calming the reactive system: low-histamine diet, single supplement introduction starting with quercetin, environmental simplification, sleep consistency, and daily nervous system practice. Advance when the four readiness markers are met—not by elapsed time alone.
- Stage 2 (months 3–8) builds foundational support: expanding the supplement protocol one compound at a time, beginning gut healing with L-glutamine and zinc carnosine, deepening nervous system practices, introducing Phase 1 recumbent exercise, and beginning hormonal assessment.
- Stage 3 (months 6–24+) addresses identified root causes directly: SIBO, mold, viral reactivation, heavy metals, hormonal correction—in order of clinical priority, with mast cell stabilization maintained as a safety net throughout. Advance to Stage 4 when root causes are either resolved or stable, flares are predictable/manageable, and baseline function is significantly improved.
- Stage 4 expands tolerance, reduces management burden, and rebuilds life—characterized by progressive reintroduction and a shift from acute management to long-term sustainable practice.
- The six most common sequencing mistakes: jumping to Stage 3 too early, introducing multiple supplements simultaneously, abandoning interventions before their timeline has elapsed, increasing restriction rather than raising the threshold, neglecting nervous system work, and pursuing aggressive die-off without mast cell stabilization.
- Consistency at 80 percent outperforms perfectionism. Missing individual practices does not undo progress. The trend over weeks and months is what matters, not daily compliance scores.
- Your protocol is a living document—the stage framework and sequencing logic are fixed, but the specific interventions within each stage belong to you and evolve as your biology reveals itself through response to treatment.

Coming Up in Chapter 26:

Even the best-designed protocol meets setbacks. Flares arrive without warning. Progress plateaus at unexpected points. The gap between the recovery trajectory you planned and the one your body is navigating can be demoralizing in ways that the science doesn't prepare you for. Chapter 26 addresses the emotional and practical reality of healing when it feels impossible—covering setbacks, flares, emotional resilience, and what it means to redefine progress in a way that honors the real complexity of this journey.

CHAPTER 26

When Healing Feels Impossible

Setbacks, Flares, Emotional Resilience, and Redefining Progress

The Month Everything Went Backwards

She had been doing so well. For three months, the trajectory had been unmistakably upward: fewer reactions, better sleep, a slowly expanding list of foods she could eat without consequence. She had started to believe—carefully, tentatively—that she was actually getting better.

Then her sister's wedding. Five days away from home, different food, different water, a hotel room that smelled of synthetic fragrance she could not escape. The flight back was brutal. The week that followed was her worst in six months.

Sitting in the rubble of that week, she did what many people with MCAS do: She concluded that she had not really been making progress at all. That the improvement had been an illusion. That she was back to square one. That this would never actually get better.

None of those conclusions were true. But they felt absolutely true, with the particular vividness that exhaustion and flares lend to catastrophic thinking. And without a framework for understanding what had actually happened—a short-term bucket overflow in an already-reactive system, not the unraveling of her recovery—she made several decisions in that distressed state that genuinely did slow her progress: stopping her supplements, abandoning her dietary protocol in a kind of defeated resignation, and avoiding her practitioner because she did not have the energy to explain how badly things had gone.

This chapter is for that week. For the setback that feels like failure. For the flare that seems to erase months of work. For the moment when everything the previous chapters describe feels not like a map but like a taunt.

✦ ✦ ✦

Understanding Setbacks and Flares

A setback is not the absence of progress. It is a feature of nonlinear recovery—and MCAS recovery is profoundly nonlinear. The trajectory of healing in this condition is not a clean upward line. It is a general upward trend containing individual dips, plateaus, reversals, and occasional dramatic crashes that look, in the moment, like total regression.

Understanding why this happens biologically reduces the catastrophic interpretation that wasted weeks of progress in the opening story. The mast cell system does not respond to triggers in a simple linear fashion. It operates with what researchers call stimulus history dependence: recent and cumulative activation events raise the baseline priming state, making the system more reactive for a period after a significant trigger exposure. Think of it like your skin after a sunburn—temporarily more reactive, even to things that normally wouldn't bother you. The wedding travel did not undo three months of healing. It temporarily raised the activation baseline through a concentrated series of unavoidable triggers—travel disruption, sleep loss, novel food environment, fragrance exposure, emotional stress—and the system's setback response was a biologically coherent reaction to an unusual load, not evidence that the foundation had dissolved.

Within two to three weeks of returning to baseline conditions, most individuals with MCAS recover their pre-setback baseline and frequently resume their prior trajectory. This is why the most important thing to do during a setback is the least emotionally satisfying: return to Stage 1 management, reduce the trigger load to the most conservative safe zone, and wait. Not giving up. Not escalating to dramatic new interventions. Just waiting, with the same disciplined consistency that built the progress in the first place.

> **The Setback Protocol:** *Return to your Stage 1 safe zone—the foods, environment, and practices that were reliable at your most stable point. Do not add anything new during a flare. Do not remove supplements that were working. Do not make protocol decisions from inside a crash. Reduce, return to basics, and reassess when the acute flare has passed.*

✦ ✦ ✦

Emotional Resilience: The Part the Science Doesn't Prepare You For

The emotional experience of chronic illness is not a side effect of MCAS. It is a dimension of it—one driven partly by the neurobiological effects of mast cell mediators on mood and cognition, and partly by the genuine psychological burden of living with an unpredictable, poorly understood condition that has cost years of ordinary life.

Brain fog, anxiety, and depression in MCAS are not purely psychological responses to difficult circumstances. As established in Chapter 9, histamine and other mast cell mediators directly disrupt neurotransmitter balance and drive neuroinflammation that impairs cognitive function and emotional regulation. During a flare, the worsening of cognitive and emotional symptoms is physiological. This matters for how those symptoms are interpreted: a thought that occurs during peak mast cell activation is not a reliable assessment of reality. The hopelessness that feels absolute at the worst moments of a crash is, in part, a symptom of the crash itself—not an objective evaluation of your prognosis.

What Actually Helps

Emotional resilience in MCAS is not about maintaining relentless positivity. It is about developing a relationship with the illness that can hold both its genuine difficulty and the genuine evidence of capacity for improvement, without either denial or catastrophe. Several specific practices support this kind of resilience.

Keep your data visible. When the current moment feels like evidence of total failure, reviewing your symptom journal from three or six months ago provides an objective baseline comparison that is more accurate than what the current flare state feels like. Most people who do this find that even their worst recent weeks are measurably better than their average state months earlier—a fact that is impossible to feel but possible to see.

Name what a setback is, not what it means. "I am having a flare triggered by travel" is a factual description. "I will never get better" is an interpretation that goes well beyond the evidence. Practicing the distinction between description and interpretation—particularly in difficult moments—is a cognitive skill that improves with practice and significantly reduces the emotional amplification of setbacks.

Maintain one or two anchors no matter what. Identify one or two practices that you will continue even in the worst flares—not the full protocol, but the smallest sustainable version. For many people this is the morning breathing practice and one confirmed safe meal per day. Maintaining any anchor during a crash preserves continuity and prevents the total abandonment of the protocol that most reliably extends recovery time.

Connect with others who understand. Isolation is one of the most consistent companions of MCAS—friends and family who have not experienced it find it difficult to fully understand, and the invisibility of the condition compounds the loneliness. Patient-led communities—Mast Cell Action, The Mastocytosis Society, Dysautonomia International, and various online forums—provide spaces where the specific experiences of MCAS and POTS are understood without explanation. These communities are not substitutes for professional support but are genuine sources of normalization, practical knowledge, and the particular comfort of being known.

✦ ✦ ✦

What the Evidence Shows

Clinical data and practitioner observations consistently demonstrate that individuals who systematically address MCAS—through the layered approach described in this book—experience meaningful improvement: fewer reactions, expanded dietary tolerance, improved sleep, better cognitive clarity, and increased quality of life. Not every person recovers identically, and timelines vary considerably. But the trajectory of this condition, when engaged with sustained, informed effort, trends toward improvement in the great majority of people who commit to the work. The section that follows asks you to reframe how you measure that improvement—not to lower your expectations, but to see the progress that is already happening.

Redefining Progress

The most destabilizing thing about MCAS recovery for most people is not the setbacks themselves—it is measuring progress against the wrong benchmark.

If progress is defined as "no longer having any reactions," most people in the early and middle stages of recovery will feel like failures most of the time—because this benchmark is too far away to function as a useful measure of where you are now. If progress is defined as "fewer reactions per week than three months ago" or "reactions that resolve in hours rather than days" or "a list of trustworthy foods that is longer than it was in January," then real progress becomes visible even during imperfect periods, because these are metrics that actually change on the timescale of MCAS recovery.

> **A More Useful Measure:** *Progress in MCAS is not the absence of reactions. It is the direction of the trend—reactions becoming less frequent, less severe, or shorter-lived over months. A single terrible week inside a months-long improvement trend is not evidence that progress has stopped. It is evidence of a bad week inside a trend that continues.*

Redefining progress also means expanding the definition of what recovery actually looks like. For many people with MCAS who have read extensively about the condition, the implicit goal is a return to the pre-illness baseline—the life they had before MCAS became a defining feature of their days. This is a reasonable aspiration, and for some it is fully achievable. But for others, the recovery that is available is something different: not a return to an earlier state, but the construction of a more informed, more sustainably managed version of life that is genuinely better in some dimensions than what preceded the illness. The awareness of what the body needs, the practices that support nervous system regulation and gut health, the intentionality around diet and environment—these are not burdens that recovery will someday allow you to put down. They are the building materials of a different kind of health.

That reframe is not resignation. It is accuracy about what sustained MCAS recovery typically produces—and accuracy about what most people who have lived through this describe, once they are far enough along the trajectory to look back with perspective—not a life from which MCAS has been erased, but a life in which MCAS taught them things about their body they could not have learned any other way, and in which they live better for knowing them.

✦ ✦ ✦

What This Means for You: Navigating the Hard Weeks

When you are in a flare: Do not make protocol decisions. Return to your Stage 1 safe zone. Reduce, do not change. Wait until the acute flare has passed before evaluating whether anything needs to be adjusted. The decisions made from inside a crash are almost universally less accurate than the ones made from a calmer state.

When you feel like you are back to zero: Open your symptom journal. Find an entry from three months ago. Compare the numbers. The feeling of being back to zero is almost never confirmed by the data—and the data is the more reliable account.

When the protocol feels impossible to maintain: Return to the 80 percent principle from Chapter 25. Identify the one or two anchors you can maintain regardless of how bad things are, and let the rest of the protocol rest temporarily. Partial maintenance is dramatically better than total abandonment, both for the physiology and for the continuity that makes restarting easier.

When the emotional weight becomes genuinely overwhelming: Professional support is appropriate and important. A therapist familiar with chronic illness, a trauma-informed practitioner, or a support group can provide the kind of sustained emotional container that friends and family, however willing, often cannot. Seeking that support is not weakness. It is accurate assessment of a genuine need.

She eventually understood what had happened during the wedding week—not as a catastrophe, but as a concentrated bucket overflow with a known cause and a predictable recovery. She returned to her safe zone. She waited. She resumed the protocol that had been working. Four weeks after the worst of the flare, she was back where she had been before the trip.

And this time, when things started improving again, she noticed something different in herself. She did not hold the improvement quite as tightly. She was less afraid of the next setback—not because she thought it would not come, but because she knew, now, that it would not erase what she had built. The trajectory was real. The setback had been real. Both could be true, and she could keep going regardless.

✦ ✦ ✦

Chapter 26 at a Glance

What to Remember:

- Setbacks are a feature of nonlinear recovery, not evidence that progress was illusory. MCAS recovery follows a general upward trend with individual dips, and most acute flares resolve within two to four weeks of returning to baseline management conditions.
- The setback protocol is to return to the Stage 1 safe zone, reduce the trigger load to the most conservative reliable baseline, and not make protocol changes from inside the crash. Reduction, not addition or abandonment.
- Cognitive and emotional symptoms worsen during flares as a direct physiological consequence of mast cell mediator effects on the brain. Hopelessness felt during a crash is partly a symptom of the crash—not a reliable assessment of prognosis.
- Progress is best measured by trend over months, not by the presence or absence of reactions in any given week. Reviewing symptom journal data from three to six months prior provides the objective perspective that flare-state cognition cannot.
- Maintaining one or two anchors during the worst periods—a morning breathing practice, one reliable safe meal—preserves continuity and prevents the full protocol abandonment that most reliably extends recovery time.
- Progress in MCAS does not always look like a return to the pre-illness baseline. For many, it looks like a more informed, more intentionally managed life that is better in measurable ways—not despite the illness, but partly because of what navigating it required learning.

Coming Up in Chapter 27:

The final chapter of this book turns toward the future—both the future of MCAS research and the future of the individuals reading this. Chapter 27 surveys the emerging science, the personalized medicine approaches on the horizon, and closes with the honest hope that this condition's story is genuinely changing: better understood, better recognized, better treated, and no longer the invisible storm it has been for so many for so long.

CHAPTER 27

The Future of MCAS Research

Emerging Theories, Personalized Medicine, and the Expanding Arc of Understanding

The Field Is Moving

Ten years ago, most physicians had never heard the term MCAS. The concept of non-clonal mast cell activation as a diagnosable clinical entity had only recently entered the peer-reviewed literature. The consensus diagnostic criteria were freshly published and already contested. Individuals who described multi-system, mediator-driven reactivity without elevated tryptase were routinely told there was nothing wrong with them, or that what was wrong was beyond conventional medicine's ability to name.

The landscape today is substantially different—and it is changing faster than at any previous point in this field's short history. MCAS is now a recognized entity in major allergy and immunology textbooks. Long COVID research has introduced the mast cell activation hypothesis to the mainstream of academic medicine, generating a wave of funding and research attention that would have been unimaginable five years ago. Patient advocacy organizations have grown rapidly, producing practitioner education resources, clinical guidelines, and referral networks that increasingly connect people with knowledgeable care. The diagnostic gap is narrowing. The therapeutic toolkit is expanding.

This chapter surveys what is coming—the emerging research directions that are most likely to reshape MCAS understanding and treatment in the years ahead, the personalized medicine approaches that will allow more precise targeting of the specific biological disruptions in each individual, and the grounds for genuine, evidence-grounded hope about where this field is heading.

✦ ✦ ✦

Emerging Theories: Where the Science Is Heading

Somatic Mutation Research and Precision Diagnosis

One of the most scientifically significant developments in MCAS research is the systematic application of next-generation genomic sequencing to mast cell populations. Dr. Lawrence Afrin and colleagues have championed the hypothesis that non-clonal MCAS is driven by acquired somatic mutations in a subset of mast cells—mutations that are too dispersed across the mast cell population and too varied in their location to be detected by standard testing, but that fundamentally alter mast cell behavior. The technology to detect these mutations at scale now exists; what is needed is the clinical research infrastructure to apply it systematically to MCAS populations and develop the biomarker signatures that would allow practitioners to identify specific mutation patterns and eventually target them with precision therapies.

Clinical trials applying comprehensive somatic mutation profiling to MCAS cohorts are a near-term research priority that could transform diagnosis within the next decade—moving from the current "symptoms plus mediator elevation plus exclusion" criteria to a molecular signature approach that identifies specific mast cell dysregulation patterns with far greater precision. This would allow not only more accurate diagnosis but the stratification of MCAS into biological subtypes that predict treatment response, much as cancer oncology has moved from anatomical staging to molecular subtyping.

The Post-Infectious MCAS Model and Long COVID

The COVID-19 pandemic produced an unintended natural experiment in mast cell biology at a scale no research trial could have generated: tens of millions of people developing post-infectious multi-system illness with a characteristic mast cell activation pattern, studied by researchers across dozens of countries with funding and urgency that infectious disease and immunology rarely attract. The resulting body of research has provided compelling evidence for the post-infectious mast cell activation model that MCAS researchers have been advancing for years—viral spike protein–mast cell interactions, mast cell mediator elevation in long COVID biopsies, the clinical overlap between long COVID and established MCAS diagnostic criteria, and the response of long COVID symptoms to mast cell–targeted interventions.[445]

This research has two significant implications for the broader MCAS field. First, it is generating mainstream academic medicine engagement with mast cell biology that is spilling over into non-COVID MCAS research, bringing resources, researchers, and credibility to a field that has historically operated at the fringe of mainstream immunology. Second, it is illuminating the post-infectious trigger mechanism in granular mechanistic detail—identifying the specific viral-mast cell receptor interactions, the persistence patterns of viral reservoirs that maintain ongoing mast cell activation, and the immune dysregulation pathways that perpetuate the condition beyond the acute infection period.[446] This mechanistic understanding will directly inform how post-infectious MCAS is identified and treated, regardless of the triggering pathogen.

The MCAS–Connective Tissue–Dysautonomia Triad: A Unified Biology

The clinical recognition that MCAS, hEDS, and POTS cluster together—established in Chapter 4—is increasingly supported by mechanistic research that points toward a unified biological explanation. Research groups in the United States, United Kingdom, and continental Europe are actively investigating the hypothesis that these three conditions share a common underlying disruption in the regulatory machinery of mast cells, connective tissue cells, and autonomic neurons—with somatic mutations, epigenetic dysregulation, and impaired cellular repair mechanisms as the upstream drivers.

If this hypothesis is confirmed through the systematic genomic and epigenomic studies currently underway, it would resolve one of the most persistent puzzles in MCAS—why these conditions co-occur so reliably and why decades of germline genetic research have failed to identify causative genes for hEDS. It would also open therapeutic pathways that address the shared upstream biology rather than each condition separately, potentially producing more complete and more durable improvement than the current condition-by-condition management approach allows.

Personalized Medicine: From Population Protocols to Individual Biology

The most transformative development in MCAS care on the horizon is the move toward genuinely personalized treatment—therapeutic decisions based on each person's specific biological profile rather than generic protocols applied to a diagnostic category. Several pillars of this personalized approach are already in development.

Metabolomic profiling—measuring the complete pattern of small metabolites in blood, urine, or tissue samples—can identify specific patterns of inflammatory mediator excess, detoxification impairment, microbiome metabolite disruption, and oxidative stress that are characteristic of individual MCAS presentations. Pairing metabolomic data with somatic mutation profiles and comprehensive microbiome sequencing will eventually allow practitioners to identify not just that a person has MCAS but which specific mediator pathways are most active, which root causes are driving those pathways, and which targeted interventions are most likely to produce benefit for that specific biological configuration.

At the therapeutic level, this means moving toward mast cell–targeted biologics—monoclonal antibodies and small molecule inhibitors directed at the specific receptor pathways most active in each individual's mast cell population. Omalizumab (anti-IgE), already used off-label for refractory MCAS (cases where people do not respond adequately to standard treatments aimed at managing the condition), represents the first generation of this approach. Ongoing research is characterizing the MRGPRX2, c-Kit, and cytokine receptor pathways as additional therapeutic targets with clinical trials in early stages. The combination of diagnostic precision (knowing exactly which pathways are dysregulated) and therapeutic precision (targeting those exact pathways) represents a fundamentally different and far more effective model of MCAS care than is currently available.

> **An Honest Note on Timelines:** *The developments described in this section are real and underway, but their translation from research finding to standard clinical practice takes years to decades. The most important implication of this emerging science for patients reading today is that the field is moving—genuinely, substantively, in the right direction. The tools available in five years will be meaningfully better than those available today. The treatments available in ten years may be transformative. This is not wishful thinking; it is a reasonable projection from the current trajectory of research activity.*

✦ ✦ ✦

Chapter 27 at a Glance

What to Remember:

- MCAS has moved from an obscure, contested concept at the fringes of immunology to a recognized, actively researched clinical entity within a single decade. The pace of change is accelerating, not slowing.
- Long COVID research has brought mainstream academic medicine, substantial funding, and global research attention to mast cell biology—generating mechanistic insights about post-infectious MCAS that will benefit the broader MCAS population far beyond COVID-related presentations.
- Somatic mutation research is the most likely path toward precision MCAS diagnosis—moving from symptom-and-exclusion criteria to molecular signatures that identify specific mast cell dysregulation patterns and predict treatment response.
- The MCAS–hEDS–POTS triad is increasingly understood as a unified biological disruption rather than three coincidentally co-occurring

conditions. Research into shared upstream mechanisms is an active priority that may yield more fundamental and durable treatments than the current condition-by-condition approach.

- Personalized medicine approaches—metabolomic profiling, comprehensive microbiome analysis, and targeted biologic therapies directed at specific receptor pathways—represent the next generation of MCAS care. The first generation (omalizumab for refractory cases) is already in clinical use; the next generations are in development.
- The tools available for MCAS diagnosis and treatment will be meaningfully better in five years and potentially transformative in ten. This is not optimism as a coping strategy—it is a reasonable projection from the current research trajectory.

✦ ✦ ✦

A Closing Word: For the Practitioners Who Care for These Patients

If you have read this book as a clinician—a physician, nurse practitioner, physician's assistant, functional medicine practitioner, physical therapist, or any of the many practitioners whose patients with MCAS have found their way to you—you already know something that this book's opening chapters describe: These patients are complex, frequently misunderstood, and extraordinarily grateful when they are seen clearly.

The clinical complexity of MCAS is real. The multi-system presentation, the variable biomarkers, the individual variability in triggers and treatment response, and the significant overlap with other conditions make it genuinely challenging to assess and manage within the constraints of conventional medical practice. The patients who reach you have often been through a long and discouraging diagnostic journey, and they arrive with a combination of exhausted hope and hard-won self-knowledge that, when met with clinical curiosity rather than skepticism, produces some of the most meaningful therapeutic partnerships in medicine.

> **For Practitioners:** *The most important clinical shift in MCAS management is moving from single-system specialist thinking to systems-level integration. These patients are not primarily dermatology patients, or gastroenterology patients, or cardiology patients. They are patients whose biology is disrupted at a level that crosses all specialty boundaries simultaneously. The practitioner who is willing to hold the whole picture—and to work collaboratively with colleagues across specialties—provides care that is qualitatively different from the best specialist care delivered in isolation.*

The natural approaches in this book are not alternatives to conventional medicine—they are complements to it. The foundational interventions that produce the most substantial and durable improvement in most people with MCAS do not come from pharmaceutical management of acute symptoms alone. They come from the careful, sustained work of reducing trigger load, healing the gut, supporting the nervous system, addressing root causes, and building the biological resilience that raises the mast cell threshold durably over time. Pharmaceutical tools have a place for managing acute reactions and providing the stability needed to do this foundational work—and the foundational work makes the pharmaceutical management more effective and often allows it to be reduced over time.

The growing body of research on MCAS—accelerated substantially by the long COVID literature—is providing the scientific foundation for this integrative approach that was previously available mainly through clinical observation. The mechanisms are increasingly characterized. The biomarker tools are improving. The therapeutic targets are being identified. The field is producing the evidence base that allows confident, evidence-informed, individualized care rather than empirical management guided primarily by case reports.

Your patients with MCAS need you to stay curious. They need you to be willing to order the functional tests that reveal what standard panels miss, to interpret results in clinical context rather than by reference range alone, to take their symptom-tracking data seriously as clinical evidence, and to accept that the pace of their recovery is governed by biology and not by willpower or compliance. They need you to hold hope for them on the days when they cannot hold it for themselves—and to hold accuracy alongside that hope, which means neither overpromising nor dismissing.

The patients who recover most substantially from MCAS do so because of a combination of factors: effective natural and medical interventions, skilled clinical guidance, their own disciplined effort, and a therapeutic relationship characterized by genuine partnership. You are the clinical cornerstone of that partnership. The work you do—seeing clearly, guiding skillfully, staying curious—changes lives in ways that deserve acknowledgment far beyond what this condition's current level of recognition allows.

The field is moving. The science is improving. The patients are getting better. You are a meaningful part of why.

✦ ✦ ✦

A Closing Word: To the Person Who Has Been Living This

You came to this book—perhaps—the way many people come to it: exhausted, frustrated, and carrying a diagnosis that finally named something you had been living with for years without a name. Or perhaps still without a firm diagnosis, but with enough recognition in these pages to believe that the unnamed thing has been found.

Either way, you have been navigating something genuinely difficult. Not difficult in the abstract, clinical way that medical language tends to describe disease—difficult in the specific, daily, accumulated way of a body that does not behave predictably, a medical system that has often not known what to do with you, and a life that has had to be built around constraints most people around you have never had to consider.

What this book has tried to offer is not a promise of cure—MCAS is too biologically complex and too individually varied for that kind of guarantee—but something more immediately useful: a framework for understanding what is happening, a toolkit of evidence-informed interventions that address the real biology, and a sequenced approach that makes it possible to act effectively rather than reactively.

The biology you have read about in these pages is real. The mechanisms are real. The interventions work—not for everyone, not completely, not immediately, but with a consistency and a reliability that justifies the effort they require. People get better from MCAS. Not everyone, not fully, not on any particular schedule—but many people, substantially, and often in ways they had given up hoping for.

The trajectory of this condition, when it is addressed systematically and with adequate support, tends toward improvement. Slowly, with setbacks, with periods where the effort feels disproportionate to the visible results—and then, gradually, with a kind of accumulating solidity. The bucket gets deeper. The threshold rises. The list of safe foods grows. The mornings become more manageable. The reactions become less frequent, less severe, less frightening. Life expands again, one careful step at a time.

> *You are not at the mercy of your mast cells. You are the person who is learning how to work with them. That shift—from patient to informed participant in your own biology—is not a small thing. It is, for many people who have been through this, the beginning of everything.*

Healing does not require perfection—it requires persistence, curiosity, and a willingness to listen to your body in a way that perhaps you were never taught to do before.

There will still be days that feel like setbacks. There will be stretches where progress is quiet enough that it is easy to miss. But if you continue to apply what you have learned—steadily, thoughtfully—you may begin to notice something subtle but profound: your body becoming less reactive, more stable, more trustworthy. Not all at once. Not in a straight line. But in a way that, over time, changes the shape of your life.

This is not a return to who you were before MCAS. It is the creation of something new—an informed, responsive relationship with your own biology. One that is built on understanding instead of fear, on strategy instead of guesswork, on partnership instead of opposition.

You are not alone in this, even if it has often felt that way. There is a growing body of knowledge, a growing number of clinicians, and a growing community of people who are learning how to navigate this condition with increasing skill and success. What once felt obscure and isolating is becoming more visible, more understood, and more manageable.

And you—by reading this, by engaging with it, by choosing to act on it—are part of that shift.

So take what is here and use it in the way that works for you. Adapt it. Move at the pace your body allows. Let progress be measured not only in symptom reduction, but in regained capacity, in increased confidence, in the quiet return of possibility.

Because that is what this work ultimately offers: not just fewer reactions, but more life. And that life—expanded, steadied, and rebuilt on your own terms—is still very much available to you.

APPENDIX A

Low-Histamine Food Quick Reference

A practical guide to foods that support mast cell calm—and the ones to approach with caution

> **How to Use This List:** *This is a starting guide, not an absolute rule book. Individual tolerance varies—a food that appears in the caution column may be fine for you in small amounts on a low-bucket day. Track your personal responses and build your own safe-food list over time. The freshness rule applies to all proteins: cook fresh, eat immediately, avoid leftovers.*

✓ PROTEINS	✓ VEGETABLES	✓ FRUITS	✓ GRAINS & STARCHES
Fresh chicken (same day)	Broccoli	Apple (with skin)	White rice (freshly cooked)
Fresh turkey (same day)	Cauliflower	Pear	Quinoa
Fresh lamb (same day)	Zucchini	Mango (not overripe)	Oats (plain, not instant)
Fresh beef (same day)	Cucumber	Blueberries (fresh/frozen)	Millet
Fresh white fish (same day / frozen-at-sea)	Carrots	Kiwi (fresh)	Sweet potato (freshly cooked)
Fresh salmon (same day / frozen-at-sea)	Green beans	Melon (not overripe)	White potato (freshly cooked)
Eggs (cage-free, freshly cooked)	Peas	Grapes (fresh)	Rice noodles
	Asparagus	Mango (ripe)	Corn tortillas (plain)
	Lettuce / romaine / butter lettuce	Banana (not overripe)	Gluten-free bread (fresh)
	Spinach (moderate — some react)	Cherries (fresh)	
	Celery	Coconut (fresh)	
	Red/yellow bell pepper	Papaya (small amounts, some react)	

✗ HIGH-HISTAMINE PROTEINS	✗ HIGH-HISTAMINE VEG	✗ HISTAMINE LIBERATORS	✗ DAO BLOCKERS / FERMENTED
Canned fish (tuna, sardines, salmon)	Tomatoes	Strawberries	Alcohol (all forms)
Smoked fish (salmon, mackerel)	Eggplant	Citrus fruits (orange, lemon, lime)	Vinegar and vinegar-based condiments
Deli meats, salami, pepperoni	Avocado (liberator for many)	Pineapple	Soy sauce, fish sauce, Worcestershire
Aged cheeses (parmesan, cheddar, brie)	Spinach (high in some)	Chocolate / cocoa	Fermented foods (sauerkraut, kimchi, kefir)
Leftovers (any cooked protein >4 hrs old)	Fermented vegetables	Egg white (raw)	Sourdough bread
Shellfish (especially canned/thawed)	Pickled vegetables	Papaya (larger amounts)	Kombucha, kefir, yogurt
Processed meats (bacon, hot dogs)	Olives (brined)	Alcohol	Black and green tea (high amounts)

The Freshness Rule—The Single Most Important Principle

Histamine accumulates over time in animal proteins under bacterial action. A piece of fresh salmon cooked and eaten immediately is a very different food, histamine-wise, from the same fish that has been sitting in a display case for two days. Cook what you need, eat it at that meal, and avoid storing cooked proteins whenever possible during stabilization.

Additional Notes

- Spices and dried herbs accumulate histamine over time—replace open spice jars after six months.
- Cooking methods matter: freshly cooked foods are safer than reheated foods, which are safer than fermented foods.
- Fermented foods—even “healthy” ones like sauerkraut, kombucha, and kefir—are high-histamine sources to avoid during stabilization.
- Vinegar-based condiments (ketchup, mustard, mayo, most salad dressings, pickles, hot sauce) are significant MCAS triggers.
- “Organic” and “natural” labels do not mean low-histamine. Some of the highest-histamine foods are organic and unprocessed (aged cheeses, cured meats, fermented foods).

APPENDIX B

Supplement Starter Guide

Introducing supplements safely—one at a time, starting low, in the right sequence

> **The Golden Rule:** *Introduce one supplement at a time. Wait 5–7 days before adding anything new. Start at the lowest dose listed. This is the only approach that tells you what is helping—and what is not.*

Supplement	Stage	Start Dose	Target Dose	Timing	Notes
Quercetin (phytosome / liposomal / dihydrate)	1	125 mg once daily	250–500 mg 2–3x daily	20–30 min before meals	First supplement to introduce; cornerstone mast cell stabilizer
Vitamin C (buffered)	1–2	250 mg once daily	500–1,000 mg 2x daily	With meals	Use calcium/magnesium ascorbate; avoid plain ascorbic acid
Magnesium glycinate	1–2	100 mg evening	200–400 mg daily	Evening, before bed	Supports mast cells, nervous system, and sleep simultaneously
Luteolin	2	100 mg once daily	100–200 mg daily	Before largest meal	CNS-penetrating; especially valuable for brain fog and neuroinflammation
Omega-3 (EPA + DHA)	2	500 mg EPA+DHA daily	1,000–2,000 mg daily	With largest fat-containing meal	Use triglyceride form or algae-based; check product freshness
Vitamin D3 + K2	2	1,000 IU daily	Per blood level testing	With fat-containing meal	Test levels first; target 50–80 ng/mL; always pair with K2 (100–200 mcg)
Vitamin B6 (P5P form)	2	10–25 mg daily	25–50 mg daily	With food	DAO cofactor + neurotransmitter support; use P5P not pyridoxine
L-Glutamine	2	1,000 mg once daily	2,500–5,000 mg daily (divided)	Between meals (empty stomach)	Gut lining repair; introduce after stabilization is established
Zinc Carnosine (PepZin GI)	2	75 mg once daily	75 mg twice daily	Before meals or bedtime	Mucosal coating and repair; long-term: supplement copper at 1–2 mg/day
DAO Enzyme	2–3	1 capsule before 1 meal	1–2 capsules before	15 min before eating	Situational—use before histamine-containing meals, not

Supplement	Stage	Start Dose	Target Dose	Timing	Notes
			histamine-risk meals		daily; porcine-derived
Probiotics (*L. rhamnosus, B. longum*)	2–3	5 billion CFU single strain	10–50 billion CFU daily multi-strain	Morning, away from antibiotics	STRAIN SELECTION IS CRITICAL – avoid *L. casei, L. reuteri, L. bulgaricus*
Milk Thistle / Silymarin (phospholipid or co-crystal complex)	3	140 mg once daily	140–420 mg daily	With meals	Liver support during detox and antimicrobial treatment phases
NAC (N-acetylcysteine)	2–3	300 mg once daily	600–1,200 mg daily	Empty stomach or 30 min before meals	Glutathione precursor; avoid with nitroglycerin; may thin mucus

How to Introduce Supplements Safely

- Begin with quercetin alone during Stage 1. Do not introduce the next supplement until quercetin is confirmed tolerated at your starting dose.
- If you react to a new supplement, reduce the dose to a fraction of the starting amount before discontinuing entirely. Many reactions are dose-related, not compound-related.
- Write the introduction date for each supplement in your symptom journal. This creates a timeline that helps identify patterns and correlations.
- Never take a new supplement for the first time on a day when you are already in a flare or have an important commitment. Give yourself a low-stakes observation window.
- Capsule fillers and excipients can cause reactions in sensitive patients. Look for products with minimal and clearly identified non-active ingredients.

Supplements to Avoid or Use With Extreme Caution in MCAS

- Probiotics containing *L. casei, L. reuteri, L. bulgaricus*, or *L. helveticus*—all are histamine producers that worsen MCAS.
- High-dose methylfolate (above 400 mcg) without careful dose titration—can cause activation symptoms in patients with MTHFR variants and histamine sensitivity.
- NAD+ precursors (niacin, NMN, NR)—can trigger flushing reactions that mimic and worsen mast cell symptoms in some individuals.
- Resveratrol at high doses—DAO inhibitor at higher concentrations despite its anti-inflammatory properties at lower doses.

APPENDIX C

Symptom Tracker Templates

Your daily data is your most powerful diagnostic tool—use it consistently

> **How to Track Effectively:** *Track daily but review weekly. Day-to-day fluctuation is noise; the weekly trend is the signal. After 4–6 weeks, patterns emerge that no specialist visit can reveal from memory alone.*

Weekly Symptom Tracker

Copy this page (***for personal use only***) and use one sheet per week. Rate each category on a 1–10 scale (1 = very low/good, 10 = very high/severe).

Date	React (1–10)	Symptoms (list, severity)	Foods Eaten (flag any new)	Triggers / Exposures	Sleep (1–10)	Stress (1–10)	Bucket Level (1–10)

Monthly Trend Summary

At the end of each month, answer these questions in your journal to track progress over time:

- ☐ Average daily reactivity score this month vs. last month: ______ vs. ______

- ☐ Number of significant reactions (7+/10) this month vs. last month: ______ vs. ______
- ☐ Number of days with no significant reactions this month: ______
- ☐ Foods or exposures newly added to safe list this month: ________________________
- ☐ Foods or exposures newly identified as triggers this month: ________________________
- ☐ Sleep quality trend: improving / stable / worsening (circle one)
- ☐ Cognitive function trend: improving / stable / worsening (circle one)
- ☐ Overall trajectory this month: clearly improving / stable / concerning (circle one)

Reaction Log — Detailed Entry

Use this format for any significant reaction (5+/10) to capture useful root-cause information:

- ☐ Date and time of reaction: ________________________________
- ☐ Symptoms and severity (1–10): ________________________________
- ☐ What was eaten in the 3 hours before: ________________________________
- ☐ Environmental exposures (fragrance, temperature, chemical): ________________________________
- ☐ Physical factors (exercise, exertion, temperature change): ________________________________
- ☐ Stress level and emotional context: ________________________________
- ☐ Sleep quality the night before (1–10): ______ Menstrual cycle day (if applicable): ______
- ☐ Estimated bucket level before the reaction (1–10): ______
- ☐ What helped: ________________________________ How long to resolve: __________________

Pattern Recognition Prompts — Review These Monthly

- Are reactions consistently worse on certain days of the week? (Possible workplace or environment trigger.)
- Are reactions consistently worse at a particular time of month? (Possible hormonal cycling — see Chapter 10.)
- Are reactions worse when you spend time in a specific building? (Possible mold or chemical exposure.)
- Do reactions improve significantly when you are away from home for more than 3 days? (Strong signal for environmental driver.)
- Do the foods that trigger you change day to day? (Confirms bucket effect — the food is not the primary driver.)
- Do reactions correlate more with stress level than with specific foods? (Points toward nervous system dimension as dominant driver.)

APPENDIX D

Questions to Ask Your Doctor

Getting the most from your medical appointments

> **Before Your Appointment:** *Print or email your symptom journal trend data to your practitioner before the visit. Objective data—not just a verbal summary of how you have been feeling—transforms the quality of the clinical conversation.*

For Any Initial MCAS Evaluation

- Based on my symptom pattern, do you think mast cell activation syndrome could explain my presentation?
- What tests would you recommend to assess for MCAS? Can we include a 24-hour urine histamine and methylhistamine alongside any serum tests?
- Is there value in drawing the mast cell mediator panel during or within two hours of a symptomatic episode, rather than at a baseline visit?
- Are you familiar with the consensus diagnostic criteria for MCAS (2011 Molderings/Afrin criteria and subsequent refinements)? How do you apply them in your practice?
- Would a therapeutic trial of an H1 and H2 antihistamine combination be a reasonable diagnostic step given my clinical picture?

For Testing and Root Cause Investigation

- Given my symptom history [describe your specific history: post-infectious onset / location-dependent symptoms / menstrual cycle variation], which root cause tests are most appropriate to prioritize?
- Can we order a full thyroid panel including TSH, free T3, free T4, reverse T3, TPO antibodies, and thyroglobulin antibodies—not just TSH?
- Can we test a four-point salivary cortisol curve rather than a single AM serum cortisol to assess my HPA axis pattern?
- Would a lactulose breath test for SIBO be appropriate given my GI symptom pattern?
- I would like to discuss mycotoxin testing. I have noticed [describe location-dependent symptoms]. What are your thoughts on ordering a urine mycotoxin panel?
- Are you familiar with MTHFR variants and their relationship to histamine metabolism? Can we include this in my genetic workup?

For Medication and Supplement Discussions

- I am currently taking the following supplements [provide list]. Are there any interactions I should be aware of with my current medications?
- I would like to try a structured H1 antihistamine trial. Which antihistamine would you recommend starting with, and what would constitute a meaningful treatment response?
- I have read about low-dose naltrexone for mast cell and immune conditions. Based on my case, is this worth discussing?
- Are you familiar with the different forms of vitamin B6 (pyridoxine vs. P5P) and their relevance to DAO enzyme function? Can we discuss which form is appropriate for me?
- If I develop significant die-off symptoms during an antimicrobial protocol, what is your protocol for managing mast cell reactions in that context?

For POTS-Specific Appointments

- Have you performed a tilt-table test or a standing heart rate test to confirm my POTS diagnosis and characterize my subtype?
- Given that MCAS and POTS are strongly associated, would you support a mast cell workup alongside my POTS evaluation?
- What are your thoughts on therapeutic salt and fluid intake for my plasma volume deficit? What targets would you recommend for my specific situation?
- Can we discuss a compression garment prescription—specifically thigh-high or waist-level coverage—rather than knee-high stockings alone?
- What is your approach to exercise prescription for people with POTS who also have significant mast cell reactivity? Are you familiar with recumbent-first reconditioning protocols?

For Ongoing Care

- How often should I schedule follow-up appointments to review my symptom tracking data and adjust the protocol?
- Who on your team is most knowledgeable about MCAS if you are not available—and are you willing to consult with other practitioners familiar with this condition if we reach the limits of your experience?
- What are the warning signs that would indicate I need an urgent evaluation rather than waiting for my next scheduled appointment?
- Are you familiar with the physician education resources from the Mastocytosis Society, Mast Cell Action, or Dysautonomia International? These may be valuable if you would like to learn more about the current state of the field.

APPENDIX E

Common Medications Used in MCAS Management

Purpose, Side Effects, and Reducing Reliance Through Natural Support

♦ ♦ ♦

Important Notice: This appendix is provided for educational purposes only. It is not a recommendation to start, stop, or change any medication without the guidance of a qualified healthcare provider. Many individuals with MCAS require pharmaceutical support during stabilization and beyond—medications are not failures of the natural approach. They are tools, and understanding them clearly is part of becoming an informed participant in your own care.

How to Use This Appendix

The medications listed here are organized by drug class and are among those most commonly prescribed for individuals managing MCAS. For each medication, you will find a plain-language description of its purpose, the most commonly reported side effects, and—where applicable—evidence-informed strategies from the book's four-stage framework (Stabilize, Support, Repair, Rebuild) that may, over time and under medical supervision, allow for a reduction in dose or reliance.

Reducing medication reliance is a reasonable long-term goal for many individuals with MCAS, but it is a goal that must be pursued carefully, sequentially, and in partnership with a knowledgeable practitioner. Attempting to taper medications before the underlying system is stable enough to support the change is one of the most common causes of preventable setbacks.

> *Key principle from Chapter 12: You cannot effectively reduce pharmaceutical support until the foundational work of stabilization has been completed. Medications hold the system steady while that work is done. Removing them prematurely is like taking down the scaffolding before the building can stand on its own.*

♦ ♦ ♦

H1 Antihistamines

H1 antihistamines block histamine from binding to H1 receptors throughout the body, reducing symptoms like itching, hives, flushing, nasal congestion, watery eyes, and some cardiovascular symptoms. They are typically among the first medications prescribed when MCAS is suspected and are often used daily rather than as needed.

Medication	Class	Primary Purpose in MCAS	Common Side Effects	Natural Reduction Strategy
Cetirizine (Zyrtec)	Second-generation H1 antihistamine	Reduces itching, hives, flushing, and nasal and eye symptoms. Less sedating than first-generation options.	Drowsiness in some individuals; dry mouth; occasional paradoxical agitation; urinary retention at higher doses.	As mast cell reactivity decreases through dietary simplification, nervous system regulation, and targeted supplementation (quercetin, vitamin C), H1 antihistamine doses may be gradually reduced in consultation with a provider. Quercetin acts on some overlapping pathways.
Loratadine (Claritin)	Second-generation H1 antihistamine	Reduces allergic and mast cell–mediated symptoms. Non-sedating for most individuals.	Headache; dry mouth; fatigue in some; less effective for some individuals than cetirizine.	Same reduction pathway as cetirizine. Dietary reduction of high-histamine foods (Chapter 13) reduces the histamine load that antihistamines are compensating for, creating space to reassess dose over time.
Fexofenadine (Allegra)	Second-generation H1 antihistamine	Broad H1 blockade; particularly useful for individuals sensitive to the sedating effects of other antihistamines.	Headache; nausea; back pain reported occasionally; grapefruit juice can significantly increase blood levels.	Consistent low-histamine lifestyle (Chapter 13) and foundational mast cell stabilizers reduce the background histamine level that requires pharmacological blockade.

Medication	Class	Primary Purpose in MCAS	Common Side Effects	Natural Reduction Strategy
Diphenhydramine (Benadryl)	First-generation H1 antihistamine	Fast-acting; frequently used for acute reactions and anaphylaxis management as part of emergency protocols.	Significant sedation; cognitive impairment; dry mouth and urinary retention; long-term use associated with anticholinergic burden—meaning long-term use can hurt memory, cause brain fog, and increase dementia risk, especially in older adults.	Typically reserved for acute use rather than daily management. Reducing the frequency of acute reactions through stabilization (Chapter 12) directly reduces the need for as-needed rescue use.
Hydroxyzine (Vistaril, Atarax)	First-generation H1 antihistamine with anxiolytic properties	Used both for MCAS symptom control and for the anxiety and sleep disruption that frequently accompany the condition.	Significant sedation; cognitive dulling; dry mouth; not appropriate for driving; dependency concerns with long-term use.	As the nervous system dimension of MCAS is addressed through vagal toning practices, breathwork, and sleep optimization (Chapter 14), pharmacological anxiolytic support may become less necessary. Magnesium glycinate supports sleep through a complementary mechanism.

◆ ◆ ◆

H2 Antihistamines

H2 receptors are concentrated in the gastrointestinal tract and on immune cells. H2 antihistamines reduce gastric acid secretion and complement H1 blockade by targeting a different receptor population. They are frequently used alongside H1 antihistamines rather than instead of them.

Medication	Class	Primary Purpose in MCAS	Common Side Effects	Natural Reduction Strategy
Famotidine (Pepcid)	H2 antihistamine	Reduces gastric acid symptoms including reflux, nausea, and abdominal burning driven by mast cell mediator release in the GI tract. Also provides additional systemic H2 receptor blockade.	Headache; constipation or diarrhea; rare liver enzyme elevation with long-term use; rebound hyperacidity if stopped abruptly. Can potentially worsen acid reflux symptoms over time because they may lead to low stomach acid levels, which can contribute to bacterial overgrowth and malabsorption issues.	Gut barrier repair work in Stage 2 (Chapter 19)—including glutamine, zinc carnosine, and dietary simplification—addresses the underlying intestinal permeability and subepithelial mast cell reactivity that drive GI symptoms. As the gut heals, acid-reducing medication needs often diminish naturally.
Ranitidine (Zantac) [Note: product recalls in several markets; verify availability with provider]	H2 antihistamine	Historically used for the same indications as famotidine; H2 blockade plus some additional mast cell effects observed in research.	Similar GI side effects to famotidine; product integrity concerns have limited availability in some regions. Can potentially worsen acid reflux symptoms over time because they may lead to low stomach acid levels, which can contribute to bacterial overgrowth and malabsorption issues.	Same reduction pathway as famotidine. Consult your healthcare provider regarding current regulatory status in your region.

♦ ♦ ♦

Mast Cell Stabilizers

Pharmaceutical mast cell stabilizers work by reducing the sensitivity of mast cells to degranulation triggers—essentially raising the activation threshold. Cromolyn sodium is the most commonly used oral mast cell stabilizer in MCAS management.

Medication	Class	Primary Purpose in MCAS	Common Side Effects	Natural Reduction Strategy
Cromolyn Sodium (Gastrocrom, NasalCrom)	Mast cell stabilizer	Reduces mast cell degranulation in the GI tract (oral form) and nasal passages (intranasal form). Used for systemic GI symptoms including cramping, diarrhea, and abdominal pain driven by mucosal mast cell activation.	Generally well tolerated; occasional nausea, headache, or diarrhea; rare hypersensitivity reactions; cost and availability can be limiting factors.	Natural mast cell stabilizers—particularly quercetin and luteolin (Chapter 16)—work through partially overlapping mechanisms and may support a gradual reduction in cromolyn dose as the underlying system stabilizes. The sequencing principle from Chapter 12 applies: natural stabilizers are introduced after a baseline is established, not as a replacement for pharmaceutical stabilization mid-crisis.
Ketotifen	Mast cell stabilizer / H1 antihistamine	Combines H1 receptor blockade with mast cell stabilizing properties. Used off-label in MCAS in regions where it is available orally.	Sedation (significant in some individuals); weight gain with longer-term use; dry mouth; rebound effects if stopped abruptly.	Similar to cromolyn: natural stabilizers and dietary approaches reduce the underlying reactivity that ketotifen compensates for. Tapering requires a stable baseline and gradual dose reduction, never abrupt cessation.

◆ ◆ ◆

Leukotriene Modifiers

Leukotrienes are a family of inflammatory mediators released by mast cells alongside histamine. Leukotriene modifiers block either leukotriene synthesis or leukotriene receptor binding, reducing a dimension of mast cell–driven inflammation that antihistamines do not address.

Medication	Class	Primary Purpose in MCAS	Common Side Effects	Natural Reduction Strategy
Montelukast (Singulair)	Leukotriene receptor antagonist	Reduces airway inflammation, asthma symptoms, and some skin and GI symptoms driven by leukotriene release. Often used when respiratory or exercise-triggered symptoms are prominent.	Neuropsychiatric effects including anxiety, depression, nightmares, and mood changes—these are FDA black box warning material and should be monitored carefully; headache; abdominal pain.	Omega-3 fatty acids (EPA/DHA) and luteolin have evidence for modulating leukotriene pathways through complementary mechanisms (Chapter 16). As inflammatory load decreases through root cause treatment (Stage 3), leukotriene-driven symptoms often diminish. Any tapering should be done slowly under medical supervision given the neuropsychiatric side effect profile.
Zafirlukast (Accolate)	Leukotriene receptor antagonist	Similar indications to montelukast; less commonly prescribed.	Headache; GI upset; rare but serious liver toxicity with long-term use; drug interactions with warfarin.	Same pathway considerations as montelukast. Liver function monitoring is important during Stage 3 detoxification work if this medication is being used concurrently.

◆ ◆ ◆

Proton Pump Inhibitors (PPIs)

PPIs reduce gastric acid production by blocking the enzyme responsible for acid secretion. They are commonly prescribed when MCAS produces significant GI symptoms including reflux, esophageal irritation, and gastric pain, but their long-term use carries meaningful implications for gut health that are particularly relevant in MCAS. Note: PPIs mask symptoms and fail to address the root cause of GERD—often low stomach acid. Betaine and pepsin, dosed and timed correctly, improve GERD by improving digestion and nutrient absorption for long-term health.

Medication	Class	Primary Purpose in MCAS	Common Side Effects	Natural Reduction Strategy
Omeprazole (Prilosec)	Proton pump inhibitor	Reduces gastric acid–driven symptoms including reflux, esophagitis, and upper GI pain.	Long-term use associated with: magnesium depletion (significant in MCAS, where magnesium is already a key support); B12 depletion; altered gut microbiome and increased risk of SIBO; calcium and iron absorption impairment; increased susceptibility to certain GI infections.	Gut healing work (Chapter 19) addresses the underlying mucosal mast cell reactivity and barrier compromise that drive acid hypersensitivity. As the gut lining heals, many individuals find acid symptoms diminish and PPI doses can be reduced. However, abrupt PPI cessation produces rebound hyperacidity—tapering must be gradual and medically supervised.
Pantoprazole (Protonix)	Proton pump inhibitor	Same indications as omeprazole; sometimes preferred due to fewer drug interactions.	Same long-term concerns as omeprazole: micronutrient depletion, microbiome disruption, rebound on cessation.	Same reduction pathway. Given that PPIs worsen SIBO risk and magnesium status—both of which are directly relevant to MCAS management—reducing PPI dependence through gut repair is a high-priority

Medication	Class	Primary Purpose in MCAS	Common Side Effects	Natural Reduction Strategy
				goal in Stage 2 and 3.

♦ ♦ ♦

Corticosteroids

Corticosteroids are potent anti-inflammatory agents used acutely in MCAS for severe flares, anaphylaxis management, and, in some cases, short-term bridging when reactivity is severely elevated. Long-term corticosteroid use in MCAS is generally discouraged due to significant side effect burden, but short-term courses remain a legitimate and sometimes necessary tool.

Medication	Class	Primary Purpose in MCAS	Common Side Effects	Natural Reduction Strategy
Prednisone / Prednisolone	Systemic corticosteroid	Broad anti-inflammatory effect across multiple mediator pathways. Used for acute severe flares, post-anaphylaxis management, and short-term symptom control when other medications are insufficient.	Short-term: elevated blood glucose, mood changes, insomnia, increased appetite, fluid retention. Long-term: adrenal suppression, osteoporosis, immune compromise, weight gain, skin thinning, cataracts.	The goal of stabilization (Chapter 12) is to reduce flare frequency and severity to the point where corticosteroid courses become rare. Adrenal support (Chapter 10) is important both during and after corticosteroid use. Any steroid taper must be medically supervised; abrupt cessation after even short courses can cause adrenal insufficiency.

♦ ♦ ♦

Epinephrine (Emergency Use)

Auto-injectable epinephrine (e.g., EpiPen) is not a daily management medication but is a life-saving emergency intervention prescribed to individuals with MCAS who are at risk of anaphylaxis. It is not a target for dose reduction—it is a safety net that every individual with moderate-to-severe MCAS should have access to and know how to use.

Medication	Class	Primary Purpose in MCAS	Common Side Effects	Natural Reduction Strategy
Epinephrine Auto-Injector (EpiPen, Auvi-Q)	Sympathomimetic / emergency anaphylaxis treatment	Reverses the life-threatening cardiovascular and airway effects of anaphylaxis through rapid adrenergic stimulation. First-line treatment for systemic anaphylactic reactions.	Tachycardia, palpitations, anxiety, pallor, and tremor immediately following injection—these are expected effects of epinephrine and not reasons to avoid using it when indicated. Always seek emergency medical evaluation after use.	Reducing anaphylaxis risk is a goal of the entire management program: stabilization, root cause treatment, dietary management, and trigger avoidance all reduce the frequency of severe reactions. However, individuals with MCAS should maintain their prescription and carry their auto-injector at all times regardless of how well-managed their condition is, because breakthrough reactions can occur.

♦ ♦ ♦

Benzodiazepines and Anxiolytics

Anxiety is one of the most common and most distressing symptoms of MCAS, driven by the direct neurological effects of mast cell mediators as well as the secondary psychological effects of living with a complex, often misunderstood chronic illness. In some cases, benzodiazepines or other anxiolytics are prescribed. Their use in MCAS warrants particular attention given their dependency potential and the availability of addressing the underlying neurological drivers of anxiety through the approaches in Chapter 14.

Medication	Class	Primary Purpose in MCAS	Common Side Effects	Natural Reduction Strategy
Lorazepam (Ativan) Clonazepam (Klonopin)	Benzodiazepine anxiolytic	Short-term anxiety relief; management of severe panic episodes; sometimes used for sleep. Some evidence for mast cell inhibitory effects at low doses in research settings.	Sedation; cognitive impairment; dependency and tolerance with regular use; withdrawal syndrome that can be severe and prolonged; increased fall risk in older individuals.	Addressing the nervous system dimension of MCAS through vagal toning, somatic practices, and limbic retraining (Chapter 14) targets the neurobiological drivers of MCAS-related anxiety more sustainably than pharmacological suppression. Tapering benzodiazepines requires a specialized, slow protocol and should never be attempted without medical guidance. Magnesium glycinate and GABA-supporting nutrients may provide complementary support during taper.

♦ ♦ ♦

Targeted Biologics and Emerging Therapies

Omalizumab (Xolair) and related biologics targeting IgE-mediated and mast cell–related pathways are increasingly used in treatment-resistant MCAS. These are typically specialist-prescribed medications used when first- and second-line approaches have been insufficient.

Medication	Class	Primary Purpose in MCAS	Common Side Effects	Natural Reduction Strategy
Omalizumab (Xolair)	Anti-IgE monoclonal antibody	Reduces mast cell activation driven by IgE-mediated pathways. Used in MCAS individuals with elevated IgE and treatment-refractory symptoms. Administered as an injection, typically monthly.	Injection site reactions; rare but serious anaphylaxis risk with injection; headache; joint pain; long-term safety profile still being characterized in MCAS-specific use.	Omalizumab addresses one upstream driver of mast cell activation but does not address root causes. The foundational work of the four-stage framework—gut healing, nervous system regulation, root cause identification and treatment—proceeds in parallel and may ultimately reduce the biological need for ongoing biologic therapy. Any changes to omalizumab dosing must be managed by the prescribing specialist.

♦ ♦ ♦

The Medication-Reduction Roadmap: Working Within the Four Stages

Many individuals with MCAS are not aiming to eliminate all medications from their management plan. The goal is more nuanced: to reduce reliance on pharmaceutical support to the minimum necessary to maintain quality of life, while the underlying drivers of reactivity are addressed. This is a different goal than simply stopping medications, and it requires a clear strategic framework.

The following maps medication reduction opportunities to the four-stage framework introduced in Chapter 12 and Chapter 25:

Stage	Medication goal
STAGE 1 Stabilize	Medication goal: maintain, not reduce. This is not the time to taper. Use your prescribed medications consistently during the 4–12 weeks of stabilization. The work of stabilization—dietary simplification, trigger removal, nervous system regulation—is building the foundation that makes reduction possible later. Attempting to taper antihistamines or stabilizers while the mast cell system is in maximum reactivity mode will likely result in setbacks. Take your medications as prescribed and focus entirely on creating the healing baseline.
STAGE 2 Support	Medication goal: natural supports begin to complement pharmaceutical ones. As quercetin, vitamin C, magnesium, gut-healing compounds, and nervous system practices build in effect, some individuals begin to notice that their symptoms are better controlled with the same or lower medication doses. This is the signal—not a reason to unilaterally reduce, but an observation to bring to your healthcare provider as the basis for a supervised, incremental taper discussion.
STAGE 3 Repair	Medication goal: supervised reduction as root causes are addressed. As SIBO is treated, viral reactivation managed, mycotoxin burden reduced, and gut barrier restored, the biological drivers of mast cell reactivity diminish. This creates genuine room for medication reduction that didn't exist before. PPI tapering as the gut heals, H1/H2 antihistamine dose reduction as dietary and supplemental histamine management matures, and cromolyn reduction as the mast cell priming state resolves—all of these become realistic conversations at this stage.
STAGE 4 Rebuild	Medication goal: minimum effective dose for long-term sustainability. Not everyone exits MCAS management free of all medication—some individuals maintain a low-dose antihistamine or mast cell stabilizer indefinitely as part of a sustainable long-term protocol. This is not failure. The goal is a medication burden that reflects your actual biology, not the maximum reactivity state you were in before the work began. For many, this means a meaningful reduction from where they started. For some, it means complete cessation.

The outcome is determined by biology and thorough root cause work, not willpower.

♦ ♦ ♦

Potential Supplement–Medication Interactions

This table provides a practical overview of potential interactions between the supplements recommended in this guide and the most commonly prescribed medications used in MCAS management. It is not an exhaustive list of all possible interactions, but rather a focused reference designed to highlight the combinations most likely to be encountered in real-world use. Individual responses can vary, and additional interactions may exist based on your full medication list, underlying conditions, and dosage levels. For this reason, this table should be used as an educational starting point—not a substitute for professional guidance. Always review your current supplements and medications with your prescribing provider or pharmacist before starting, stopping, or combining any therapies.

Supplement	Medication(s)	What Happens	Why It Matters (Simple Explanation)	What to Do
Omega-3 (EPA/DHA)	Montelukast (Singulair)	Acts on similar inflammation pathways	Both reduce leukotrienes (inflammation chemicals)	Usually safe, but monitor symptoms when adjusting meds
Quercetin	H1 antihistamines (e.g., cetirizine, loratadine)	Works on overlapping histamine pathways	May enhance antihistamine effect	Can support gradual dose reduction (with doctor guidance)
Vitamin C	H1 antihistamines	Supports histamine breakdown	May reduce need for higher medication doses over time	Safe combo; track symptom improvement
Vitamin C	PPIs (omeprazole, pantoprazole)	PPIs may interfere with absorption	PPIs may deplete vitamin C or decrease supplemental absorption; Supplement helps offset depletion	Often beneficial combination
Luteolin	Mast cell stabilizers (e.g., cromolyn, ketotifen); proton pump inhibitors	Similar mast cell–calming effects; PPIs may interfere with absorption	Adds to stabilization effect	May help reduce medication need later (not during flare)
Magnesium glycinate	Benzodiazepines / sedating antihistamines	Adds calming/sedating effect	Can increase drowsiness	Use at night; be cautious with daytime sedation

Supplement	Medication(s)	What Happens	Why It Matters (Simple Explanation)	What to Do
	(diphenhydramine, hydroxyzine)			
Magnesium glycinate	PPIs (omeprazole, pantoprazole)	PPIs lower magnesium levels	Supplement helps offset depletion	Often beneficial combination
DAO enzyme	Histamine-related meds (antihistamines)	Works in gut, meds work systemically	Complementary, not conflicting	Safe to combine
Milk thistle (silymarin)	Many medications (general caution)	Affects liver detox pathways	May alter how drugs are processed	Use caution; discuss with doctor if on multiple meds
Probiotics	PPIs (omeprazole, pantoprazole)	May alter probiotic effectiveness (mixed evidence)	PPIs may neutralize digestive, immunity, and other benefits	Take probiotics at least 2 hours after PPIs

♦ ♦ ♦

Practical Guidance for Discussing Medications with Your Healthcare Provider

Being an informed, active participant in your medication management requires knowing what questions to ask. The following prompts may help structure conversations with your prescribing physician or MCAS-knowledgeable practitioner:

1. "What is the minimum effective dose of this medication for my current symptom pattern, and how will we know when that has changed?"
2. "Which of my current medications would you suggest we consider tapering first, once stabilization is achieved, and what would the protocol look like?"
3. "Are there any natural supplements I am taking or considering that interact with my current medications?"
4. "What symptom threshold or duration of stability would indicate I am ready to attempt a supervised taper?"
5. "What is the correct way to stop this medication if needed—should it be tapered, and over what timeframe?"

♦ ♦ ♦

A final word on medications and identity: Many individuals with MCAS carry a sense of shame or failure around needing pharmaceutical support—especially when pursuing a natural healing approach. This is worth examining honestly. Medications are not the enemy to natural healing. In a highly reactive mast cell system, they are a tool to help make natural healing possible. The four-stage framework does not ask you to choose between them. It asks you to use them wisely, sequence them correctly, and work steadily toward a place where you need the minimum necessary to live well. That is a worthy and realistic goal.

APPENDIX F

Glossary of Terms

Key concepts from the book, defined plainly

Medical terminology can make an already complex condition feel more inaccessible than it needs to be. This glossary provides plain-language definitions for the key terms used throughout the book, listed alphabetically. For deeper exploration of any concept, the chapter references in the definition point you to the relevant discussion.

Term	Definition
Anaphylaxis	A severe, potentially life-threatening allergic reaction involving multiple body systems. In MCAS, anaphylactic-level events can occur without IgE-mediated allergy and may not always involve the classic triggers.
Autonomic nervous system	The branch of the nervous system that controls involuntary functions including heart rate, blood pressure, digestion, and sweating. Divided into the sympathetic (fight-or-flight) and parasympathetic (rest-and-digest) branches.
Baroreceptors	Pressure-sensitive sensors in blood vessel walls and the heart that detect changes in blood pressure and relay signals to the brainstem to trigger compensatory cardiovascular responses.
Beta-caryophyllene (BCP)	A sesquiterpene compound found in black pepper, copaiba, and other plants. A CB2 receptor agonist with anti-inflammatory and pain-modulating properties relevant to MCAS.
Biogenic amines	A group of naturally occurring compounds including histamine, tyramine, putrescine, and cadaverine, produced by bacterial action on amino acids in food. Competitive inhibitors of DAO clearance.
Biofilm	A protective matrix of polysaccharides, proteins, and DNA produced by communities of microorganisms that adhere to surfaces. Biofilm-enclosed bacteria are highly resistant to antibiotics and immune clearance.
Butyrate	A short-chain fatty acid produced by colonic bacteria fermenting dietary fiber. Primary energy source for colonocytes; supports gut barrier integrity and has anti-inflammatory epigenetic effects.
CB2 receptor	Cannabinoid receptor type 2, expressed on immune cells including mast cells. CB2 agonism reduces mast cell mediator release and suppresses NF-κB-driven inflammation.
Cholinergic anti-inflammatory pathway	A neural circuit through which the vagus nerve directly suppresses inflammation by releasing acetylcholine, which binds to alpha-7 nicotinic receptors on mast cells and macrophages.

Term	Definition
Chromogranin A	A protein released from secretory cells including mast cells and enteroendocrine cells; used as a supportive marker for mast cell activation when other mediators are equivocal.
CRH (Corticotropin-releasing hormone)	A peptide hormone released by the hypothalamus in response to stress; activates the HPA axis and is a direct non-IgE mast cell activator.
Cytokines	Signaling proteins released by immune cells that coordinate immune responses. Mast cells release cytokines including TNF-alpha, IL-6, and IL-33 that drive systemic inflammation.
DAO (Diamine oxidase)	The primary enzyme responsible for breaking down histamine in the gut lumen before absorption. Produced by intestinal enterocytes; activity is reduced by gut inflammation, alcohol, and certain medications.
Degranulation	The process by which mast cells release the contents of their granules — including histamine, tryptase, heparin, and other mediators — in response to an activation signal.
DIM (Diindolylmethane)	A compound derived from the breakdown of indole-3-carbinol in cruciferous vegetables; supports phase 2 liver estrogen metabolism toward less reactive metabolites.
Dysautonomia	A general term for dysfunction of the autonomic nervous system, encompassing POTS and other conditions of impaired autonomic regulation of cardiovascular and other functions.
Epigenetics	Changes in gene expression that do not involve alterations to the underlying DNA sequence. Influenced by diet, stress, toxin exposure, and lived experience; plays a significant role in MCAS vulnerability.
Estrobolome	The community of gut bacteria that produce enzymes capable of metabolizing estrogens; influences circulating estrogen levels and the risk of estrogen-driven mast cell sensitization.
Glymphatic system	The brain's waste-clearance system, which operates primarily during deep sleep, flushing inflammatory debris and neurotoxic proteins through channels surrounding blood vessels.
HαT (Hereditary alpha-tryptasemia)	A genetic trait caused by duplication of the TPSAB1 gene, producing elevated baseline tryptase levels and amplified mast cell reactivity. Present in approximately 4–7% of Northern Europeans.
HLA-DR	Human leukocyte antigen DR; a gene involved in immune recognition. Certain HLA-DR variants (approximately 25% of

Term	Definition
	the population) impair mycotoxin clearance, increasing susceptibility to mold illness.
HNMT (Histamine N-methyltransferase)	The enzyme responsible for breaking down histamine inside cells and in systemic circulation, through methylation. Dependent on adequate SAM produced through the methylation cycle.
HPA axis	The hypothalamic-pituitary-adrenal axis; the central hormonal control system for the stress response. Chronic HPA dysregulation contributes to impaired cortisol response and mast cell priming.
HRV (Heart rate variability)	The natural variation in the interval between heartbeats. A measure of autonomic flexibility and vagal tone; improved by consistent nervous system practices; directly correlates with mast cell regulation capacity.
Intestinal permeability (leaky gut)	A state in which tight junctions between intestinal epithelial cells are disrupted, allowing bacteria, food proteins, and endotoxins to enter the bloodstream and activate subepithelial mast cells.
IgE	Immunoglobulin E; an antibody class that mediates classical allergic responses by binding to high-affinity receptors on mast cells and triggering degranulation upon re-exposure to the sensitizing allergen.
Leukotrienes	Lipid mediators synthesized by mast cells and other immune cells; potent inflammatory compounds involved in airway constriction, mucus production, and vascular permeability.
Limbic system retraining	A neuroplasticity-based approach that uses directed mental practices to interrupt habitual threat-response neural pathways and establish new patterns associated with safety; used for chronic illness with significant nervous system sensitization.
LPS (Lipopolysaccharide)	A component of the outer membrane of gram-negative bacteria. When LPS translocates across a leaky gut barrier, it activates subepithelial mast cells via toll-like receptor 4 (TLR-4).
MCAS (Mast Cell Activation Syndrome)	A condition in which mast cells activate inappropriately, releasing mediators in response to triggers that should not cause a significant immune response, producing multi-system symptoms.
Mediators	Chemical compounds released by mast cells during activation, including histamine, tryptase, prostaglandins, leukotrienes, and

Term	Definition
	cytokines. Different mediators produce different downstream effects across multiple organ systems.
Methylation	A fundamental biochemical process in which a methyl group is added to a molecule, controlling gene expression, detoxification, histamine clearance (via HNMT), and neurotransmitter production.
MRGPRX2	Mas-related G protein-coupled receptor X2; a receptor on mast cells that responds to neuropeptides (including substance P) and certain medications, triggering non-IgE mast cell activation.
MTHFR	Methylenetetrahydrofolate reductase; an enzyme in the methylation cycle. Common genetic variants (C677T, A1298C) reduce enzyme efficiency, impairing histamine clearance, detoxification, and folate metabolism.
Mycotoxins	Toxic secondary metabolites produced by certain mold species. Distinguished from mold spores; responsible for the most significant biological damage in mold illness through mast cell activation and organ toxicity.
NF-κB	Nuclear factor kappa B; a master transcription factor that upregulates the expression of inflammatory genes. Inhibited by quercetin, luteolin, curcumin, and other mast cell–stabilizing natural compounds.
NRF2	Nuclear factor erythroid 2-related factor 2; a master regulator of antioxidant gene expression. Activated by sulforaphane, EGCG, curcumin, and NAC; protects against the oxidative stress that primes mast cells.
Orthostatic intolerance	Difficulty maintaining adequate blood pressure and heart function when upright. Encompasses POTS, classical orthostatic hypotension, and related forms of impaired cardiovascular compensation for standing.
POTS (Postural Orthostatic Tachycardia Syndrome)	A form of dysautonomia in which heart rate increases excessively (≥30 bpm) upon standing due to impaired autonomic compensation for gravitational blood pooling. Strongly associated with MCAS.
Prostaglandins	Lipid mediators derived from arachidonic acid and released by activated mast cells. Prostaglandin D2 (PGD2) is particularly relevant to MCAS, producing vasodilation, airway constriction, and sleep disruption.
RAAS (Renin-angiotensin-aldosterone system)	The hormonal system that regulates blood volume and vascular resistance through sodium and water retention. Mast cell

Term	Definition
	tryptase interacts with RAAS components, contributing to the plasma volume depletion of POTS.
Resonance frequency breathing	A breathing technique performed at approximately 5–6 breaths per minute that maximizes heart rate variability and baroreflex sensitivity; the gold standard autonomic retraining practice.
Rosmarinic acid	A polyphenolic compound found in herbs of the mint family (rosemary, basil, perilla, lemon balm); simultaneously inhibits COX-2 and 5-LOX, providing dual prostaglandin and leukotriene suppression.
SIBO (Small Intestinal Bacterial Overgrowth)	A condition in which bacteria establish significant colonies in the small intestine, producing histamine and other biogenic amines that contribute to chronic histamine excess independent of dietary intake.
Silymarin	The standardized extract from milk thistle seed (Silybum marianum); hepatoprotective compound that stabilizes liver cell membranes, scavenges free radicals, and supports phase 2 detoxification.
Small-fiber neuropathy	Damage to small unmyelinated nerve fibers that regulate autonomic and sensory function. Documented in MCAS and POTS; contributes to the impaired vascular innervation of neuropathic POTS.
Somatic mutation	An acquired genetic change that occurs in an individual cell during a person's lifetime rather than being inherited. In MCAS, somatic mutations in mast cell subpopulations may alter their behavioral programming.
Tryptase	A serine protease stored in mast cell granules; the most clinically accessible mast cell activation biomarker. Elevated in systemic mastocytosis; often normal in MCAS, making its absence insufficient to rule out the condition.
Tight junctions	Protein structures (including occludin, claudin, and ZO-1) that seal the spaces between intestinal epithelial cells, preventing translocation of bacteria and food proteins across the gut barrier.
TLR (Toll-like receptor)	Pattern recognition receptors on mast cells that detect pathogen-associated molecular patterns. TLR-4 activation by LPS and TLR-2 activation by bacterial lipoproteins are primary non-IgE mast cell activation pathways.
Vagus nerve	The tenth cranial nerve; the primary channel of parasympathetic nervous system activity. Mediates the cholinergic anti-inflammatory pathway that directly suppresses mast cell activity through acetylcholine release.

Term	Definition
Venous return	The flow of blood back to the heart from the peripheral circulation. Adequate venous return is essential for cardiac output; gravitational pooling reduces venous return upon standing, precipitating POTS.

This glossary covers the terms most frequently used throughout this book. The field of MCAS research is evolving rapidly; for the most current terminology and diagnostic criteria, consult the Mastocytosis Society (mastocytosis.org), Mast Cell Action (mastcellaction.org), and the Dysautonomia International clinical resources (dysautonomiainternational.org).

References

[1] Moon TC, Defus AD, Kulka M. Mast Cell Mediators: Their Differential Release and the Secretory Pathways Involved. *Front Immunol.* 2014 Nov 14;5:569.
[2] Oettgen HC. Mast cells in food allergy: Inducing immediate reactions and shaping long-term immunity. *JACI.* 2023 Jan;151(1):21-25.
[3] EDS.clinic. Triggers of Mast Cell Activation. Accessed March 19, 2026 from: https://www.eds.clinic/articles/triggers-of-mcas-and-mcad.
[4] Miller CS, Palmer RF, Dempsey TT, et al. Mast cell activation may explain many cases of chemical intolerance. *Enviro Sci Eur.* 2021 Nov;33(129).
[5] The Institute for Functional Medicine. Mast Cells and Stress: The Mind-Body Connection. Accessed March 19, 2026 from: https://www.ifm.org/articles/mast-cells-stress-mind-body-connection/
[6] Zierau O, Zenclussen AC, Jensen F. Role of female sex hormones, estradiol and progesterone, in mast cell behavior. *Front Immunol.* 2012 Jun 19;3:169.
[7] Munoz-Cruz S, Mendoza-Rodriguez Y, Nava-Castro KE, et al. Gender-Related Effects of Sex Steroids on Histamine Release and FcεRI Expression in Rat Peritoneal Mast Cells. *J Immunol Res.* 2015 Apr 20;2015:351829.
[8] Conway AE, Verdi M, Shaker MS, et al. Beyond Confirmed Mast Cell Activation Syndrome: Approaching Patients With Dysautonomia and Related Conditions. *JACI.* 2024 Jul;12(7)):1738-50.
[9] Asadi S, Alysandratos KD, Angelidou A, et al. Substance P (SP) induces expression of functional corticotropin-releasing hormone receptor-1 (CRHR-1) in human mast cells. *J Invest Dermatol.* 2012 Feb;132(2):324-9.
[10] Kaag S, Lorentz A. Effects of Dietary Components on Mast Cells: Possible Use as Nutraceuticals for Allergies? *Cells.* 2023;12(22):2602.
[11] Krausfeldt LE, Cao V, Rodrigues R, et al. Evidence for dysbiosis in the gut microbiome of patients with systemic mastocytosis. *J Allergy Clin Immunol.* Published online October 9, 2025.
[12] Hu KK, Bruce MA, Butte MJ. Spatiotemporally and Mechanically Controlled Triggering of Mast Cells using Atomic Force Microscopy. *Immunol Res.* 2014 May;58(0):211–217.
[13] Alsaleh NB, Mendoza RP, brown JM. Exposure to silver nanoparticles primes mast cells for enhanced activation through the high-affinity IgE receptor. *Toxicol Appl Pharmacol.* 2019 Sep 5;382:114746.
[14] Kempuraj D, Asadi S, Zhang B, et al. Mercury induces inflammatory mediator release from human mast cells. *J Neuroinflammation.* 2010 Mar 11;7:20.
[15] Talkington J, Nickell SP. Borrelia burgdorferi Spirochetes Induce Mast Cell Activation and Cytokine Release. *Infect Immun.* 1999 Mar;67(3):1107–1115.
[16] Berrich M, Kieda C, Grillon C, et al. Differential Effects of Bartonella henselae on Human and Feline Macro- and Micro-Vascular Endothelial Cells. *PLoS One.* 2011 May 27;6(5):e20204.
[17] Hoek KL, Cassell GH, Duffy LB, et al. Mycoplasma pneumoniae-induced activation and cytokine production in rodent mast cells. *J Allergy Clin Immunol.* 2002 Mar;109(3):470-6.
[18] Cole W. Is It Long COVID Or Mast Cell Activation Syndrome? Breaking Down the Connection. Accessed March 19, 2026 at: https://drwillcole.com/long-covid-and-mcas-breaking-down-connection.
[19] Kuhl U, Lassner D, Wallaschek N, et al. Chromosomally integrated human herpesvirus 6 in heart failure: prevalence and treatment. *Eur J Heart Fail.* 2015 Jan;17(1):9-19.
[20] Schmiedeke JK, Hartmann AK, Ruckenbrod T, et al. The Anti-apoptotic Murine Cytomegalovirus Protein vMIA-m38.5 Induces Mast Cell Degranulation. *Front Cell Infect Microbiol.* 2020 Aug 25;10:439.

---

[21] Afrin LB. Weinstock LB, Molderings GJ. Covid-19 hyperinflammation and post-Covid-19 illness may be rooted in mast cell activation syndrome. *Int J Infect Dis.* 2020 Sep 10;100:327–332.
[22] Valent P, Akin C, Arock M. Reversible Elevation of Tryptase Over the Individual's Baseline: Why is It the Best Biomarker for Severe Systemic Mast Cell Activation and MCAS? *Curr Allergy Asthma Rep.* 2024 Feb 3;24(3):133–141.
[23] Gonzalez-de-Olano D, Navaroo-Navarro P, Munoz-Gonzalez JI, et al. Clinical impact of the TPSAB1 genotype in mast cell diseases: A REMA study in a cohort of 959 individuals. *Allergy.* 2024 Mar;79(3):711-723.
[24] Luskin KT, White AA, Lyons JJ. The Genetic Basis and Clinical Impact of Hereditary Alpha-Tryptasemia. *J Aller Clin Immunol In Pract.* 2021 Jun;9(6):2235-42.
[25] Gonzalez-de-Olano D, Navaroo-Navarro P, Munoz-Gonzalez JI, et al. Clinical impact of the TPSAB1 genotype in mast cell diseases: A REMA study in a cohort of 959 individuals. *Allergy.* 2024 Mar;79(3):711-723.
[26] Vernino S, Bourne KM, Stiles LE, et al. Postural Orthostatic Tachycardia Syndrome (POTS): Priorities for Specialized Care, Education, and Research. *Auton Neurosci.* 2021 Jun 5;235:102828.
[27] Stahlberg M, Reistam U, Fedorowski A, et al. Post-COVID-19 Tachycardia Syndromes: A Distinct Clinical Entity? *Am J Med.* 2021 Aug 11;134(12):1451–1456.
[28] Weinstock LB, Brook JB, Walters AS, et al. Mast cell activation syndrome is frequently associated with postural orthostatic tachycardia syndrome and Ehlers-Danlos syndrome. *J Personalized Med.* 2021;11(9):912.
[29] Raj SR. The Postural Tachycardia Syndrome (POTS): Pathophysiology, Diagnosis & Management. *Indian Pacing Electrophysiology J.* 2006 Apr 1;6(2):84-99. (Updated through 2024 in clinical practice guidelines).
[30] Weinstock LB, Brook JB, Walters AS, et al. Characterization of Mast Cell Activation Syndrome (MCAS): An International Survey of 4,000 Patients. *J Pers Med.* 2021;11(9):912.
[31] Raj SR, Biaggioni I, Yamhure PC, et al. Postural orthostatic tachycardia syndrome: Low plasma volume and early rise in plasma renin activity in the standing position. *Hypertension.* 2005;46(3):615-620.
[32] Tinkle B, Castori M, Berglund B, et al. Hypermobile Ehlers-Danlos syndrome (a.k.a. Ehlers-Danlos syndrome Type III and Ehlers-Danlos syndrome hypermobility type): Clinical description and natural history. *Am J Med Genet C Semin Med Genet.* 2017;175(1):48-69.
[33] Castori M, Tinkle B, Levy H, et al. A framework for the classification of joint hypermobility and related conditions. *Am J Med Genet C Semin Med Genet.* 2017 Mar;175(1):148-57.
[34] Atuesta-Rodriguez AJ, Medina-Velasquez YF, Motta O, et al. Association between Postural Orthostatic Tachycardia Syndrome and Joint Hypermobility. *Case Rep Cardiol.* 2021 Apr 28;2021:8875003.
[35] Roma M, Marden CL, De Wandele I, et al. Postural tachycardia syndrome and other forms of orthostatic intolerance in Ehlers-Danlos syndrome. *Autonomic Neurosci Bas Clin.* 2018 Dec;215:89-96.
[36] Weinstock LB, Brook JB, Walters AS, et al. Characterization of Mast Cell Activation Syndrome (MCAS): An International Survey of 4,000 Patients. *J Pers Med.* 2021;11(9):912.
[37] The Ehlers-Danlos Society. The Ehlers-Danlos Society. The Road to 2026: A Path Toward Progress. Accessed March 20, 2026 from: https://www.ehlers-danlos.com/road-to-2026/.
[38] Aziz Q, Harris LA, Goodman BP, et al. AGA Clinical Practice Update on GI Manifestations and Autonomic or Immune Dysfunction in Hypermobile Ehlers-Danlos Syndrome: Expert Review. *Clin Gastroenterol Hepatol.* 2025;23(8):1291-1302.
[39] McNeil BD, Pundir P, Meeker S, et al. Identification of a mast-cell-specific receptor crucial for pseudo-allergic drug reactions. *Nature.* 2015 Mar 12;519(7542):237-41.
[40] Ye D, Xhang Y, Zhao X, et al. MRGPRX2 gain-of-function mutation drives enhanced mast cell reactivity in chronic spontaneous urticaria. *JACI.* 2025 Jul;156(1):159-70.
[41] Mousavizadeh R, Waugh CM, McCormack RG, et al. MRGPRX2-mediated mast cell activation by substance P from overloaded human tenocytes induces inflammatory and degenerative responses in tendons. *Sco Reports.* 2024 Jun 12;14(13540).
[42] Shirvani P, Shirvani A, Holick MF. Decoding the Genetic Basis of Mast Cell Hypersensitivity and Infection Risk in Hypermobile Ehlers-Danlos Syndrome. *Curr Issues Mol Biol.* 2024 Oct 16;46(10):11613-29.
[43] Monaco A, Choi D, Uzun S, et al. Association of mast-cell-related conditions with hypermobile syndromes: a review of the literature. *Nature.* 2022;70:419-31.

[44] Afrin LB. *Never Bet Against Occam: Mast Cell Activation Disease and the Modern Epidemics of Chronic Illness and Medical Complexity*. Sisters Media, 2016.
[45] Afrin LB. Presentation, Diagnosis, and Management of Mast Cell Activation Syndrome. In: Mast Cells: Methods and Protocols. *Mast Cells*. 2013 Apr;1220:155-232.
[46] Molderings GJ, Brettner S, Homann J, Afrin LB. Mast cell activation disease: a concise practical guide for diagnostic workup and therapeutic options. *Deutsche Medizinische Wochenschrift*. 2014;139:1523-34.
[47] Hakim A, Wandele ID, O'Callaghan C, et al. Chronic fatigue in Ehlers-Danlos syndrome—Hypermobile type. *AJMG*. 2017 Mar;175(1):175-80.
[48] De Wandele I, Rombaut L, Leybaert L, et al. Dysautonomia and its underlying mechanisms in the hypermobility type of Ehlers-Danlos syndrome. *Semin Arthritis Rheum*. 2014;44(1):93–100.
[49] Castori M, Celletti C, Camerota F. Ehlers-Danlos syndrome hypermobility type: a possible unifying concept for various functional somatic syndromes. *Rheumatol Int*. 2013;33(3):819–821.
[50] Clauw DJ. Fibromyalgia: A Clinical Review. *JAMA*. 2014;311(15):1547–1555.
[51] Leone CM, Di Stefano G, Celletti C, et al. Central sensitization as the mechanism underlying pain in joint hypermobility syndrome/Ehlers–Danlos syndrome, hypermobility type. *Eur J Pain*. 2016;20(8):1319–1325.
[52] Skaper SD, Facci L, Giusti P. Mast cells, glia and neuroinflammation: partners in crime? Neurosci Biobehavior Rev. 2017 Aug;79:119-33.
[53] Institute of Medicine (now National Academy of Medicine). *Beyond Myalgic Encephalomyelitis/Chronic Fatigue Syndrome: Redefining an Illness*. National Academies Press, 2015.
[54] Theoharides TC, Tsilioni I, Ren H. Recent advances in our understanding of mast cell activation—or should it be mast cell mediator disorders? *Expert Rev Clin Immunol*. 2019 Jun;15(6):639-656.
[55] Komaroff AL, Lipkin WI. Insights from ME/CFS may help unravel the pathogenesis of post-acute COVID-19 syndrome. 2021 Jun 7;27(9):895–906.
[56] Komaroff AL, Lipkin WI. Insights from myalgic encephalomyelitis/chronic fatigue syndrome may help unravel the pathogenesis of postacute COVID-19 syndrome. *Trends in Molecular Medicine*. 2021 Jun 7;27(9):895–906.
[57] Wisk LE, L'Hommedieu M, Roldan KD. Variability in Long COVID Definitions and Validation of Published Prevalence Rates. *JAMA Netw Open*. 2025 Aug 12;8(8):e2526506.
[58] Halas RG, Vaduva DMB, Radulescu M, et al. Long COVID Prevalence and Risk Factors: A Systematic Review and Meta-Analysis of Prospective Cohort Studies. 2025 Nov;13(12):2859.
[59] Weinstock LB, Brook JB, Walters AS, et al. Mast cell activation symptoms are prevalent in Long-COVID. *Int J Infect Diseases*. 2021 Nov;112:103-110.
[60] Budnevsky AV, Avdeev SN, Kosanovic D, et al. Involvement of Mast Cells in the Pathology of COVID-19: Clinical and Laboratory Parallels. *Cells*. 2024 Apr 19;13(8):711.
[61] Dorward DA, Russell CD, Um IH, et al. Tissue-specific immunopathology in fatal COVID-19. *Am J Respiratory Critical Care Med*. 2020;203(2).
[62] Motta Junior JDS, et al. Mast cells in alveolar septa of COVID-19 patients: a pathogenic pathway that may link interstitial edema to immunothrombosis. *Front Immunol*. 2020;11.
[63] Zhang S, Xu CL, Wang J, et al. Spike proteins of coronaviruses activate mast cells for degranulation via stimulating Src/PI3K/AKT/Ca2+ intracellular signaling cascade. *J Virol*. 2025 Apr 30;99(5):e00078-25.
[64] Theoharides TC, Alysandratos KD, Angelidou A, et al. Mast cells and inflammation. *Biochim Biophys Acta*. 2012 Jan;1822(1):21-33.
[65] Javan MR, Akhlaghi M, Hormozi A, et al. Mast cells in autoimmune disease: Unveiling their multifaceted roles and therapeutic potential. *Hum Immunol*. 2025 Jul;86(4):111334.
[66] Afrin LB. Presentation, Diagnosis, and Management of Mast Cell Activation Syndrome. In: Mast Cells: Methods and Protocols. *Methods Mol Biol*. 2015;1220:405–438.
[67] Wang E, Ganti T, Vaou E, et al. The relationship between mast cell activation syndrome, postural tachycardia syndrome, and Ehlers–Danlos syndrome. *Allergy Asthma Proc*. 2021 May 1;42(3):243-246.
[68] Fratzl P. (Ed.). *Collagen: Structure and Mechanics*. Springer, 2008.
[69] Hynes RO. The extracellular matrix: not just pretty fibrils. *Science*. 2009;326(5957):1216–1219.
[70] Tinkle B, Castori M, Berglund B, et al. Hypermobile Ehlers–Danlos syndrome (a.k.a. Ehlers–Danlos syndrome Type III and Ehlers–Danlos syndrome hypermobility type): Clinical description and natural history.
Am J Med Genet C Semin Med Genet. 2017 Mar:48-69.

[71] Gregersen PK, Olsson LM. Recent advances in the genetics of autoimmune disease. *Annu Rev Immunol.* 2009;27:363-91.
[72] Galli SJ, Gaudenzio N, Tsai M. Mast cells in inflammation and disease: Recent Progress and Ongoing Concerns. *Nat Rev Immunol.* 2020 Apr 26:38:49-77.
[73] Piliponsky AM, Acharya M, Shubin NJ. Mast Cells in Viral, Bacterial, and Fungal Infection Immunity. *Int J Mol Sci.* 2019 Jun 12;20(12):2851.
[74] Felitti VJ, Anda RF, Nordenberg D, et al. Relationship of Childhood Abuse and Household Dysfunction to Many of the Leading Causes of Death in Adults: The Adverse Childhood Experiences (ACE) Study. *Am J Prev Med.* 1998;14(4):245–258.
[75] Gunnar MR, Quevedo K. The neurobiology of stress and development. *Annu Rev Psychol.* 2007;58:145–173.
[76] Danese A, Pariante CM, Caspi A, et al. Childhood maltreatment predicts adult inflammation. *PNAS.* 2007 Jan;104(4):1319–1324.
[77] Thayer JF, Sternberg EM. Beyond heart rate variability: vagal regulation of allostatic systems. *Ann N Y Acad Sci.* 2006 Nov;1088:361-72.
[78] Theoharides TC, Cochrane DE. Critical role of mast cells in inflammatory diseases and the effect of acute stress. *J Neuroimmunol.* 2004 Jan;146(1–2):1–12.
[79] Maintz L, Novak N. Histamine and histamine intolerance. *Am J Clin Nutr.* 2007;85(5):1185–1196.
[80] Reese I, Ballmer-Weber B, Beyer K, et al. German guideline for the management of adverse reactions to ingested histamine. *Allergo J Int.* 2017 Feb;26:72-79.
[81] Maintz L, Novak N. Histamine and histamine intolerance. *Am J Clin Nutr.* 2007;85(5):1185–1196.
[82] Theoharides TC, Cochrane DE. Critical role of mast cells in inflammatory diseases and the effect of acute stress. *J Neuroimmunol.* 2004 Jan;146(1–2):1–12.
[83] Maintz L, Novak N. Histamine and histamine intolerance. *Am J Clin Nutr.* 2007;85(5):1185–1196.
[84] Vally H, Misso NL. Adverse reactions to the sulphite additives. *Gastroenterol Hepatol Bed Bench.* 2012 Winter;5(1):16–23.
[85] Fasano A. Leaky gut and autoimmune diseases. *Clin Rev Allergy Immunol.* 2012;42:71-78.
[86] Sapone A, Bai JC, Ciacci C, et al. Spectrum of gluten-related disorders: consensus on new nomenclature and classification. BMC Med. 2012;10(13).
[87] Marino M, Mele E, Viggiano A, et al. Pleiotropic Outcomes of Glyphosate Exposure: From Organ Damage to Effects on Inflammation, Cancer, Reproduction and Development. *Int J Mol Sci.* 2021 Nov 22;22(22):12606.
[88] Lehman PC, Cady N, Ghimire S, et al. Low-dose glyphosate exposure alters gut microbiota composition and modulates gut homeostasis. *Environ Toxicol Pharmacol.* 2023 May 15;100:104149.
[89] Afrin LB. Presentation, Diagnosis, and Management of Mast Cell Activation Syndrome. In: Mast Cells: Methods and Protocols. *Methods Mol Biol.* 2015;1220:405–438.
[90] Theoharides TC, Cochrane DE. Critical role of mast cells in inflammatory diseases and the effect of acute stress. *J Neuroimmunol.* 2004 Jan;146(1–2):1–12.
[91] Irwin MR, Opp MR. Sleep health: reciprocal regulation of sleep and innate immunity. *Nat Rev Immunol.* 2017;17(12):745–753.
[92] Afrin LB. Presentation, Diagnosis, and Management of Mast Cell Activation Syndrome. In: Mast Cells: Methods and Protocols. *Methods Mol Biol.* 2015;1220:405–438.
[93] Kritas SK, Gallenga CE, Ovidio CD, et al. Impact of mold on mast cell-cytokine immune response. *J Biol Regul Homeost Agents.* 2018 Jul-Aug;32(4):763-768.
[94] Makrufadi F, Peng SW, Chung KF, et al. Extreme temperatures modulate gene expression in the airway epithelium of the lungs in mice and asthma patients. *Front Med Sec Pulmonary Med.* 2025 Apr;12.
[95] Wang R, Yin X, Zhang H, et al. Effects of a Moderately Lower Temperature on the Proliferation and Degranulation of Rat Mast Cells. *J Immunol Res.* 2016 Apr 18;2016:8439594.
[96] Mastcellsunited.com. MCAS and EMFs: Do they matter? Accessed March 20, 2026 from https://mastcellsunited.com/2017/12/14/mcas-and-emfs-do-they-matter/.
[97] Bircham D. Mast Cell Activation: MCAS and Environmental Pollution - The Toxic Truth. Accessed March 20, 2026 from: https://www.mastcellaction.org/assets/_/2025/04/21/daed2066-372f-4aa1-91bd-10a4d23ab98a/mcas-and-environmental-pollution-the-toxic-truth.pdf?v=1.
[98] Zaitsu M, Narita S, Lambert KC, et al. Estradiol activates mast cells via a non-genomic estrogen receptor-α and calcium influx. *J Immunol.* 2007;178(5): 2920–2927.
[99] Landucci E, Laurino A, Cinci L, et al. Thyroid Hormone, Thyroid Hormone Metabolites and Mast Cells: A Less Explored Issue. *Front Cell Neurosci.* 2019 Mar 29;13:79.

[100] Papa V, Li Pomi F, Gioacchino MD, et al. Mast Cells and Microbiome in Health and Disease. *IMR Press.* 2025 Mar 20.
[101] Barcik W, Wawrzyniak M, Akdis CA, O'Mahony L. Immune regulation by histamine and histamine-secreting bacteria. Curr Opin Immunol. *2017 Oct:48:108-113.*
[102] Dahlin JS, Hallgren J. Mast cell progenitors: Origin, development and migration to tissues. *Mol Immunol.* 2015 Jan;63(1):9-17.
[103] Camilleri M. Leaky gut: mechanisms, measurement and clinical implications in humans. *Gut.* 2019 Aug;68(8):1516-1526.
[104] Bischoff SC, Barnara G, Buurman W, et al. Intestinal permeability--a new target for disease prevention and therapy. *BMC Gastroenterol.* 2014 Nov 18:14:189.
[105] Seethaler B, Basari M, Neyrinck AM, et al. Biomarkers for assessment of intestinal permeability in clinical practice. *Am J Physiol-Gastrointestinal Liver Physiol.* 2024;321(11):G11-G17.
[106] Wallon C, Yang P–C, Keita AV, et al. Corticotropin-releasing hormone regulates macromolecular permeability via mast cells in human colonic mucosa. *Gut.* 2008;57(1):50–58.
[107] Peng L, Zhong-Rong L, Green RS, et al. Butyrate enhances the intestinal barrier by facilitating tight junction assembly via activation of AMPK. *J Nutr.* 2009 Sep;139(9):1619–1625.
[108] Levy M, et al. Dysbiosis and the immune system. *Nature Rev Immunol.* 2017 Mar;17(4):219–232.
[109] Chassaing B, Koren O, Goodricj JK, et al. Dietary emulsifiers impact the mouse gut microbiota promoting colitis and metabolic syndrome. *Nature.* 2015 Mar 5;519(7541):92–96.
[110] Fasano A.Zonulin and its regulation of intestinal barrier function: the biological door to inflammation.
Physiol Rev. 2011 Jan;91(1):151-75.
[111] Patel S, Behera R, Swanson GR, et al. Alcohol and the intestine. *Biomolecules.* 2015 Oct 14;5(4):10.3390.
[112] Bishehsari F, Magno E, Swanson G, et al. Alcohol and gut-derived inflammation. *Alcohol Res.* 2017;38(2):163–171.
[113] Bjarnason I, Peters TJ. Intestinal permeability, non-steroidal anti-inflammatory drug enteropathy and inflammatory bowel disease: an overview. *Gut.* 1989 Nov;30(Spec No):22-28.
[114] Wallace JL. NSAID gastropathy and enteropathy: distinct pathogenesis likely necessitates distinct prevention strategies. *Br J Pharmacol.* 2012 Jan;165(1):67-74.
[115] Imhann F, Bonder MJ, Vila AV, et al. Proton pump inhibitors affect the gut microbiome. *Gut.* 2016 May;65(5):740-8.
[116] Bischoff SC, Barnara G, Buurman W, et al. Intestinal permeability--a new target for disease prevention and therapy. *BMC Gastroenterol.* 2014 Nov 18:14:189.
[117] Turner JR. Intestinal mucosal barrier function in health and disease. *Nat Rev Immunol.* 2009 Nov;9(11):799–809.
[118] Akbari P, Barber S, Varasteh S, et al. The intestinal barrier as an emerging target in the toxicological assessment of mycotoxins. *Archives Toxicol.* 2016 Jul;91:1007-1029.
[119] Allain T, Amat CB, Motta JP, et al. Interactions of Giardia sp. with the intestinal barrier: Epithelium, mucus, and microbiota. *Tissue Barriers.* 2017 Jan 3;5(1):e1274354.
[120] Bischoff SC, Barnara G, Buurman W, et al. Intestinal permeability--a new target for disease prevention and therapy. *BMC Gastroenterol.* 2014 Nov 18:14:189.
[121] Turner JR. Intestinal mucosal barrier function in health and disease. *Nat Rev Immunol.* 2009 Nov;9(11):799–809.
[122] Bilgic HK, Bek M, Kleuskens M, et al. Mast cells in digestive diseases: New insights to keep them under control. *Pharmacol Res.* 2026 Jan;223:108069.
[123] Musa MA, Kabir M, Hossain MI, et al. Measurement of intestinal permeability using lactulose and mannitol with conventional five hours and shortened two hours urine collection by two different methods: HPAE-PAD and LC-MSMS. *PLoS One.* 2019 Aug 8;14(8):e0220397.
[124] Fasano A. Intestinal Permeability and its Regulation by Zonulin: Diagnostic and Therapeutic Implications. *Clin Gastroenterol Hepatol.* 2012 Aug 16;10(10):1096–1100.
[125] Fasano A. All disease begins in the (leaky) gut: role of zonulin-mediated gut permeability in the pathogenesis of some chronic inflammatory diseases. *F1000Res.* 2020 Jan 31;9:F1000 Faculty Rev-69. [Version 1]
[126] Massier L, Chakaroun R, Kovacs P, et al. Blurring the picture in leaky gut research: how shortcomings of zonulin as a biomarker mislead the field of intestinal permeability. *Gut.* 2020 Oct 9;70(9):1801–1802.

[127] González-Quintela A, Alonso M, Campos J, et al. Determinants of serum concentrations of lipopolysaccharide-binding protein (LBP) in the adult population: the role of obesity. *PLoS One.* 2013;8(1):e54600.
[128] Vreugdenhil AC, Snoek AMP, van 't Veer C. et al. (2003). LPS-binding protein circulates in association with apoB-containing lipoproteins and enhances endotoxin-LDL/VLDL interaction. *J Clin Invest.* 2001 Jan 15;107(2):225–234.
[129] Bischoff SC, Barnara G, Buurman W, et al. Intestinal permeability--a new target for disease prevention and therapy. *BMC Gastroenterol.* 2014 Nov 18:14:189.
[130] Sender R, Fuchs S, Milo R. Revised estimates for the number of human and bacteria cells in the body. *PLOS Biology.* 2006;14(8):e1002533.
[131] Fiorani M, del Vecchio LE, Dargenio P, et al. Histamine-producing bacteria and their role in gastrointestinal disorders. *Exp Rev Gastroenterol Hepatol.* 2023 Jul 6;17(7):709-18.
[132] Thomas CM,Hong T, van Pijkeren JP, et al. Histamine derived from probiotic Lactobacillus reuteri suppresses TNF via modulation of PKA and ERK signaling. *PLoS ONE.* 2012;7(2):e31951.
[133] Mazzoli R, Pessione E. The neuro-endocrinological role of microbial glutamate and GABA signaling.
Front Microbiol. 2016 Nov;7(1934).
[134] Wunderlichová L, Bunkova L, Koutny M, et al. Formation, degradation, and detoxification of putrescine, cadaverine, and histamine by foodborne bacteria. *Comp Rev Food Sci Food Safety.* 2014 Aug;3(5):1010–1033.
[135] Ozogul F. Production of biogenic amines by Morganella morganii, Klebsiella pneumoniae and Hafnia alvei using a rapid HPLC method. *Eur Food Res Tech.* 2004 Aug 25;219:465-69.
[136] Kalhotka L, Manga I, Prichystalova J, et al. Decarboxylase activity test of the genus Enterococcus isolated from goat milk and cheese. *Acta Vet Brno.* 2012;81:145-51.
[137] Wisniewski P, Barbieri F. Molecular Identification and Biogenic Amine Production Capacity of Enterococcus faecalis. *Int J Mol Sci.* 2025 Oct 28;26(21):10480.
[138] Oksaharju A, Kankainen M, Kekkonen RA, et al. Probiotic Lactobacillus rhamnosus downregulates FCER1 and HRH4 expression in human mast cells. *World J Gastroenterol.* 2011 Feb 14;17(6):750–759.
[139] Liu Y, Zhou X, Ye W, et al. Effect of Lactobacillus rhamnosus LZ260E on allergic symptoms and intestinal microbiota in β-lactoglobulin–sensitized mice. *J Funct Foods.* 2024 Feb;113:106045.
[140] Thomas CM, Hong T, van Pijkeren JP, et al. Histamine derived from probiotic Lactobacillus reuteri suppresses TNF via Modulation of PKA and ERK Signaling. *PLoS One.* 2012 Feb 22;7(2):e31951.
[141] Landete JM, Ferrer S, Pardo I. Biogenic amine production by lactic acid bacteria, acetic bacteria and yeast isolated from wine. *Food Control.* 2007 Dec;18(12):1569-74.
[142] Xia B, Zhang R, Wang X, et al. Lactobacillus plantarum modulates intestinal homeostasis through tryptophan metabolism-AhR signaling axis. *J Future Foods.* 2025 Oct 25. Online ahead of print.
[143] Kung HF, Lee YC, Huang YL, et al. Degradation of Histamine by Lactobacillus plantarum Isolated from Miso Products. *J food Protect.*
[144] Abdulqadir R, Engers J, Al-Sadi R. Role of Bifidobacterium in Modulating the Intestinal Epithelial Tight Junction Barrier: Current Knowledge and Perspectives. *Curr Develop Nutr.* 2023 Dec;7(12):102026.
[145] Yang Y, Song X, Wang G, et al. Understanding Ligilactobacillus salivarius from Probiotic Properties to Omics Technology: A Review. 2024;13(6):895.
[146] Kalkan AE, BinMowyna MN, Raposo A, et al. Beyond the Gut: Unveiling Butyrate's Global Health Impact Through Gut Health and Dysbiosis-Related Conditions: A Narrative Review. *Nutrients.* 2025 Apr 9;17(8):1305.
[147] Cortes M, Olate P, Rodriguez R, et al. Human Microbiome as an Immunoregulatory Axis: Mechanisms, Dysbiosis, and Therapeutic Modulation. *Microorganisms.* 2025;13(9):2147.
[148] Dicks LMT. Gut Bacteria and Neurotransmitters. *Microorganisms.* 2022 Sep 14;10(9):1838.
[149] Hou Y, Li J, Ying S. Tryptophan Metabolism and Gut Microbiota: A Novel Regulatory Axis Integrating the Microbiome, Immunity, and Cancer. *Metabolites.* 2023 Nov 20;13(11):1166.
[150] Staller K, Olen O, Soderling J, et al. Mortality risk in irritable bowel syndrome: results from a nationwide, prospective cohort study. *Am J Gastroenterol.* 2020 May;115(5):746–755.
[151] Lee KN, Lee OY. The Role of Mast Cells in Irritable Bowel Syndrome. *Gastroenterol Res Pract.* 2016 Dec 28;2016:2031480.

[152] Wouters MM, Vicario M, Santos J. The role of mast cells in functional GI disorders. *Gut.* 2015;65(1):155-68.
[153] Aguilera-Lizarranga J, Hussein H, Boeckxstens GE. Immune activation in irritable bowel syndrome: what is the evidence? *Nat Rev Immunol.* 2022;22:674-86.
[154] Calderone RA, Fonzi WA. Virulence factors of Candida albicans. *Trends Microbiol.* 2001 Jul;9(7):327-35.
[155] Mayer FL, Wilson D, Hube B. Candida albicans pathogenicity mechanisms. *Virulence.* 2013 Jan 9;4(2):119–128.
[156] Gow NAR, van de Veerdonk FL, Brown AJP, et al. Candida albicans morphogenesis and host defence: discriminating invasion from colonization. *Nature Rev Microbiol.* 2012;10(2):112–122.
[157] Tillonen J, Homann N, Rautio M, et al. Role of yeasts in the salivary acetaldehyde production from ethanol among risk groups for ethanol-associated oral cavity cancer. *Alcoholism Clin Exp Res.* 1999 Aug;23(8):1409-15.
[158] Droracel.ai. Does Small Intestine Fungal Overgrowth (SIFO) theoretically increase acetaldehyde levels? Accessed March 23, 2026 from: https://www.droracle.ai/articles/792998/does-small-intestine-fungal-overgrowth-sifo-theoretically-increase-acetaldehyde.
[159] Alemany-Fortes M, Bori J, Muguerza B, et al. Diamine oxidase deficiency implications for health, current management, and future directions in the treatment of histamine intolerance: A review. *Int J Biol Macromol.* 2025 Oct;327(Pt 1):147130.
[160] Schnedl WJ, Schenk M, Lackner S, et al. Diamine oxidase supplementation improves symptoms in patients with histamine intolerance. *Food Sci Biotechnol.* 2019 May 24;28(6):1779–1784.
[161] Geng ZH, Zhu Y, Li QL, et al. Enteric Nervous System: The Bridge Between the Gut Microbiota and Neurological Disorders. *Front Aging Neurosci.* 2022 Apr 19;14:810483.
[162] Planchette A, Gantar I, Scholler J, et al. enGLOW 3D microscopy of the enteric nervous system in cleared human and mouse gut. *Commun Biol.* 2026 Feb;9(357).
[163] Mohebali N, Weigel M, Hain T, et al. Faecalibacterium prausnitzii, Bacteroides faecis and Roseburia intestinalis attenuate clinical symptoms of experimental colitis by regulating Treg/Th17 cell balance and intestinal barrier integrity. *Biomed Pharmacol.* 2023 Nov;167:115568.
[164] Galli SJ, Tsai M, Piliponsky AM. The development of allergic inflammation. *Nature.* 2008;454:445–454.
[165] Theoharides TC, Alysandratos KD, Angelidou A, et al. Mast cells and inflammation. *Biochim Biophys Acta.* 2012 Jan;1822(1):21-33.
[166] U.S. Centers for Disease Control and Prevention. Lyme Disease. Accessed March 23, 2026 from: https://www.cdc.gov/lyme/signs-symptoms/chronic-symptoms-and-lyme-disease.html?CDC_AAref_Val=https://www.cdc.gov/lyme/postlds/index.html.
[167] Talkington J, Nickell SP. Borrelia burgdorferi Spirochetes Induce Mast Cell Activation and Cytokine Release. *Infect Immun.* 1999 Mar;67(3):1107–1115.
[168] No author listed. Lyme Neuroborreliosis. Accessed March 23, 2026 from: https://www.sciencedirect.com/topics/pharmacology-toxicology-and-pharmaceutical-science/lyme-neuroborreliosis.
[169] Rocha SC, Velasquez CV, Aquib A, et al. Transmission Cycle of Tick-Borne Infections and Co-Infections, Animal Models and Diseases. *Pathogens.* 2022 Nov 8;11(11):1309.
[170] Deng H, Pang Q, Zhao B, et al. Molecular Mechanisms of Bartonella and Mammalian Erythrocyte Interactions: A Review. *Front Cell Infect Microbiol.* 2018 Dec 12;8:431.
[171] Vumbaco N. Bartonella and Mast Cell Activation Syndrome (MCAS). Accessed March 23, 2026 from: https://www.battlingbartonellosis.com/post/mast-cell-activation-syndrome.
[172] Delaney S, Robveille C, Maggi RG, et al. Bartonella species bacteremia in association with adult psychosis. *Front Psychiatry.* 2024 Jun 7;15:1388442.
[173] Beydon M, Rodriguez C, Karras A, et al. Bartonella and Coxiella infections presenting as systemic vasculitis: case series and review of literature. *Rheumatology (Oxford).* 2022 May 30;61(6):2609-2618.
[174] Maluki A, Breitschwerdt E, Bemis L, et al. Imaging analysis of Bartonella species in the skin using single-photon and multi-photon (second harmonic generation) laser scanning microscopy. *Clin Case Rep.* 2020 Jul 19;8(8):1564-1570.
[175] Chen F, Fu S, Jiang J-f, et al. Persistent human babesiosis with low-grade parasitemia, challenges for clinical diagnosis and management. *Heliyon.* 2024 Nov 3;10(22):e39960.
[176] Merck Manual Professional Version. Ehrlichiosis and Anaplasmosis. Accessed March 23, 2026 from: https://www.merckmanuals.com/professional/infectious-diseases/rickettsiae-and-related-organisms/ehrlichiosis-and-anaplasmosis.

[177] Cohen JI. Herpesvirus latency. *J Clin Invest.* 2020 Jul 1;130(7):3361-3369.
[178] Damiana B, Kenney SC, Raab-Traub N. Epstein-Barr Virus (EBV): Biology and Clinical Disease. *Cell.* 2022 Sep 15;185(20):3652–3670.
[179] Ruiz-Pablos M, Paiva B, Zabaleta A. Epstein–Barr virus-acquired immunodeficiency in myalgic encephalomyelitis—Is it present in long COVID? *J Translational Med.* 2023 Sep;21(633).
[180] Realegeno S, Pandey U. Human Herpesvirus 6 Infection and Diagnostics. *Clin Microbiol Newsletter.* 2022 May;44(9):83-90.
[181] Bolle LD, Naesens L, Clercq ED. Update on Human Herpesvirus 6 Biology, Clinical Features, and Therapy. *Clin Microbiol Rev.* 2005 Jan;18(1):217–245.
[182] Piotrowski SL, Allnutt MA, Johnson K, et al. Herpesvirus genome integration in whole-genome sequences of dementia and control cohorts. *Alzheimers Dement.* 2026 Mar;22(3):e71047.
[183] Mariani M, Zimmerman C, Rodriguez P, et al. Higher-Order Chromatin Structures of Chromosomally Integrated HHV-6A Predict Integration Sites. *Front Cell Infect Microbiol.* 2021 Feb 26;11:612656.
[184] Zhang E, Bell AJ, Wilkie GS, et al. Inherited Chromosomally Integrated Human Herpesvirus 6 Genomes Are Ancient, Intact, and Potentially Able To Reactivate from Telomeres. *J Virology.* 2017 Oct;91(22).
[185] Clark DA. Clinical and laboratory features of human herpesvirus 6 chromosomal integration. *Clin Microbiol Infect.* 2016 Apr;22(4):333-9.
[186] Varani S, Pandini MP. Cytomegalovirus-induced immunopathology and its clinical consequences. *Herpesviridae.* 2011 Apr 7;2:6.
[187] Mihalic A, Zeleznjak J, Lisnic B, et al. Immune surveillance of cytomegalovirus in tissues. *Cell Mol Immunol.* 2024 Aug;21:959-81.
[188] Gandhi MK, Khanna R. Human cytomegalovirus: clinical aspects, immune regulation, and emerging treatments. *Lancet Infect Dis.* 2004 Dec;4(12):725-38.
[189] Costerton JW, Stewart PS, Greenberg EP. Bacterial biofilms: a common cause of persistent infections. *Science.* 1999;284(5418):1318–1322.
[190] Stewart PS, Costerton JW. Antibiotic resistance of bacteria in biofilms. *Lancet.* 2001;358(9276):135–138.
[191] Thakur A, Mikkelsen H, Jungersen G. Intracellular Pathogens: Host Immunity and Microbial Persistence Strategies. *J Immunol Res.* 2019 Apr 14;2019:1356540.
[192] Galli SJ, Tsai M. Mast cells in allergy and infection: versatile effector and regulatory cells in innate and adaptive immunity. *Eur J Immunol.* 2010 Jul;40(7):1843–1851.
[193] Proal AD, VanElzakker MB. Pathogens accelerate features of human aging: A review of molecular mechanisms. *Ageing Res Rev.* 2025 Dec;112:102865.
[194] Abraham SN, St John AL. Mast cell–orchestrated immunity to pathogens. *Nature Rev Immunol.* 2010 Jun;10(6):440–452.
[195] Talkington J, Nickell SP. Borrelia burgdorferi induces mast cell activation and cytokine release. *Infect Immunity.* 2001;69(11):6936–6942.
[196] Kritas SK, Gallenga CE, Ovidio CD, et al. Impact of mold on mast cell-cytokine immune response. *J Biol Regul Homeost Agents.* 2018 Jul-Aug;32(4):763-768.
[197] Adhikari M, Negi B, Kaushik N, et al. T-2 mycotoxin: toxicological effects and decontamination strategies. *Oncotarget.* 2017 Feb 16;8(20):33933–33952.
[198] Benkerroum N. Chronic and Acute Toxicities of Aflatoxins: Mechanisms of Action. *Int J Environ Res Public Health.* 2020 Jan 8;17(2):423.
[199] Zhou Y, Chen W, Feng S, et al. Ochratoxin A-induced mitochondrial pathway apoptosis and ferroptosis by promoting glycolysis. *Apoptosis.* 2025 Jun;30(5-6):1440-1452.
[200] Pestka JJ. Deoxynivalenol: mechanisms of action, human exposure, and toxicological relevance. *Arch Toxicol.* 2010 Sep;84(9):663–679.
[201] Mehrzad J, Bahari A, Basmami MR, et al. Data on environmentally relevant level of aflatoxin B 1 - induced human dendritic cells' functional alteration. *Data Brief.* 2018 Apr 30;18:1576–1580.
[202] Kipkoech G, Jepkorir M, Kamau S, et al. Immunomodulatory effects of aflatoxin B1 (AFB1) and the use of natural products to ameliorate its immunotoxic effects: A review. *Open Res Afr.* 2025 Feb 7:6:22.
[203] Petzinger E, Ziegler K. Ochratoxin A from a toxicological perspective. J Vet Pharmacol Ther. 2000 Apr;23(2):91–98.
[204] Assunção R, et al. Challenges in risk assessment of multiple mycotoxins in food. *World Mycotoxin J.* 2016 Nov;9(5):791-811.

[205] Traherne JA. Human MHC architecture and evolution: implications for disease association studies. *Int J Immunogenet.* 2008 Apr;35(3):179–192.
[206] Shoemaker RT, MD. *Surviving mold: life in the era of dangerous buildings.* Baltimore, MD: Otter Bay Books; 2010.
[207] Chariewicz AE, Omeljaniuk WJ, Garley M, et al. Mercury Exposure and Health Effects: What Do We Really Know? *Int J Mol Sci.* 2025;26(5):2326.
[208] Kempuraj D, Asadi S, Zhang B, et al. Mercury induces inflammatory mediator release from human mast cells. *J Neuroinflammation.* 2010 Mar 11;7:20.
[209] Pounds JG, Long GJ, Rosen JF. Cellular and molecular toxicity of lead in bone. *Environ Health Perspect.* 1991 Feb;91:17–32.
[210] Goyer RA. Toxic effects of metals. In: Klaassen CD (ed). *Casarett and Doull's Toxicology: The Basic Science of Poisons.* 8th ed. McGraw-Hill; 2013.
[211] Flora SJ, Gupta D, Tiwari A. Toxicity of lead: a review with recent updates. *Interdisciplinary Toxicol.* 2012;5(2):47–58.
[212] Zahoor SM, Ishaq S, Ahmed T. Neurotoxic effects of metals on blood brain barrier impairment and possible therapeutic approaches. *Vitam Horm.* 2024:126:1-24.
[213] Liu JT, Dong MH, Chen LW, et al. Microglia and astroglia: the role of neuroinflammation in lead toxicity and neuronal injury in the brain. *Neuroimmunol Neuroinflamm.* 2015 Jul;2:156980.
[214] Chen G, Han B, Nan W, et al. Cadmium Tolerance and Detoxification Mechanisms of Lentinula edodes: Physiology, Subcellular Distribution, and Chemical Forms. *Microorganisms.* 2025 Jan;13(1):62.
[215] Hutchinson LM. Inorganic Arsenite Inhibits Allergic Signal Transduction in Mast Cells. Thesis. Accessed March 23, 2026 from: https://digitalcommons.library.umaine.edu/etd/660/.
[216] Krystel-Whittemore M, Dileepan KN, Wood JG. Mast cell: a multi-functional master cell. *Front Immunol.* 2016;6:620.
[217] Cadez T, Kolic D, Sinko G, et al. Assessment of four organophosphorus pesticides as inhibitors of human acetylcholinesterase and butyrylcholinesterase. *Sci Reports.* 2021;11(21586).
[218] Cunha Ignacio AD, Reis Guerra AMD, de Souza-Silca TG, et al. Effects of glyphosate exposure on intestinal microbiota, metabolism and microstructure: a systematic review. *Food Funct.* 2024 Jul 29;15(15):7757-7781.
[219] Mertens M, Hoss S, Neumann G, et al. Glyphosate, a chelating agent—relevant for ecological risk assessment? *Environ Sci Eur.* 2018;30:2.
[220] Dalamaga M, Kounatidis D, Tsinilgiris D, et al. The Role of Endocrine Disruptors Bisphenols and Phthalates in Obesity: Current Evidence, Perspectives and Controversies. *Int J Mol Sci.* 2024 Jan 4;25(1):675.
[221] McCall JR, Sausman KT, Mead RN. Per- and polyfluoroalkyl substances (PFAS) alter immune responses from THP-1 human monocytes. *Environ Toxicol Pharmacol.* 2026 Mar;122:104938.
[222] Noyes TS, Abington LM, 't Evre TJ, et al. Per and polyfluoroalkyl substances affect thyroid hormones for people with a history of exposure from drinking water. *Sci Rep.* 2025 Apr;15(12502).
[223] Hananeh WM, Ghbari FAA, Rukibat RA, et al. Effects of fake and original perfumes on the presence, numbers, and distribution of mast cells in selected tissues in rats. *Open Vet J.* 2021 Jun 6;11(2):277–282.
[224] Ma Q. Role of nrf2 in oxidative stress and toxicity. *Annu Rev Pharmacol Toxicol.* 2013:53:401-26.
[225] Tracey KJ. The inflammatory reflex. *Nature.* 2002;420(6917):853–859.
[226] Wessler I, Kirkpatrick CJ. Acetylcholine beyond neurons: the non-neuronal cholinergic system in humans.
Br J Pharmacol. 2008;154(8):1558–1571.
[227] Arnsten AFT. Stress signalling pathways that impair prefrontal cortex structure and function. *Nature Rev Neuroscience.* 2009;10(6):410–422.
[228] Cao J, Papadopoulou N, Kempuraj D, et al. Human mast cells express corticotropin-releasing hormone (CRH) receptors and CRH leads to selective secretion of vascular endothelial growth factor. *J Immunol.* 2005 Jun 15;174(12):7665-75.
[229] Kempuraj D, Papadppoulou NG, Lytinas M, et al. Corticotropin-Releasing Hormone and Its Structurally Related Urocortin Are Synthesized and Secreted by Human Mast Cell. *Endocrinol.* 2004 Jan;145(1):43-48.
[230] Shonkoff JP, Boyce WT, McEwen BS. Neuroscience, molecular biology, and the childhood roots of health disparities: building a new framework for health promotion and disease prevention. *JAMA.* 2009;301(21):2252–2259.

[231] Hughes K, Bellis MA, Hardcastle KA, et al. The effect of multiple adverse childhood experiences on health: a systematic review and meta-analysis. *The Lancet Public Health*. 2017;2(8):e356–e366.
[232] Turecki G, Meaney MJ. Effects of the social environment and stress on glucocorticoid receptor gene methylation: a systematic review. *Biol Psych*. 2016;79(2):87–96.
[233] Giridharan VVm De Quevedo CEB, Petronilho F. Microbiota-gut-brain axis in the Alzheimer's disease pathology - an overview. *Neurosci Res*. 2022 Aug;181:17-21.
[234] Borovikova LV, Ivanova S, Zhang M, et al. Vagus nerve stimulation attenuates the systemic inflammatory response to endotoxin. *Nature*. 2000 May 25;405(6785):458–462.
[235] McNeil BD, Pundir P, Meeker S, et al. Identification of a mast-cell-specific receptor crucial for pseudo-allergic drug reactions. *Nature*. 2015 Mar 12;519(7542):237–41.
[236] Gour N, Dong X. The MRGPR family of receptors in immunity. 2024 Jan 9;57(1):28-39.
[237] Subramanian H, Gupta K, Ali H. Roles of Mas-related G protein–coupled receptor X2 on mast cell–mediated host defense, pseudoallergic drug reactions, and chronic inflammatory diseases. *J Allergy Clin Immunol*. 2016 Sep;138(3):700–710.
[238] Steinhoff MS, von Mentzer B, Geppetti P, et al. Tachykinins and their receptors: contributions to physiological control and the mechanisms of disease. *Physiol Rev*. 2014 Jan;94(1):265–301.
[239] Subramanian H, Gupta K, Ali H. Roles of Mas-related G protein–coupled receptor X2 on mast cell–mediated host defense, pseudoallergic drug reactions, and chronic inflammatory diseases. *J Allergy Clin Immunol*. 2016 Sep;138(3):700–710.
[240] Grigorev IP, Korzhevskii DE. Mast Cells in the Vertebrate Brain: Localization and Functions. 2021;57:16-32.
[241] Weinstock LB, Brook JB, Walters AS, et al. Mast cell activation symptoms are prevalent in Long-COVID. *Int J Infect Diseases*. 2021 Nov;112:103-110.
[242] Theoharides TC, Kempuraj D, Tagen M, et al. Mast cells, brain inflammation and autism. *Eur J Pharmcol*. 2015 May;778:96-102.
[243] van der Kolk BA. Clinical implications of neuroscience research in PTSD. *Ann N Y Acad Sci*. 2006 Jul:1071:277-93.
[244] Xie L, Kang H, Xu Q, et al. Sleep drives metabolite clearance from the adult brain. *Science*. 2013 Oct 18;342(6156):373-7.
[245] Zondek D, Bromberg YM. Endocrine allergy: I. Allergic sensitivity to endogenous hormones. *J Allergy*. 1945 Jan;16(1):1-16.
[246] Zierau O, Zenclussed AC, Jensen F. Role of female sex hormones, estradiol and progesterone, in mast cell behavior. *Front Immunol*. 2012 Jun 18;3.
[247] Landucci E, Laurino A, Cinci L, et al. Thyroid Hormone, Thyroid Hormone Metabolites and Mast Cells: A Less Explored Issue. *Front Cell Neurosci*. 2019 Mar 29;13:79.
[248] Zaitsu M, Narita SI, Lambert KC, et al. Estradiol activates mast cells via a non-genomic estrogen receptor-α and calcium influx. *Mol Immunol*. 2007 Mar;44(8):1977-85.
[249] Zaitsu M, Narita SI, Lambert KC, et al. Estradiol activates mast cells via a non-genomic estrogen receptor-α and calcium influx. *Mol Immunol*. 2007 Mar;44(8):1977-85.
[250] Schmidt G, Owman C, Sjoberg NO. Histamine induces ovulation in the isolated perfused rat ovary. *J Reprod Fertil*. 1986 Sep;78(1):159-66.
[251] Bodis J, Tinneberg HR, Schwarz H, et al. The effect of histamine on progesterone and estradiol secretion of human granulosa cells in serum-free culture. *Gynecol Endocrinol*. 1993 Dec;7(4):235-9.
[252] Zwahlen M, Stute P. Impact of progesterone on the immune system in women: a systematic literature review. *Arch Gynecol Obstet*. 2024 Jan;309(1):37-46.
[253] Landucci E, Laurino A, Cinci L, et al. Thyroid Hormone, Thyroid Hormone Metabolites and Mast Cells: A Less Explored Issue. *Front Cell Neurosci*. 2019 Mar 29;13:79.
[254] Bacarri GC, Falvo S, Lanni A, et al. Mast Cell Population and Histamine Content in Hypothyroid Rat Tissues. *Animals (Basel)*. 2022 Jul 20;12(14):1840.
[255] Finotto S Mekori YA, Metcalfe DD. Glucocorticoids decrease tissue mast cell number by reducing the production of the c-kit ligand, stem cell factor, by resident cells: in vitro and in vivo evidence in murine systems. *J Clin Invest*. 1997 Apr;99(7):1721-28.
[256] Cain DW, Cidlowski JA. Immune regulation by glucocorticoids. *Nat Reviews*. 2017 Feb;17:233-47.
[257] Rhen T, Cidlowski JA. Antiinflammatory Action of Glucocorticoids — New Mechanisms for Old Drugs. *New Engl J Med*. 2025 Oct;353:1711-23.
[258] Prall SP, Muehlenbein MP. Chapter Four - DHEA Modulates Immune Function: A Review of Evidence. *Vitamins Hormones*. 2018;108:125-44.

[259] Zhang J, Shi GP. Mast cells and metabolic syndrome. *Biochimia Biophysica Acta (BBA) – Mol Basis Dis.* 2012 Jan;1822(1):14-20.
[260] Lessman E, Grochowy G, Weingarten L, et al. Insulin and insulin-like growth factor-1 promote mast cell survival via activation of the phosphatidylinositol-3-kinase pathway. *Exp Hematol.* 2006 Nov;34(11):1532-41.
[261] Laffont S, Blanquart E, Savignac M, et al. Androgen signaling negatively controls group 2 innate lymphoid cells. *J Exp Med.* 2017;214(6):1581–1592.
[262] Guhl S, Atruc M, Zuberbier T, et al. Testosterone exerts selective anti-inflammatory effects on human skin mast cells in a cell subset dependent manner. *Exp Dermatol.* 2012 Nov;21(11):878-80.
[263] Fehervaru Z. Mast cells in autoimmune disease. *Natur Immunol.* 2018;19(316).
[264] Park SL, Kim MS, Kim TH. Gut Microbiome and Estrogen. *J Menopausal Med.* 2025 Jul 3;31(2):95–101.
[265] Ezhilarason D. Critical role of estrogen in the progression of chronic liver diseases. *Hepatobiliary Pancreatic Dis Int.* 2020 Oct;19(5):429-34.
[266] Fenneman AC, Bruinstroop E, Nieuwdorp M, et al. A Comprehensive Review of Thyroid Hormone Metabolism in the Gut and Its Clinical Implications. *Thyroid.* 2023 Jan;33(1):32-44.
[267] Brighton J. PMDD in Autistic Women: Symptoms, Causes & Effective Solutions. Accessed March 24, 2026 from: https://drbrighten.com/autistic-women/.
[268] Duelo A, Comas-Baste O, Sanchez-Perez S, et al. Pilot Study on the Prevalence of Diamine Oxidase. *Nutrients.* 2024 Apr 12;16(8):1142.
[269] Marin EF, Marcolin LC, Melero LM, et al. The Prevalence of Single Nucleotide Polymorphisms of the AOC1 Gene Associated with Diamine Oxidase (DAO) Enzyme Deficiency in Healthy Newborns: A Prospective Population-Based Cohort Study. *Genes (Basel).* 2025 Jan 24;16(2):141.
[270] Schalich K, Rajagopala S, Das S, et al. Intestinal epithelial cell-derived components regulate transcriptome of Lactobacillus rhamnosus G. *Front Microbiol.* 2023 Jan;13:01-11.
[271] Grootens J, Ungerstedt JS, Ekoff M, et al. Single-cell analysis reveals the KIT D816V mutation in haematopoietic stem and progenitor cells in systemic mastocytosis. *eBioMedicine.* 2019 Apr 8;43:150–158.
[272] Akin C, Valent P, Metcalfe DD. Mast cell activation syndrome: Proposed diagnostic criteria. *J Allergy Clin Immunol.* 2010 Dec;126(6):P1099-1104.
[273] Jackson CW, Pratt CM, Rupprecht CP, et al. Mastocytosis and Mast Cell Activation Disorders: Clearing the Air. *Int J Mol Sci.* 2021 Oct 19;22(20):11270.
[274] Afrin LB. Presentation, Diagnosis, and Management of Mast Cell Activation Syndrome. In: Mast Cells Methods and Protocols. *Methods Mol Biol.* 2015;1220:405–438.
[275] U.S. National Institute of Allergy and Infectious Diseases. Hereditary Alpha Tryptasemia and Hereditary Alpha Tryptasemia Syndrome FAQ. Accessed March 24, 2026 from: https://www.niaid.nih.gov/research/hereditary-alpha-tryptasemia-faq.
[276] Lyons JJ, Yu X, Hughes JD, et al. Elevated basal serum tryptase identifies a multisystem disorder associated with increased TPSAB1 copy number. *Nat Genet.* 2016 Dec;48(12):1564-1569.
[277] Lyons JJ. Hereditary alpha tryptasemia: genotyping and associated clinical features. *Immunol Allergy Clin North Am.* 2018 Jun 9;38(3):483–495.
[278] Lyons JJ, Yu X, Hughes JD, et al. Elevated basal serum tryptase identifies a multisystem disorder associated with increased TPSAB1 copy number. *Nat Genet.* 2016 Dec;48(12):1564-1569.
[279] Luskin KT, White AA, Lyons JJ. The Genetic Basis and Clinical Impact of Hereditary Alpha-Tryptasemia. *J Aller Clin Immunol In Pract.* 2021 Jun;9(6):2235-42.
[280] National Library of Medicine. MTHFR gene. Accessed March 24, 2026 from: https://medlineplus.gov/genetics/gene/mthfr/.
[281] Frosst P, Blom HJ, Milos R, et al. A candidate genetic risk factor for vascular disease: a common mutation in methylenetetrahydrofolate reductase. *Nat Genet.* 1995 May;10(1):111-3.
[282] Botto LD, Yang Q. 5,10-Methylenetetrahydrofolate reductase gene variants and congenital anomalies: a HuGE review. *Am J Epidemiol.* 2000 May;151(9):862-77.
[283] Wicken B, Bamforth F, Li Z, et al. Geographical and ethnic variation of the 677C>T allele of 5,10 methylenetetrahydrofolate reductase (MTHFR): findings from over 7000 newborns from 16 areas world wide. *J Med Genet.* 2003 Aug;40(8):619-25.
[284] Younesian S, Mohammadi MH, Younesian O, et al. DNA methylation in human diseases. *Heliyon.* 2024 Jun 15;10(11):e32366.

[285] Ostaiza-Cardenas J, Tobar AC, Costa SC, et al. Epigenetic modulation by life–style: advances in diet, exercise, and mindfulness for disease prevention and health optimization. *Front Nutr.* 2025 Aug 21;12:1632999.
[286] Abdul QA, Yu BP, Chung HY, et al. Epigenetic modifications of gene expression by lifestyle and environment. *Arch Pharm Res.* 2017 Nov;40(11):1219-1237.
[287] Caporali S, Russo S, Leist M, et al. Interplay between genes and social environment: from epigenetics to precision medicine. *Cell Death Discovery.* 2025;11(293).
[288] Torres-Alegria J, Baccarelli A, Bollati V. Epigenetics and lifestyle. *Epigenomics.* 2011 Jun;3(3):267–277.
[289] Sanchez-Perez S, Comas-Baste O, Veciana-Nogues MT, et al. Low-Histamine Diets: Is the Exclusion of Foods Justified by Their Histamine Content? *Nutrients.* 2021 Apr 21;13(5):1395. doi: 10.3390/nu13051395.
[290] Ozogul F. Production of biogenic amines by Morganella morganii, Klebsiella pneumoniae and Hafnia alvei using a rapid HPLC method. *Eur Food Res Tech.* 2004 Aug 25;219:465-69.
[291] Engevik KA, Hazzard A, Puckett B, et al. Phylogenetically diverse bacterial species produce histamine. *System Appl Microbiol.* 2024 Sep;47(5):126539.
[292] Altafini A, Roncada P, Guerrini A, et al. Development of Histamine in Fresh and Canned Tuna Steaks Stored under Different Experimental Temperature Conditions. *Foods.* 2022 Dec;11(24):4034.
[293] Tahmouzi S, Ghasemlou M, Alibadi FS, et al. HISTAMINE FORMATION AND BACTERIOLOGICAL QUALITY IN SKIPJACK TUNA (KATSUWONUS PELAMIS): EFFECT OF DEFROSTING TEMPERATURE. *J Food Proc Preserv.* 2012 Mar.
[294] Morrow JD, Margolies GR, Rowlnad J, et al. Evidence That Histamine Is the Causative Toxin of Scombroid-Fish Poisoning. *N Engl J Med.* 1991 Mar 14;324:716-20.
[295] del Rio B, Fernandez M, Redruello B, et al. New insights into the toxicological effects of dietary biogenic amines. *Food Chem.* 2024 Mar;435:137558.
[296] Pircher A, Bauer F, Paulsen P. Formation of cadaverine, histamine, putrescine and tyramine by bacteria isolated from meat, fermented sausages and cheeses. *Nature Link.* 2006;226:225-31.
[297] Turna NS, Chung R, McIntyre L. A review of biogenic amines in fermented foods: Occurrence and health effects. *Heliyon.* 2024 Jan 17;10(2):e24501.
[298] FSA Panel on Biological Hazards. Scientific opinion on risk based control of biogenic amine formation in fermented foods. *EFSA Journal.* 2011;9(10):2393.
[299] Karr T, Guptha LS, Bell K, et al. Oxalates: Dietary Oxalates and Kidney Inflammation: A Literature Review. *Integr Med (Encinitas).* 2024 May;23(2):36-44.
[300] Rechenauer T, Raithel M, Gotze T, et al. Idiopathic Mast Cell Activation Syndrome With Associated Salicylate Intolerance. *Front Pediatr.* 2018 Mar 27;6:73.
[301] Gerritsen RJS, Band GPH. Breath of Life: The Respiratory Vagal Stimulation Model of Contemplative Activity. *Front Hum Neurosci.* 2018 Oct 9;12:397.
[302] Huberman Lab. Physiological sigh. Accessed March 24, 2026 from: https://ai.hubermanlab.com/s/cCSj1L7a.
[303] Huang X, Sun X, Wang Q, et al. Structural insights into the diverse actions of magnesium on NMDA receptors. *Neuron.* 2025 Apr 2;113(7):1006-1018.e4.
[304] Lehrer P, Kaur K, Sharma A, et al. Heart Rate Variability Biofeedback Improves Emotional and Physical Health and Performance: A Systematic Review and Meta Analysis. *Appl Psychophysiol Biofeedback.* 2020 Sep;45(3):109-129.
[305] Fournie C, Chouchou F, Dalleau G, et al. Heart rate variability biofeedback in chronic disease management: A systematic review. *Complement Ther Med.* 2021 Aug;60:102750.
[306] Vann-Adibe S, Tsui HKH, Zhou HQ, et al. Efficacy and Methodology of Remote Heart Rate Variability Biofeedback Interventions for Mental Health: A Systematic Review and Meta-Analysis. *Appl Psychophysiol Biofeedback.* 2025 Nov 27.
[307] Carta MG, Cossu G, Primavera D, et al. Heart Rate Variability Biofeedback Efficacy on Fatigue and Energy Levels in Fibromyalgia: A Secondary Analysis of RCT NCT0412183. *J Clin Med.* 2024 Jul;13(14):4005.
[308] Zhang P. The Role of Diet and Nutrition in Allergic Diseases. *Nutrients.* 2023 Aug 22;15(17):3683.
[309] Calder PC, Ahluwalia N, Brouns F, et al. Dietary factors and low-grade inflammation in relation to overweight and obesity. *Br J Clin Pharmacol.* 2017;83(4):640–652.
[310] Makki K, Deehan EC, Walter J, et al. The Impact of Dietary Fiber on Gut Microbiota in Host Health and Disease. *Cell Host Microbe.* 2018;23(6):705–715.

[311] Jafarinia M, Hosseini MS, Kasiri N, et al. Quercetin with the potential effect on allergic diseases. *Allergy Asthma Clin Immunol.* 2020 May 14;16:36.
[312] Tsilioni I, Theharides T. Luteolin Is More Potent than Cromolyn in Their Ability to Inhibit Mediator Release from Cultured Human Mast Cells. *Int Arch Allergy Immunol.* 2024;185(8):803-809.
[313] Kempuraj D, Madhappan B, Christodoulou S, et al. Flavonols inhibit proinflammatory mediator release, intracellular calcium ion levels and protein kinase C theta phosphorylation in human mast cells. *Br J Pharmacol.* 2005;145(7):934–944.
[314] Theoharides TC, Kempuraj D, Tagen M, et al. Differential release of mast cell mediators and the pathogenesis of inflammation. *Clin Ther.* 2012;34(4):e1–e15.
[315] Mlcek J, Jurikova T, Skrovankova S, et al. Quercetin and Its Anti-Allergic Immune Response. *Molecules.* 2016;21(5):623.
[316] Calder PC. Omega-3 fatty acids and inflammatory processes: from molecules to man. *Biochem Soc Trans.* 2017;45(5):1105–1115.
[317] Mlcek J, Jurikova T, Skrovankova S, et al. Quercetin and Its Anti-Allergic Immune Response. *Molecules.* 2016;21(5):623.
[318] Manach C, Williamson G, Morand C, et al. Bioavailability and bioefficacy of polyphenols in humans. I. Review of 97 bioavailability studies. *Am J Clin Nutr.* 2005;81(1 Suppl):230S–242S.
[319] Johnston CS. The antihistamine action of ascorbic acid. *Subcell Biochem.* 1996;25:189–213.
[320] Calder PC. Omega-3 fatty acids and inflammatory processes: from molecules to man. *Biochem Soc Trans.* 2017;45(5):1105–1115.
[321] Calder PC. n-3 polyunsaturated fatty acids, inflammation, and inflammatory diseases. *Am J Clin Nutr.* 2006;83(6 Suppl):1505S–1519S.
[322] Theoharides TC, Stewart JM, Hatziagelaki E, et al. Brain "fog," inflammation and obesity: key aspects of neuropsychiatric disorders improved by luteolin. *Front Neurosci.* 2015;9:225.
[323] Nielsen FH. Magnesium deficiency and increased inflammation: current perspectives. *J Inflamm Res.* 2018;11:25–34.
[324] Theoharides TC, Tsilioni I, Bawazeer M. Mast Cells, Neuroinflammation and Pain in Fibromyalgia Syndrome. *Front Cell Neurosci.* 2019 Aug;13:353.
[325] Liu MC, Xiao HQ, Brown AJ, et al. Vitamin D contributes to mast cell stabilization. *Eur J Allergy Clin Immunol.* 2017 Aug;72(8):1184-92.
[326] Nani A, Murtaza B, Khan AS, et al. Antioxidant and Anti-Inflammatory Potential of Polyphenols Contained in Mediterranean Diet in Obesity: Molecular Mechanisms. *Molecules.* 2021;26(4):985.
[327] Singh BN, Shankar S, Srivastava RK. Green tea catechin, epigallocatechin-3-gallate (EGCG): mechanisms, perspectives and clinical applications. *Biochem Pharmacol.* 2011 Dec 15;82(12):1807–1821.
[328] Aggarwal BB, Harikumar KB. Potential therapeutic effects of curcumin, the anti-inflammatory agent, against neurodegenerative, cardiovascular, pulmonary, metabolic, autoimmune and neoplastic diseases. *Int J Biochem Cell Biol.* 2009 Jul 9;41(1):40–59.
[329] Mlcek J, Jurikova T, Skrovankova S, et al. Quercetin and Its Anti-Allergic Immune Response. *Molecules.* 2016;21(5):623.
[330] Kempuraj D, Castellani ML, Petrarca C, et al. Inhibitory effect of quercetin on tryptase and interleukin-6 release, and histidine decarboxylase mRNA transcription by human mast cell-1 cell line. *Clin Exp Med.* 2006 Dec;6(4):150-6.
[331] Manach C, Scalbert A, Morand C, et al. Polyphenols: food sources and bioavailability. *Am J Clin Nutr.* 2004 May;79(5):727–747.
[332] Theoharides TC, Conti P. Mast cells: the Jekyll and Hyde of tumor growth. *Trends Immunol.* 2004 May;25(5):235–241.
[333] Theoharides TC, Stewart JM, Hatziagelaki E, et al. Brain "fog," inflammation and obesity: key aspects of neuropsychiatric disorders improved by luteolin. *Front Neurosci.* 2015;9:225.
[334] Charriere K, Schneider V, Perrignon-Sommet M, et al. Exploring the Role of Apigenin in Neuroinflammation: Insights and Implications. 2024 May;25(9):5041.
[335] McKay DL, Blumberg JB. A review of the bioactivity and potential health benefits of chamomile tea (Matricaria recutita L.). *Phytother Res.* 2006;20(7):519–530.
[336] Dinda B, Dinda M, Kulsi G, et al. Therapeutic potentials of baicalin and its aglycone, baicalein against inflammatory disorders. *Eur J Med Chem.* 2017;131:68–80.
[337] Osakabe N, Yasuda A, Natsume M, et al. Rosmarinic acid inhibits epidermal inflammatory responses: anticarcinogenic effect of Perilla frutescens extract in the murine two-stage skin model. *Carcinogenesis.* 2004;25(4):549–557.

338 Takano H, Osakabe N, Sanbongi C, et al. Extract of Perilla frutescens enriched for rosmarinic acid inhibits seasonal allergic rhinoconjunctivitis in humans. *Exp Biol Med (Maywood).* 2004;229(3):247–254.
339 Schapowal A. Randomised controlled trial of butterbur and cetirizine for treating seasonal allergic rhinitis. *BMJ.* 2002 Jan 19;324(7330):144.
340 Merk J, Boonen G, Butterweck V, et al. Efficacy and Safety of Petasites hybridus Leaf Extract Ze 339 for the Treatment of Allergic Rhinitis. *Adv Respir Med.* 2025;93(3):13.
341 KSM-66 Ashwagandha. Research on KSM-66. Accessed March 25, 2026 from https://www.ksm66ashwagandhaa.com/science.php.
342 Kerry. Sensoril Ashwagandha Research Studies. Accessed March 25, 2026 from: https://supplements.kerry.com/proactive-health/womens-health/sensoril/sensoril-clinical-studies/.
343 Darbinyan V, Aslanyan G, Amroyan E, et al. Clinical trial of Rhodiola rosea L. extract SHR-5 in the treatment of mild to moderate depression. *Nord J Psychiatry.* 2007;61(5):343-8.
344 Shevtsov VA, Zholus BI, Shervarly VI, et al. A randomized trial of two different doses of a SHR-5 Rhodiola rosea extract versus placebo and control of capacity for mental work. *Phytomed.* 2003;10(2-3):95-105.
345 Shoba G, Joy D, Joseph T, et al. Influence of piperine on the pharmacokinetics of curcumin in animals and human volunteers. *Planta Med.* 1998;64(4):353–356.
346 Osakabe N, Yasuda A, Natsume M, et al. Rosmarinic acid inhibits epidermal inflammatory responses: anticarcinogenic effect of Perilla frutescens extract in the murine two-stage skin model. *Carcinogenesis.* 2004;25(4):549–557.
347 Osakabe N, Yasuda A, Natsume M, et al. Rosmarinic acid inhibits epidermal inflammatory responses: anticarcinogenic effect of Perilla frutescens extract in the murine two-stage skin model. *Carcinogenesis.* 2004;25(4):549–557.
348 Liu ZS, Truong TTT, Bortolasci CC, et al. The potential of baicalin to enhance neuroprotection and mitochondrial function in a human neuronal cell model. *Mol Psychiatry.* 2024 Mar 19;29(8):2487–2495.
349 Dinda B, Dinda M, Kulsi G, et al. Therapeutic potentials of baicalin and its aglycone, baicalein against inflammatory disorders. *Eur J Med Chem.* 2017;131:68–80.
350 Yoshida K, Takabayashi T, Kaneko A, et al. Baicalin suppresses type 2 immunity through breaking off the interplay between mast cell and airway epithelial cell. *J Ethnopharm.* 2021 Mar;267:113492.
351 Wang F, Xu Z, Ren L, et al. GABA A receptor subtype selectivity underlying selective anxiolytic effect of baicalin. *Neuropharmacology.* 2008 Dec;55(7):1231-7.
352 Sell CS. On the unpredictability of odor. *Angew Chem Int Ed Engl.* 2006;45(38):6254–6261.
353 Kim HM, Cho Sh. Lavender oil inhibits immediate-type allergic reaction in mice and rats. *J Pharm Pharmacol.* 1999 Feb;51(2):221-26.
354 Bohm C, Wiessler AL, Janzen D, et al. Modulatory effect of various essential oils on different GABAA receptor subtypes present in the central nervous system. *Phtomed Plus.* 2025 Aug;5(3):100852.
355 Tarumi W, Shinohara K. The Effects of Essential Oil on Salivary Oxytocin Concentration in Postmenopausal Women. *J Altern Complement Med.* 2020 Mar;26(3):226-230.
356 Tyagi V, Singh VK, Sharma PK, et al. Essential oil-based nanostructures for inflammation and rheumatoid arthritis. *J Drug Del Sci Technol.* 2020;60:101983.
357 Toprak Ç, Ergin Özcan P, Demirbolat İ, et al. The effect of lavender and bergamot oil applied via inhalation on the anxiety level and sleep quality of surgical intensive care unit patients. *Explore (NY).* 2024 Sep-Oct;20(5):102991.
358 Gertsch J, Leonti M, Raduner S, et al. Beta-caryophyllene is a dietary cannabinoid. *Proc Natl Acad Sci U S A.* 2008;105(26):9099–9104.
359 Blain EJ, Ali AY, Duance VC. Boswellia frereana (frankincense) suppresses cytokine-induced matrix metalloproteinase expression and production of proinflammatory molecules in articular cartilage. *Phytother Res.*2010 jun;24(6):905-12.
360 Mikhaeil BR, Maatooq GT, Badira FA, et al. Chemistry and immunomodulatory activity of frankincense oil. *Z Naturforsch C.* 2003 Mar-Apr;58(3-4):230-38.
361 Rufino AT, Ribeiro M, Judas F, et al. Anti-inflammatory and chondroprotective activity of (+)-α-pinene: structural and enantiomeric selectivity. *J Nat Prod.* 2014 Feb;77(2):264-69.
362 Neves A, Rosa S, Goncalves J, et al. Screening of five essential oils for identification of potential inhibitors of IL-1- induced Nf-kappaB activation and NO production in human chondrocytes: characterization of the inhibitory activity of alpha-pinene. *Planta Med.* 2010 Feb;76(3):303-08.
363 Chen SX, Xiang JY, Han JX, et al. Essential Oils from Spices Inhibit Cholinesterase Activity and Improve Behavioral Disorder in AlCl3 Induced Dementia. *Chem Biodivers.* 2022 Jan;19(1):e202100443.

[364] Lee KB, Cho E, Yang YS. Changes in 5-hydroxytryptamine and cortisol plasma levels in menopausal women after inhalation of clary sage oil. *Phytother Res.* 2014 Nov;28(11):1599-605.
[365] Bakkali F, Averbeck S, Averbeck D, et al. Biological effects of essential oils – A review. *Food Chem Toxicol.* 2008;46(2):446–475.
[366] McKemy DD. How cold is it? TRPM8 and TRPA1 in the molecular logic of cold sensation. *Mol Pain.* 2005;1:16.
[367] McNeil BD, Pundir P, Meeker S, et al. Identification of a mast-cell-specific receptor crucial for pseudo-allergic drug reactions. *Nature.* 2015;519(7542):237–241.
[368] Burkhard PR, Burkhardt K, Haenggeli CA, et al. Plant-induced seizures: reappearance of an old problem. *J Neurol.* 1999;246(8):667–670.
[369] Millet Y, Tognetti P, Lavaire-Perlovisi M, et al. Experimental study of the toxic convulsant properties of commercial preparations of essences of sage and hyssop (author's transl). *Rev Electroencephalogr Neurophysiol Clin.* 1979 Jan-Mar;9(1):12–18.
[370] Loos HM, Schreiner L, Karacan B. A systematic review of physiological responses to odours with a focus on current methods used in event-related study designs. *Int J Psychophysiol.* 2020;158:143–157.
[371] Xu L, Han Y, Chen X, et al. Molecular mechanisms underlying menthol binding and activation of TRPM8 ion channel. *Natur Commun.* 2020 Jul;11(3790).
[372] Domocos D, Follansbee T, Nguyen A, et al. Cinnamaldehyde elicits itch behavior via TRPV1 and TRPV4 but not TRPA1. *Itch.* 2020 Jul-Sep;5(3):e36.
[373] Hashimoto M, Takahashi K, Ohta T. Inhibitory effects of linalool, an essential oil component of lavender, on nociceptive TRPA1 and voltage-gated Ca2+ channels in mouse sensory neurons. *Biochem Biophys Rep.* 2023 Jul;34:101468.
[374] Hashiesh HM, Sharma C, Goyal SN, et al. Pharmacological Properties, Therapeutic Potential and Molecular Mechanisms of JWH133, a CB2 Receptor-Selective Agonist. *Front Pharmacol.* 2021 Jul;12.
[375] Rakotoarivelo V, Mayer TZ, Simand M, et al. The Impact of the CB2 Cannabinoid Receptor in Inflammatory Diseases: An Update. *Molecules.* 2024;29(14):3381.
[376] Koulivand PH, Khaleghi Ghadiri M, Gorji A. Lavender and the nervous system. *Evid Based Complement Alternat Med.* 2013;2013:681304.
[377] Sayorwan W, Siripornpanich V, Piriyapunyaporn T, et al. The effects of lavender oil inhalation on emotional states, autonomic nervous system, and brain electrical activity. *J Med Assoc Thai.* 2012;95(4):598–606.
[378] Schuwald AM, Noldner M, Wilmes T, et al. Lavender Oil-Potent Anxiolytic Properties via Modulating Voltage Dependent Calcium Channels. *PLoS One.* 2013 Apr 29;8(4):e59998.
[379] Wang J, Zhang L, Hou X. Efficacy of rifaximin in treating with small intestine bacterial overgrowth: a systematic review and meta-analysis. *Expert Rev Gastroenterol Hepatol.* 2021 Dec;15(12):1385-1399.
[380] Low K, Hwang L, Hua J, Zhu A, Morales W, Pimentel M. A combination of rifaximin and neomycin is most effective in treating irritable bowel syndrome patients with methane on lactulose breath test. *J Clin Gastroenterol.* 2010 Sep;44(8):547-550.
[381] Sun D, Courtney HS, Beachey EH. Berberine sulfate blocks adherence of Streptococcus pyogenes to epithelial cells, inhibits DNA and protein synthesis, and prevents infection in vivo. *Antimicrob Agents Chemother.* 1988;32(9):1370–1374.
[382] Kosalec I, Jembrek MJ, Vlainic J. The Spectrum of Berberine Antibacterial and Antifungal Activities. *Nature Link.* 2022 Feb:119-32.
[383] Zhang H, Wei J, Xue R, et al. Berberine lowers blood glucose in type 2 diabetes mellitus patients through increasing insulin receptor expression. *Metabolism.* 2010;59(2):285–292.
[384] Duda-Madej A, Viscardi S, Labaz JP, et al. Berberine in Bowel Health: Anti-Inflammatory and Gut Microbiota Modulatory Effects. 2025 Dec;26(24):12021.
[385] Gao J, Guo H, Zhu L, et al. IDDF2025-ABS-0189 New choice for small intestinal bacterial overgrowth: an RCT comparing berberine and rifaximin. *Gut.* 2025 Jul;74(Suppl 3):A1-A437.
[386] AGA. BERBERINE IS NOT INFERIOR TO RIFAXIMIN IN TREATMENT OF SMALL INTESTINAL BACTERIAL OVERGROWTH: AN INTERIM ANALYSIS OF THE BRIEF-SIBO RCT STUDY. Accessed March 26, 2026 from: https://eposters.ddw.org/ddw/2024/ddw-2024/413770/huai-zhu.guo.berberine.is.not.inferior.to.rifaximin.in.treatment.of.small.html?f=listing%3D0%2Abrowseby%3D8%2Asortby%3D1%2Asearch%3Dsibo https://eposters.ddw.org/ddw/2024/ddw-2024/413770/huai-

zhu.guo.berberine.is.not.inferior.to.rifaximin.in.treatment.of.small.html?f=listing%3D0%2Abrowseby%3D8%2Asortby%3D1%2Asearch%3Dsibo.
[387] Busquet M, Calsamiglia S, Ferret A, Carro MD, Kamel C. Effect of garlic oil and four of its compounds on rumen microbial fermentation. *J Dairy Sci.* 2005;88(12):4393–4404.
[388] Rathod NB, Kulawik P, Ozogul F, et al. Biological activity of plant-based carvacrol and thymol and their impact on human health and food quality. *Trends Food Sci Technol.* 2021 Oct;116:733-48.
[389] Marchese A, Orhan IE, Dagalia M, et al. Antibacterial and antifungal activities of thymol: A brief review of the literature. *Food Chem.* 2016 Nov;210:402-14.
[390] Alammar N, Wang L, Saberi B, et al. The impact of peppermint oil on the irritable bowel syndrome: a meta-analysis of the pooled clinical data. *BMC Complement Altern Med.* 2019 Jan 17;19:21.
[391] da Nobrega Alves D, Monteiro AFM, Andrade PN, et al. Docking Prediction, Antifungal Activity, Anti-Biofilm Effects on Candida spp., and Toxicity against Human Cells of Cinnamaldehyde. *Molecules.* 2020 Dec 16;25(24):5969.
[392] Efthymakis K, Neri M. The role of Zinc L-Carnosine in the prevention and treatment of gastrointestinal mucosal disease in humans: a review. *Clinics Res Hepatol Gastroenterol.* 2022 Aug-Sep;46(7):101954.
[393] Murray MT. Glycyrrhiza glabra (Licorice). *Textbook of Natural Medicine.* 2020 Jul 10:641–647.e3.
[394] Langmead L, Feakins RM, Goldthorpe S, et al. Randomized, double-blind, placebo-controlled trial of oral aloe vera gel for active ulcerative colitis. *Aliment Pharmacol Ther.* 2004;19(7):739–747.
[395] Langmead L, Rampton DS. *Review article: complementary and alternative therapies for inflammatory bowel disease. Aliment Pharmacol Ther.* 2006;23(3):341–349.
[396] Liu C, Cui Y, Pi F, et al. Extraction, purification, structural characteristics, biological activities and pharmacological applications of acemannan, a polysaccharide from Aloe vera: A review. *Molecules.* 2019;24(8):1554.
[397] Walia R, Chaudhuri SR, Dey P. Reciprocal interaction between gut microbiota and aloe-emodin results in altered microbiome composition and metabolism of aloe-emodin. *Food Biosci.* 2025 Aug;70:107061.
[398] Oksaharju A, Kankainen M, Kekkonen RA, et al. Probiotic Lactobacillus rhamnosus downregulates FCER1 and HRH4 expression in human mast cells. *World J Gastroenterol.* 2011 Feb 14;17(6):750–759.
[399] Schwelberger HG. Histamine intolerance: a metabolic disease? *Inflamm Res.* 2010;59(Suppl 2):S219–S221.
[400] Maintz L, Novak N. Histamine and histamine intolerance. *Am J Clin Nutr.* 2007;85(5):1185–1196.
[401] Honzawa Y, Nakase H, Matsuura M, et al. Clinical significance of serum diamine oxidase activity in inflammatory bowel disease. *J Crohns Colitis.* 2011;5(6):551–556.
[402] Phillips TD, Sarr AB, Grant PG. Selective chemisorption and detoxification of aflatoxins by phyllosilicate clay. *Nat Toxins.* 1995;3(4):204–213.
[403] Avantaggiato G, Havenaar R, Visconti A. Assessment of the multi-mycotoxin-binding efficacy of a carbon/aluminosilicate-based product in an in vitro gastrointestinal model. *J Agric Food Chem.* 2007;55(12):4810–4819.
[404] Bhattacharyya KG, Gupta SS. Adsorption of a few heavy metals on natural and modified kaolinite and montmorillonite: a review. *Adv Colloid Interface Sci.* 2008;140(2):114–131.
[405] Carretero MI. Clay minerals and their beneficial effects upon human health. A review. *Appl Clay Sci.* 2002;21(3-4):155–163.
[406] Cervini-Silva J, Nieto-Camancho A, Kaufhould S, et al. The anti-inflammatory activity of bentonites. *Appl Clay Sci.* 2015 Dec;118:56-60.
[407] Eliaz I, Hotchkiss AT, Fishman ML, Rode D. The effect of modified citrus pectin on urinary excretion of toxic metals. *Phytother Res.* 2006;20(10):859–864.
[408] Dongowski G, Lorenz A. Intestinal absorption of heavy metals in rats is reduced by dietary pectin. *J Nutr Biochem.* 1998;9(6):349–354.
[409] Eliaz I, Raz A. Pleiotropic Effects of Modified Citrus Pectin. *Nutrients.* 2019 Nov 1;11(11):2619.
[410] Zhang T, Sun G, Shuai M et al. Purification, chemical analysis and inhibitory effects on galectin-3 of enzymatic pH-modified citrus pectin. *Food Chem X.* 2021 Nov 23;12:100169.
[411] Shoemaker RC, House DE. A time-series study of sick building syndrome: chronic, biotoxin-associated illness from exposure to water-damaged buildings. *Neurotoxicol Teratol.* 2005;27(1):29–46.
[412] Genuis SJ, Birkholz D, Rodushkin I, Beesoon S. Blood, urine, and sweat (BUS) study: monitoring and elimination of bioaccumulated toxic elements. *Arch Environ Contam Toxicol.* 2011;61(2):344–357.

[413] Sears ME, Kerr KJ, Bray RI. Arsenic, Cadmium, Lead, and Mercury in Sweat: A Systematic Review. *J Environ Public Health.* 2012 Feb 22;2012:184745.
[414] Genuis SJ, Beesoon S, Lobo RA, Birkholz D. Human elimination of phthalate compounds: blood, urine, and sweat (BUS) study. ScientificWorldJournal. 2012;2012:615068.
[415] Grady H. IMMUNOMODULATION THROUGH CASTOR OIL PACKS. *J Naturopathic Med.*
[416] Rowell LB. Human Cardiovascular Control. New York: Oxford University Press; 1993.
[417] Raj SR. Postural tachycardia syndrome (POTS). *Circulation.* 2013;127(23):2336–2342.
[418] Raj SR, Biaggioni I, Yamhure PC, et al. Renin-aldosterone paradox and perturbed blood volume regulation underlying postural tachycardia syndrome. *Circulation.* 2005;111(13):1574–1582.
[419] Stewart JM. Common syndromes of orthostatic intolerance. *Pediatrics.* 2013;131(5):968–980.
[420] Furlan R, Jacob G, Snell M, et al. Chronic orthostatic intolerance: a disorder with discordant cardiac and vascular sympathetic control. *Circulation.* 1998;98(20):2154–2159.
[421] Rah SR, Fedorowski A, Sheldon RS. Diagnosis and management of postural orthostatic tachycardia syndrome. *CMAJ.* 2022 Mar 14;194(10):E378–E385.
[422] Low PA, Novak V, Spies JM, et al. Cerebrovascular regulation in the postural orthostatic tachycardia syndrome (POTS). *Am J Med Sci.* 199 Feb;317(2):124-33.
[423] Jacob G, Costa F, Shannon JR, et al. The neuropathic postural tachycardia syndrome. *N Engl J Med.* 2000;343(14):1008–1014.
[424] Steinberg RS, Dicken W, Cutchings A. Narrative Review of Postural Orthostatic Tachycardia Syndrome: Associated Conditions and Management Strategies. *US Cardiol Rev.* 2023;17:e13.
[425] Safavi-Naeini P, Razavi M. Postural Orthostatic Tachycardia Syndrome. *Tex Heart Inst J.* 2020 Feb 1;47(1):57–59.
[426] Nakamura T, Maeda S, Horiguchi K, et al. PGD2 deficiency exacerbates food antigen-induced mast cell hyperplasia. *Nature Commun.* 2015 Jul;6(7514).
[427] Roberts LJ 2nd, Sweetman BJ, Lewis RA, et al. Increased production of prostaglandin D2 in patients with systemic mastocytosis. *N Engl J Med.* 1980;303(24):1400–1404.
[428] Benarroch EE. Postural tachycardia syndrome: a heterogeneous and multifactorial disorder. *Mayo Clin Proc.* 2012;87(12):1214–1225.
[429] DiNicolantonio JJ, O'Keefe JH, Wilson W. Subclinical magnesium deficiency: a principal driver of cardiovascular disease and a public health crisis. *Open Heart.* 2018;5(1):e000668.
[430] Raj SR. Postural tachycardia syndrome (POTS). *Circulation.* 2013;127(23):2336–2342.
[431] Figueroa JJ, Basford JR, Low PA. Preventing and treating orthostatic hypotension: as easy as A, B, C. *Cleve Clin J Med.* 2010;77(5):298–306.
[432] Wieling W, van Dijk N, Thijs RD, et al. Physical countermeasures to increase orthostatic tolerance. *J Intern Med.* 2015;277(1):69–82.
[433] Streeten DH, Anderson GH Jr. Delayed orthostatic intolerance. *Arch Intern Med.* 1992;152(5):1066–1072.
[434] Raj SR, Biaggioni I, Yamhure PC, et al. Renin-aldosterone paradox and perturbed blood volume regulation underlying postural tachycardia syndrome. *Circulation.* 2005;111(13):1574–1582.
[435] Raj SR, Biaggioni I, Yamhure PC, et al. Renin-aldosterone paradox and perturbed blood volume regulation underlying postural tachycardia syndrome. *Circulation.* 2005;111(13):1574–1582.
[436] Fu Q, Vangundy TB, Shibata S, Auchus RJ, Williams GH, Levine BD. Menstrual cycle affects renal-adrenal and hemodynamic responses during prolonged standing in the postural tachycardia syndrome. *Hypertension.* 2010;56(1):82–90.
[437] Bourne KM, Chew DS, Stiles LE, et al. Compression garments for orthostatic intolerance and postural tachycardia syndrome: a systematic review. *Clin Auton Res.* 2021;31(3):385–395.
[438] Smit AAJ, Halliwill JR, Low PA, Wieling W. Pathophysiological basis of orthostatic hypotension in autonomic failure. *J Physiol.* 1999;519(Pt 1):1–10.
[439] Goessl VC, Curtiss JE, Hofmann SG. The effect of heart rate variability biofeedback training on stress and anxiety: a meta-analysis. *Psychol Med.* 2017 Nov;47(15):2578–2586.
[440] Sikiric P, Seiwerth S, Rucman R, et al. Stable gastric pentadecapeptide BPC 157: novel therapy in gastrointestinal tract. *Curr Pharm Des.* 2011;17(16):1612–1632.
[441] Sikiric P, Seiwerth S, Brcic L, et al. Revised Robert's cytoprotection and adaptive cytoprotection and stable gastric pentadecapeptide BPC 157. *Curr Pharm Des.* 2010;16(10):1224–1234.
[442] Fu Q, Levine BD. Exercise and Non-Pharmacological Treatment of POTS. *Auton Neurosci.* 2018 Jul 4;215:20–27.

[443] Fu Q, Vangundy TB, Shibata S, Auchus RJ, Williams GH, Levine BD. Exercise training versus propranolol in the treatment of the postural orthostatic tachycardia syndrome. *Circulation*. 2011 Apr 19;123(14): 1504–1512.
[444] Howden EJ, Fu Q, Shibata S, et al. Cardiovascular responses to exercise training in patients with postural orthostatic tachycardia syndrome. *J Physiol.* 2015 Jan 15;593(2):349–363.
[445] Afrin LB, Weinstock LB, Molderings GJ. Covid-19 hyperinflammation and post-Covid-19 illness may be rooted in mast cell activation syndrome. *Int J Infect Dis.* 2020 Nov;100:327–332.
[446] Kempuraj D, Selvakumar GP, Ahmed ME, et al. COVID-19, mast cells, cytokine storm, psychological stress, and neuroinflammation. *Neurosci.* 2020 Aug;26(5-6):402–414.

INDEX

D

E

I

L

M

N

O

P

Q

R

S

T

V

W

Z

www.ingramcontent.com/pod-product-compliance
Lightning Source LLC
LaVergne TN
LVHW080041170826
845677LV00024B/1328

* 9 7 9 8 9 8 8 7 2 0 6 9 0 *